Civil War
Hospital Newspapers

ALSO BY IRA SPAR

*New Haven's Civil War Hospital:
A History of Knight U.S. General Hospital, 1862–1865*
(McFarland, 2014)

Civil War Hospital Newspapers

*Histories and Excerpts
of Nine Union Publications*

IRA SPAR, M.D.

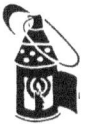

McFarland & Company, Inc., Publishers
Jefferson, North Carolina

LIBRARY OF CONGRESS CATALOGUING-IN-PUBLICATION DATA

Names: Spar, Ira, 1943– author, editor.
Title: Civil War hospital newspapers : histories and excerpts of nine Union publications / Ira Spar.
Description: Jefferson, North Carolina : McFarland & Company, Inc., Publishers, 2017. | Includes bibliographical references and index.
Identifiers: LCCN 2017022188 | ISBN 9781476665603 (softcover : acid free paper) ∞
Subjects: LCSH: United States—History—Civil War, 1861–1865—Press coverage. | United States—History—Civil War, 1861–1865—Hospitals. | United States—History—Civil War, 1861–1865—Sources.
Classification: LCC E609 .S69 2017 | DDC 973.7/76—dc23
LC record available at https://lccn.loc.gov/2017022188

BRITISH LIBRARY CATALOGUING DATA ARE AVAILABLE

ISBN (print) 978-1-4766-6560-3
ISBN (ebook) 978-1-4766-2529-4

© 2017 Ira Spar. All rights reserved

No part of this book may be reproduced or transmitted in any form or by any means, electronic or mechanical, including photocopying or recording, or by any information storage and retrieval system, without permission in writing from the publisher.

On the cover: *inset:* A ward in Armory Square Hospital, Washington, D.C., between 1861 and 1865 (Library of Congress); *background: The Voice of the Soldier,* Sloan U.S. Army General Hospital, Montpelier, Vermont (courtesy of Vermont State Library)

Printed in the United States of America

McFarland & Company, Inc., Publishers
Box 611, Jefferson, North Carolina 28640
www.mcfarlandpub.com

Table of Contents

Preface	1
Introduction	3
One. *Hospital Register*	9
Two. *Armory Square Hospital Gazette*	47
Three. *The Soldiers' Journal*	77
Four. *The Cripple*	111
Five. *The Crutch*	135
Six. *Hammond Gazette*	157
Seven. *The Cartridge Box*	171
Eight. *Knight Hospital Record*	192
Nine. *Voice of the Soldier*	217
Conclusions	221
Appendices	
I. Union General Hospitals, December 1864	235
II. Department of Washington, December 1864	235
III. Department of Pennsylvania	236
IV. Middle Department Hospitals	236
V. Department of the East	236
VI. Hospital Newspapers	237
Chapter Notes	238
Bibliography	244
Index	245

Preface

A recent meeting of the Hartford Medical Society had as guest speaker a former governor and senator who was asked why America never had a single-payer, universal health care system. As president I took the initiative to re-acquaint the audience with *New Haven's Civil War Hospital,* a recently published account of the federal government's efforts to provide health care for the flood of sick and wounded soldiers resulting from the Civil War. Starting virtually from scratch, 192 hospitals with 120,000 beds were created. "Lincoln-care" paid $3.50 a week for each bed filled, along with rent and salaries of all their employees including doctors, nurses, apothecaries, cooks and clerks.

Their self-published newspaper, *Knight Hospital Record,* provided a major source of unpublished and unvarnished material. Its poems have been transcribed and divided by subject and can be found on the Hartford Medical Society Library web site. I have since located eight other hospital newspapers illustrating the differences and similarities of each facility along with the hopes, goals and experiences of their soldiers. Some of the newspapers are in poor condition and can be read only in digital form, while others required on-site reading or are available on the net.

Hospital literature is an unreported and unique body of work consisting of prose, poetry and reportage; they were "selfies" written and edited by those who experienced war as it occurred. Convalescents, soldiers in the field, surgeons, medical students, chaplains and women volunteers provide insight on the health care system and the life of a soldier, designed to be shared with peers and the general public.

Each chapter describes the founding and evolution of a hospital and its role in providing health care through its closing. Each newspaper is summarized, selecting relevant material divided by subject matter, including romance and marriage, battlefield experience, health care, humor, disability, religion, patriotism, politics, and the treatment of prisoners. The soldier's life is dissected from the struggle to be warm in winter and dry in spring, to surviving fever or a hive of air-born iron missiles.

Relationships with blacks, Irish, Confederates, sweethearts, and family are explored. Chaplains provide sermons supporting the war effort while cautioning against drink, tobacco and profanity. The white-hot anger after Lincoln's assassination still radiates from black-draped columns written 150 years ago. The public's horrified disgust from pictures and stories of returning, emaciated Union prisoners translated into demand for justice and revenge. The needs of disabled veterans were of keen interest. Who would hire them? Who would marry them? The inability of political parties to compromise and solve problems and their lack of civility was far more vexing in a murderous civil war than in today's Washington. Supplemental material includes letters from hospital patients and, for the West Philadelphia Hospital, a collection of orders composed and printed by the hospital chief of staff giving insight as to hospital administration of that era, including the importance of medical records, physician behavior and patient outcome studies.

Burning issues of their day are still with us, just as costly and unresolved. As a Civil War-era correspondent pointed out, "those who live at a distance from the state of actual warfare can never know or appreciate its real horror." My experience as a Vietnam War surgeon and student of medical history leads me to the same conclusion. Brackets were placed around comments following medical stories intended to represent a twenty-first-century surgeon's insight into nineteenth-century medical events.

Introduction

With the bombing of Fort Sumter on April 12, 1861, an epidemic of war fever broke out across America. Both sides predicted a quick victory: their soldiers braver, more skilled in the science of warfare, and God and justice on their side. Down Broadway in New York and across many a small town green, the steady drone of soldier boots was accompanied by a chorus of speech-making and the flutter of silk Tiffany and plain cotton flags. The ladies hugged and kissed their menfolk farewell amidst the strains of fife and drum.

Initially enthusiasm was the rule. Even New England bankers were eager, willing and able to finance the uniforms and armaments of regiments yet to be formed. Within 48 hours of the explosions in Charleston Harbor, Governor William Buckingham of Connecticut had bank pledges for half a million dollars delivered by telegram or hand, with the promise of the same amount in six months if the war had not ended, which of course it would. All strove to contribute, be it doctors, ministers, mothers and wives.

The excitement and enthusiasm soon gave way to the consequences of modern warfare and 700,000 deaths; the proportional equivalent today of seven million, more than all previous and subsequent American wars combined. The level of health care required for the sick and wounded was unprecedented. For the Union alone endured 1.1 million cases of malaria, 41,000 deaths from diarrhea dysentery, and 35,000 amputations. One hundred ten military surgeons in the entire army pre-war evolved to 10,000, and 40 army hospital beds nationwide grew to 120,000 in 192 military hospitals regulated and funded by the federal government. Military hospitals were divided into 16 departments as the federal government took charge in providing health care (see Appendix I).[1]

In the nineteenth century, patients were treated at home and not at "pest" hospitals generally reserved for the homeless and indigent. The Lincoln administration realized change was necessary but was reluctant to build facilities in the North, fearing soldiers sent home would not return to the battlefield. Their concern was real, as only one of three resumed field duty. Some died, some were disabled by disease or wounds, and others found the safety of being near home irresistible. Placing large convalescent facilities near the battlefield risked being overrun or shelled with disastrous consequences. With an eye to the next election, there was political virtue in showing all was being done for the health and welfare of our soldiers. They deserve and would get the best hometown food, clean air, and state-of-the-art health care where loved ones could visit and contribute.

The army's antiquated medical department was headed by an 82-year-old Surgeon General who opposed medical education and took pride in returning money to the federal government. The seniority system determined promotion, allowing him to serve in place for 26 years until his death. Accomplishing major transformation in the midst of a cataclysmic civil war required radical surgery. The Lincoln administration installed 33-year-old William Hammond. His task was to modernize a medical department designed for a garrison army and not modern war. In just 18 months, major changes were instituted stressing education with the start of a national medical library, a national pathology center, and formal examinations for entering army surgeons designed to exclude the incompetent.

Providing health care for any society is a complex matter. Oliver Wendell Holmes Senior, dean of Harvard Medical School and father of the future Supreme Court Justice wounded at Antietam, stated that health care delivery was impacted not just by the science of medicine but also by politics, religion, philosophy, and economics. At the outbreak of the Civil War, there was no practical experience in large-scale health care; "most of our volunteer medical officers knew nothing of military hospitals small or large."[2] The initial arrangement of regimental camp health care delivered in tents was replaced by larger divisional organizations where teams of surgeons pooled an ever increasing base of experience in deciding who received surgery and when.

The first facilities were in Washington D.C., where hotels, colleges, infirmaries, warehouses, and churches were transformed into hospitals. Temporary hospitals were established in private residences, the Capital building, the Patent Office and St. Elizabeth's Insane Asylum. With the Peninsula campaign in the spring of 1862, barrack buildings near Washington and Baltimore were converted to hospitals wards.[3]

Surgeon General Hammond, who was keen on the military hospital experience in Europe, recommended ridge-ventilated, wooden pavilion buildings. Fresh air, proper ventilation and exposure to sunlight were thought essential to treatment of disease or trauma, as demonstrated in the Crimean War by the British Army and reported worldwide by Florence Nightingale. Assistant surgeon Lewis Eastman noted on April 1, 1862: "it is very difficult in ordinary buildings used as hospitals to secure ventilation without exposing the inmates to injurious drafts of air. This difficulty is avoided in the building of ridge ventilation, which keeps the air constantly pure without exposing anyone to unpleasant or dangerous drafts."[4] The problem with this construction was pointed out by surgeon George Oliver in October 1862. "These buildings though well adapted for use in warm weather do not afford sufficient protection from the cold of winter for sick and wounded men. The ridge ventilators having no sash or shutter to close, the wind, rain and snow penetrate to an extent unbearable by the patients."[5] Vents placed near the floor permitted easy entrance of small, unwelcome visitors. Vermin and other creatures came and went, producing no discernible health benefits.

Ventilation in the summer was non-existent, hand-powered fans offered slight improvement, but for stifling heat rolling up tent flaps worked best. Crowded wards with wound infections produced hospital-wide gangrene. Hospitals tents were set aside for treatment of gangrenous wounds and for contagious diseases such as smallpox.

Mass transportation in the nineteenth century was by water or rail. The ability to move large numbers of patients by ship or train made hospital location critical. Though the existence of bacteria and anti-sepsis was unknown, the importance of sanitation was part of the armamentaria of every successful general. Building hospitals on contaminated soil or wetlands was to be strictly avoided. The site needed to be well-drained to accommodate buildings with septic systems. The grounds needed to be elevated and remote from sources of malaria, and most important have access to clean water. Water supply would be either piped in from a local town or from spring, reservoir or well. Sometimes water was brought in by wagon and rainwater used as well.

In order to gain efficiency and improve patient outcomes, federal regulations were formally issued as to where and how military hospitals should be built, as well as recommendations about proper staffing. There would be full examination and approval by a medical inspector and ultimately the Surgeon General.[6]

One-story, detached pavilions averaging 130 by 24 feet would comprise each ward with beds for 50 to 100 patients each. Structures for general administration, dining room, kitchen, laundry, quartermaster, knapsack house, guardhouse, quarters for female nurses, chapel, operating room and dead room were to be connected by covered walks with floors but without sides. Buildings were to be 30 feet apart for proper ventilation. They could be arranged in echelon as a V, circle, parallel, oblong or elliptical.

There were separate kitchens for ordinary and other diets. The Quartermaster Corps ran the Knapsack House with two-foot,[2] individual pigeon holes for each patient, holding their belongings. Autopsy was performed in the Dead House, whose location next to the operating room was out of sight and earshot of the wards. Quarters for female nurses, both civilian volunteers and Catholic sisters, were in detached buildings. The chapel also served as a library and reading room. Usually situated near the administrative building was the water supply: a large tank supplied by well or spring and powered by pumps and steam engines providing hot water for kitchen, laundry and bathing facilities.[7]

The importance of immediate disposal of human waste descends from biblical times. If water supply was adequate, water closets were installed at the ward's end, separated by a wall to segregate foul odors. Ventilation of these units depended on the ingenuity and skill of local officials. Some privies were built a distance from the wards in slit trenches to be filled with peat moss or other available materials daily. Those with limited water supply used pits or vaults instead of movable boxes.

Each hospital had its own police department to discourage desertion and anti-social behavior. Each had its own fire department that performed fire drills and conducted patrols. Axes, fire buckets and rubber hoses for attachment to water closets were kept on every ward. Hospitals with tarred paper and wards massed together were a fire risk.

The chaplain offered services on the Sabbath and bible classes and lectures during the week. He also had responsibility for the cemetery, post office, reading room and library, assisted by ladies' societies and convalescents. Charitable contributions and hospital newspaper sales were sources of funding for items in the library.

The surgeon in charge had full and complete military command over the persons and property connected with the hospital and was held responsible and accountable for both. The executive officer was in charge of administration, record keeping, clerks and orderlies, issued orders and conducted general correspondence. The army demanded daily, weekly and monthly reports, and in triplicate, concerning records of admission, register of inpatients, casualties, furloughs, deaths, discharges and transfers, and financial statements of hospital funds and property.

Each ward had an assistant surgeon who might be assigned to cover two or three other wards. The medical officer of the day had 24 hour duty to admit patients, prescribe medications and diet, inspect meals and enforce discipline. They were responsible for medical and surgical care, policing of ward, care of property, morning and evening rounds, keeping diet and prescription books, giving a morning report to the executive officer, and recommending return to duty, furlough, discharge, or transfer to Invalid Corps. In the absence of the physician, care was assumed by the ward master. Eager and ready medical cadets [students] were employed as clerks and wound dressers under the supervision of the ward physician, receiving experience, room and board but no pay.

Recovering convalescents became clerks, cooks and nurses. There was no substitute for a visiting mother, sister or loving wife in providing care. In some facilities, particularly those with Catholic populations, sisters of religious orders provided the best in skilled nursing, having the unique distinction of previous training. In the Victorian age, contact between the sexes was viewed with suspicion.

Convalescent patients performed guard duty, freeing up others for the battlefield. Fourteen-foot fences were built to discourage sojourners from making pilgrimages home or to Canada. A thousand-bed hospital required 20 ward masters, 40 to 100 nurses, six cooks, ten assistant cooks, five laundry workers, and 25 more for the bakery, blacksmith, painting, carpentry, dispensary, knapsack storerooms, administrative offices and cemetery. The average ratio of support personnel was 200 employees per thousand beds.[8]

The Department of Washington was the largest of 16, containing 25 hospitals of which 17 were in the capital city, including the Armory Square Hospital, whose newspaper was the *Armory Gazette*. There were six hospitals in or around Alexandria, Virginia, initially organized in abandoned dwellings, warehouses, churches, and seminaries. Both *The Soldiers' Journal*, published in Augur U.S. Army General Hospital, and *The Cripple* at the 3rd Division U.S. Army General Hospital, originated in that locale. Point Lookout, Maryland, several miles south of Baltimore, was the location of Hammond U.S. Army General Hospital and the *Hammond Gazette*. The total number of hospital beds for the Department was 21,146 (see Appendix II).[9]

Eleven hospitals were established in Philadelphia, the first opening in June 1861. The campaign of 1862 by the Army of the Potomac forced speedy conversion of a railroad depot, coach factory, silk factory, and arsenal into hospital facilities. The largest Union hospital was Satterlee U.S. Army General Hospital, with 3,519 beds and the first hospital newspaper, the *Hospital Register*. There were seven other hospitals in the Department of Pennsylvania, with a total bed capacity of 18,709. The military hospital in York, Pennsylvania, published *The Cartridge Box* (see Appendix III).[10]

The Middle Department included Baltimore, where hotels and warehouses were converted to hospitals. In Annapolis, buildings of the Naval Academy and grounds of the Agricultural Society were converted to the U.S. Army General Hospital, Division No. 1, that issued its newspaper, *The Crutch* (see Appendix IV).[11]

The Department of the East included 25 hospitals, whose beds totaled 14,289. In New Haven were the Knight U.S.A. General Hospital and its paper, the *Knight Hospital Record*. In Montpelier, Vermont, were Sloan U.S. Army General Hospital and the *Voice of the Soldier* (see Appendix V).[12]

The newspaper is the first draft of history. The very next issue and those that follow are revisions that create society's notion of "truth." This was not modern "gotcha" journalism, though relations with the press were sometimes stormy.

The importance of the print media was emphasized by Abraham Lincoln in his lectures on *Discoveries and Inventions* in 1858–1859.[13] "Man is not the only animal who labors; but he is the only one who improves his workmanship." Writing was a great invention, enabling conversation with the dead and absent unborn. Printing allowed communication of thought in a timeless fashion, leading to new invention years later. Thousands of copies could be cheaply printed, exposing facts and ideas for the many and not just the few. Discoveries, invention and improvements would follow. The educable could be emancipated, thus eliminating "slavery of the mind" while breaking its shackles, leading to freedom of thought and the advance of civilization. The only obstacle was "a real downright old-fogyism" that smothers the intellect and energies of man. "Public sentiment" was critical; with it "nothing can fail; without it nothing can succeed."

A revolution in technology made possible rapid dissemination of information. The American continent was crisscrossed with telegraph wires from Maine to Texas and Massachusetts to Kansas and as far as the Rocky Mountains, connecting over 6,000 cities and villages. The first telegraph line began operation in 1844 between Washington and Baltimore and spread rapidly. By 1860 there were 50,000 miles of telegraph wire with over 1,400 stations employing 10,000 operators and clerks. Each year the increasingly popular and lucrative wire delivered 5,000,000 messages and $2,000,000.[14]

It was much faster and cheaper than the mail or Pony Express. The hospital newspaper in New Haven described the amazement of an elderly lady who received a yellow envelope responding to her message in just a few hours. She proclaimed, "All the way from Wheeling Virginia and the waifer's still wet. That's an awkward looking box but it can travel like pisen."[15]

In Europe, with the exception of Great Britain, the telegraph was under the control of governments and restricted to the wealthier classes because if its high toll rates. In America it was open to all, the lines mostly privately owned.

From Boston to New York and New York to Boston, 2,800 words an hour were transmitted. On April 19, 1865, the day of Lincoln's funeral, over nine wires, 85,000 words were transmitted between Washington and New York, between 7 p.m. and 1 a.m. over 14,000 words per hour.

The advance in technology, including steam-driven printing presses, dramatically increased the ability to cheaply print thousands of copies an hour. America was a literate nation of 25 million, with poetry and general reading a common practice. On the eve of war, there were 4,000 newspapers and periodicals, 176 of which were in New York City.[16]

Because of the ease in transportation, local papers were offered for sale in other towns and states, aided by cheap mailing rates. Newsboys hawked broadsheet dailies and weeklies fresh off the newly arrived train. Direct sales were stimulated by dodgy headlines and opinions camouflaged as scandalous "news" engineered to capture public interest. *Harper's Weekly* was launched in 1857, carrying crisp lithographic reproductions, often copied from photographs of recent events, enthralling its 200,000 subscribers nationwide. The best-selling *New York Herald* sold 30,000 copies a day. Weekly and quarterly magazines on military history and events were printed in New York and disseminated to soldiers everywhere.

Politics and journalism were joined at the hip, heart and brain. New Haven, like most towns, had papers representing both opposition parties: the *Palladium* for the Republicans and the *Register* for the Democrats. Impartial reporting was not stressed.

The copperhead dailies assailed the Lincoln administration on every level, declaring the draft unnecessary and illegal, bringing accusations of financial and moral corruption, portraying them as incompetent and dictatorial, while advocating pro-slavery status for most of the continent and urging cessation of hostilities. The nation was better off divided and at peace. Papers supporting the administration accused the Democrats of treason and those who preached such infamy traitors. In the presidential election year 1864, more than 30 newspaper offices were attacked by mobs, organized and not. The writ of *habeas corpus* was suspended. Numerous publishers, editors, and reporters were arrested, imprisoned and offices closed for business. That "Congress shall make no law abridging the freedom of speech or of the press" went on sabbatical. Pro-peace newspapers were banned from the U.S. mails. Telegraphs, though privately owned, were censored. The notion that the duty of a newspaper is to print the news and "raise hell" was for the administration incongruous and counter-productive with the perilous times.

Of the 192 Union hospitals created during the Civil War, 19 had their own newspaper. Nine have been located, with the number of issues ranging from one to 96, and are the focus of this book. They were printed in one long sheet and by folding in half created four pages. One briefly had eight pages, and two were large format. Some had skilled artwork adorning their mast heads, with occasional illustrations and others showing varying quality in print and content (see Appendix VI).

Each chapter describes the creation and evolution of a hospital and its role in providing health care. Choice, relevant material from each newspaper is summarized and divided by subject matter: humor, romance and marriage, religion, sacrifice and patriotism, race and ethnic relations, medical treatment, daily soldier life, battlefield experience, politics, ill treatment of prisoners of war, Lincoln, and prospects for the disabled. Hospitals exchanged newspapers, experiences and points of view. The writers were knowledgeable participants reporting what they saw and felt.

The largest hospital produced the first, longest running and best newspaper—well written in broadsheet format, with lithographic illustrations. The story of the *Hospital Register* follows.

ONE

Hospital Register

The army hospital in West Philadelphia rested in a bucolic locale believed "eminently healthy," 200 feet above and 250 yards from a water source, the Mill Creek. The air was "free from mephitic odors or pestilential malaria," a feature considered essential for good health. This was an ideal location with "pure country air," shade trees on well-drained soil, near a railroad and major river. Sixteen acres of high ground and all its buildings were intended to be owned permanently by the federal government. It opened June 9, 1862, and within 40 days seven of the 34 buildings were completed.[1] It would have shocked the original occupants that closure would be August 3, 1865, over 60,000 patients later.

Today a five-block area from 40th to 44th Streets and Spruce to Pine is bounded by Clark Park, with tall, elegant, leafy trees whose shade now protects baby carriages. It was bordered by Woodland Cemetery, founded in the 1830s and filled with elaborate marble and stone tombstones from which the Schuylkill River is now barely visible. Rows of upscale town houses, a Veterans' Hospital complex, University Medical school and hospital, and a College of Pharmacy founded in 1830 complete the surroundings. The largest of all Union hospitals became a diverse, modern medical complex.

Horse-drawn wagons conveyed the wounded and sick from the river, while others were floated on rafters along Mill Creek. Pipes drained the effluent from a catch basin connecting runoff from kitchens, bathtubs and laundries. Ten-inch clay pipes were buried below the frost level to a sink which drained into a small river. The sink was closed over with earth and was 100 yards from the hospital.[2]

There was a boiler and engine house which furnished hot water distributed by iron pipes from kitchens and laundries. Despite state-of-the-art engineering, water shortages still occurred, as reported in the *Hospital Register*:

> The federal government pays water bills from 24th ward of Philadelphia whose supply regularity is humbug. Complaints are continually made in newspapers and elsewhere that *the supply of water is always uncertain* and often deficient in private houses and in the hospital where an abundant supply is the first essential. Three thousand sick and wounded are without water despite being in sight of the Schuylkill River and a giant "Stand Pipe" and yet such is the fact. Frequently there is no water at all in the hospital. It is almost constantly scarce. Last week it was hauled in barrels. We need 130,000 gallons daily. It has been a nuisance for a month. We are getting a new steam pump to suck water from pipes but if that fails then what?[3]

In 1862, Dr. William Hammond of Maryland ordered the creation of a military hospital in Philadelphia as part of a national health care system for returning sick and wounded soldiers. In May 1863, the hospital's original name changed from West Philadelphia

Hospital to honor the "the faithful and meritorious services" of the most senior surgeon in the army who had been bypassed for Surgeon General.

General Richard Sherwood Satterlee (1796–1880) was born in Herkimer County, New York, of Puritan ancestors; his father was a Connecticut Major in the Revolutionary War. He began the practice of medicine in civilian life in 1818, becoming military assistant surgeon in 1822, and served in the Black Hawk, Seminole and Mexican Wars. Just prior to and during the Civil War, he was assigned attending surgeon and medical purveyor of New York City, responsible for purchase and issuing materials worth millions. He was praised for economy and fidelity and received promotions to colonel and brigadier general, retaining this position throughout the war, and retiring in 1869.[4] The nursing staff was headed by Lady Superior Sister Gonzaga of the Sisters of Charity, first organized in Paris in 1576. Twenty-two Sisters arrived as the hospital opened, rose to 41 in number, with over 100 serving over the hospital's life. By all accounts, these women were providential gifts who required no pay and bare living expenses. They were in charge of donations, delivering medicine prescribed by surgeons and prepared by apothecaries, and providing special diets.[5]

The types of diet (full, half, low and extra) were considered a form of treatment or tonic. Red or white tickets were issued determining who got "extra," which on a daily basis meant milk, vegetables, butter and eggs. On Sunday and Wednesday the "extra" menu was steak and chicken, on Monday and Thursday mutton chops and oysters, on Tuesday, Friday and Saturday, steak, chicken and oysters. Sister Gonzaga handled the logistics well and was charged with their administration.[6]

The surgeon in charge was Isaac Israel Hayes, recently returned from Arctic exploration. His first printed order was a call to duty of all medical officers and hospital attendants assigned as of June 7, 1862. Grand rounds with ward inspection would be held every Sunday at 9 a.m. The "parade" would include ward officers, officer of the day, steward and chief ward master, chief cook, chief druggist, and commander of the Guard, with every soldier and person on duty at their assigned post in waiting. If unable to attend, a replacement was required.

He had an extensive support staff, including an executive officer, assistant executive officer, two chaplains, chief of quartermaster, chief of commissary, a pathologist, and separate commander of guards, officers of Veterans Reserve Corps and hospital detachment. In September 1862, Assistant Surgeon John S. Billings was appointed executive

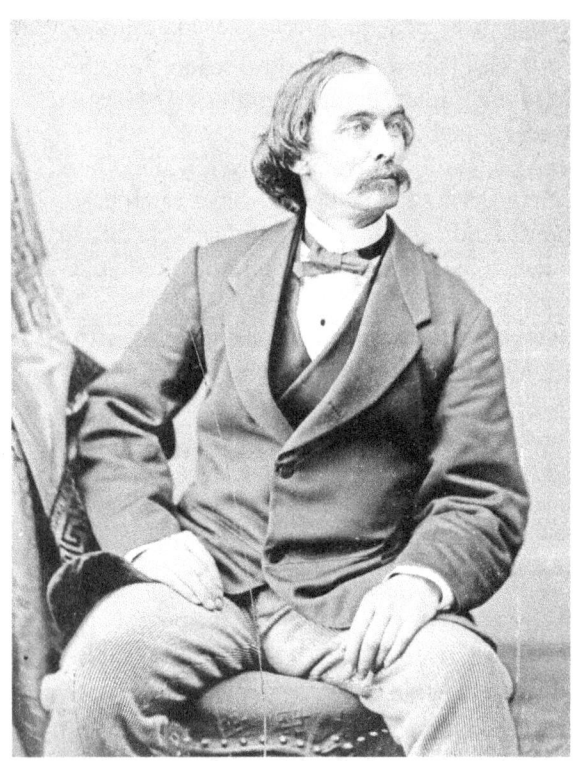

Isaac Israel Hayes. Arctic explorer and chief of staff, Satterlee Hospital. 1862–1865 (Library of Congress).

officer to clarify lines of command and improve efficiency, accountability and discipline. He received all reports and papers connected with administration and business affairs, reports from surgeons, stewards, ward masters, officers and NCOs, certificates of disability and all matters dealing with discharge of soldiers and assignments of cadets.

There were 34 wards; A through Z, XX, OK, 1–5, and Camp 5. All surgical cases were moved to wards F, D and Q. Diseases of the eye and ear went to ward M. Each surgeon was assigned a ward, often two and sometimes four. Each visiting surgeon was assigned one assistant surgeon and one cadet. They were expected to wear uniform on duty and aid in organizing and enforcing hospital sanitary rules and discipline thought essential for a military establishment. Individual ward inspections described uneven living conditions such as: "individually wretchedly kept, badly kept, clerks not responsible, mostly correct, carelessly and improperly kept, neat but imperfect, and excused."[7]

Keeping appropriate medical records was necessary to evaluate patient outcomes. Collecting data to evaluate efficacy of treatment and administration demanded accuracy and uniformity to make comparisons. Initial record keeping was minimal to none. Case book and prescription books were created for each ward, one page per patient. The listing included bed number, full name, rank, company and regiment, marital status, age, nativity, date of admission, concise statement of nature of disease, principal symptoms and general history of case, plan of treatment, and cause of death or injury. Changes in treatment including new symptoms were eventually added. If the patient died, he was crossed out with a red line and the same page continued for the bed's next occupant.

Absence of trauma records needed remedy. "Surgeons are requested to report to this office either from notes or from memory all cases of surgical operation performed in their wards. As of late much negligence has existed in regard recording treatment and transfer." Tabular statements about surgical operations, injuries rendering them necessary and the results with full accounts of the more interesting cases were established. Every case involving loss of life or limb was reportable to the surgeon in charge, who directed a consultation of not less than three surgeons.[8]

The Surgeon General issued gunshot wound forms to be pasted on the inside of each ward book for reference: site of wound, character, how received, nature of missile, treatment by amputation, resection or simple dressing, involvement of shaft, joint or tendons, result and remarks. For amputation were it primary (within 48 hours) or secondary (after 30 days), the results and any remarks were recorded. Other categories included wounds of the head, face, neck, chest, abdomen, back, perineum, genital and urinary, upper extremity, lower extremity, arteries, large nerves, sword, bayonet, miscellaneous, burns, and explosions.

Surgical reports were to be more comprehensive: full description of injured parts, constitutional state of patient at time of surgery, amount of hemorrhage, number of ligatures, duration of procedure, and anesthetic agent used and its effects. The report should include a full account of treatment and progress from day to day, complications, eventual disposition, and cause of death and post mortem with name and rank of operator.

Behavioral problems were not limited to the foot soldier but included the medical staff, prompting Surgeon Hayes to make new ground rules, starting November 1863.

> The business of the Hospital is seriously embarrassed in consequence of the systematic absence of several of the medical officers in direct violation of existing orders. Many seem to imagine that their duty is done when they register their names, walk through their wards and without asking permission to be absent notify the executive officer that this or that doctor will substitute them for the

remainder of the day. Such officers are a useless expense to the government. Hereafter medical officers will remain in the hospital at all hours of the day and night unless specially excused by the surgeon in charge, upon written application stating clearly the necessity of such absence. If granted, a substitute must be obtained and in no case can the same officer be substituted in two wards at the same time.[9]

Rounds were to be made twice daily, at 9 a.m. by surgeons and between 4 and 6 p.m. by cadets, who visited the sick before breakfast as well. Surgeons needed written approval to be absent ward, needed to get a replacement before leaving, and could not leave at night. Resident surgeon and cadet could not be absent at the same time. The surgeon's private quarters were not for socializing with the ladies. The executive officer would keep attendance records including arrival and departure of all visiting physicians. Medical officers wrote prescriptions but were admonished to "not interfere with druggists in any way and on no occasion go behind the pharmacy counter."[10]

Each issue of the hospital newspaper listed the names of medical cadets, quartermaster, steward, postmaster, baggage master, chief ward master, chief clerk, chief female nurse, chief printer, chief or carpenter, and chief engineer. Each ward also had a Sister of Charity, ward master, three nurses and a medical cadet. In times of peak use, skilled local physicians rendered assistance to the resident surgeons, a feature only large cities could offer. The University of Pennsylvania Medical Department had seven emeritus professors and seven faculty doctors available for service. The school session of 1863–1864 started the first Monday of October and ended the first of March. [Cadaver dissection was done only in cool weather.] Their previous session held 319 students, of whom 78 graduated.

The medical library run by a cadet was maintained in the resident surgeon room. Three books could be removed at a time for one week and were accessible at all times for medical staff on duty. If lost or destroyed, the borrower was charged the original value. A course of lectures on military medicine, surgery and hygiene for the instruction of the cadets was inaugurated by Dr. Joseph Leidy on Tuesday and Friday during lunch hour. Medical education would be stressed nationwide, initiated and encouraged by the Surgeon General's Office.

The Reverend Nathaniel West, hospital chaplain, praised its 41 surgeons and 33 medical cadets for "advances made in science of surgery, medical treatment and improvements of the sanitary condition of the hospital. A competent mind that heads any complex establishment will work wonders."[11]

Although there were no schools to train apothecaries, experienced personnel compounded and dispensed 3,500 prescriptions daily. Chemists working in a laboratory prepared pills, plasters, potions, and syrups. It was compared in appearance and quality to a first-class city drugstore. Department head Dr. Samuel Fries, an experienced pharmacist, had four chemists in the laboratory and five in the dispensary.

By December 1864, there were 3,519 beds, of which 2,464 were occupied. The federal government paid $4 a week for each bed filled. Wards holding 70 patients could double capacity. After the battle of Bull Run, wounded arrived by the hundreds. After Gettysburg, the hospital population exceeded 6,000, with the largest monthly admissions July 1863 at 4,062, requiring hundreds of additional tents on open grounds for the overflow. Deaths that August averaged one a day. From Satterlee's opening on June 9, 1862, through May 27, 1864, there were 12,773 admissions and 260 deaths, a mortality rate of just 2.2 percent.

The largest and most elegant of hospital constructions included flower beds and a 400-seat chapel. There were two parallel groupings of 14 one-story pavilions separated

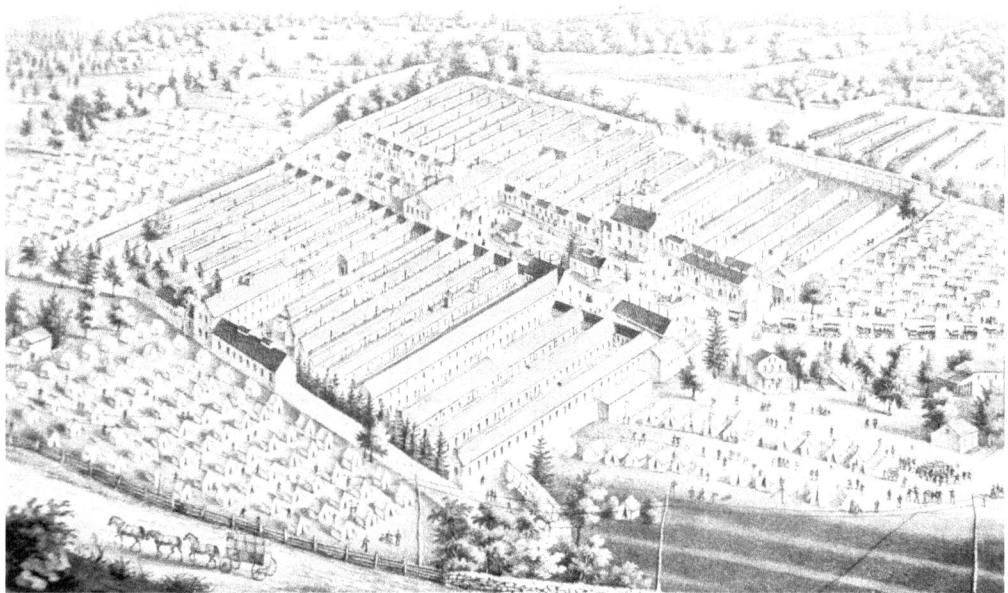

Satterlee U.S. Army General Hospital, West Philadelphia. Chromolithograph (author's collection).

by a two-story administration building and courtyard. Each ward was 167 feet long, 24 feet wide and 13 feet high. The corridors running east to west were 900 feet in length. On each side were 15 windows, six by eight feet. At one end were two rooms for the Ward master and female nurses (Sisters of Charity). At the opposite end was a water closet with a cast-iron trough 12'3" long, the accumulations let off every hour through a three-inch discharge pipe into a general sewer by elevating a lever.[12]

The closeness of each building (21 feet) and the narrow width separating the groupings were not repeated elsewhere for fire safety. Two-inch hoses were supplied in the water closets for emergencies, and trained fire fighters were in readiness. Two large water tanks held 40,000 gallons and the means of extinguishing fire anywhere on site. The fear of fire was no illusion, the *Armory Square Hospital Gazette* reporting an event at Lincoln Hospital in Washington. "Last night at midnight an alarm of fire was sounded on 4th St., East and C St., North. The cause of the alarm was burning of Ward C of Lincoln Hospital which communicated with Ward 8 and spread towards 10 and 12 all of which were consumed. The fire started in the room formerly occupied by the sisters and is believed to be the work of an incendiary as no fire had been in the building for a long time."[13] There was no mention of casualties. Many towns and villages had no fire departments. Wooden buildings and factories laden with grease and oil became total conflagrations in minutes. Death and destruction were frequent events.

Dr. Hayes issued a series of detailed orders to prevent such an accident. Fire rounds were started in October 1862. Three patients per ward took three-hour shifts from 9 p.m. to 5 a.m. A cook was on duty in the kitchen and storerooms for the same vigil. A druggist, officers, ward masters, clerks, sisters, surgeons, cadets and sergeants of the guard checked their respective work areas in the same time slots. The officer of the day then checked the inspectors to be certain proper investigations were made.

Sound alarm came from a sentry firing his rifle and shouting "fire!" Engineers manned the pumps and officers assembled in the surgeon's room, awaiting orders. A fire brigade was formed of the most reliable convalescent patients, 28 detachments of 6–12 men each. They had fire axes, buckets and attached hose. The goal was to preserve order among patients, allow no one to leave wards, remain quiet and await orders. Only the wounded would be escorted out. Periodic drills were announced in advance with day and time, expecting all participants to be at their station and ready.

Bathtubs were filled with water every night and fire buckets filled and ready. In December 1863, Hayes ordered all stoves to be opened at taps and kept open until reveille. If a stove went out, it would not be re-lighted under any circumstances. "Use no more wood than necessary and the stove need not be red-hot or coals piled above fire bricks."[14]

By January 1865, there were seven acres of flooring and an enclosure adjacent to the office of Dr. Hayes adorned with a fountain producing towering jets of water and populated with gold fish and one statuesque white swan. The second floor of administration had rooms for officers and one for visiting surgeons.

A formal department of engineering was in charge of machinery, water pipes, water tanks, water closets, gas pipes, steam pipes, boilers, fire apparatus and lightning rods to ensure the safety and effectiveness of this system. Each washroom had a cast-iron receiver for washing hands and face, and a cast-iron bathtub with hot and cold water. Each kitchen had a large range, two large cooking stoves, and three boilers, each holding 60 gallons. Despite the closeness of the wards, air circulation was considered good, reasonably cool in summer, and for winter 200 coal-powered stoves provided heat. The buildings were plastered for insulation purposes. Natural gas from the Philadelphia Works provided light. There was also a tank house, barber shop, carpentry shop, news depot, sutler store, blacksmith shop, paint shop, fire and police company, library and reading room with piano and large vases with many species of gold fish.

Officers and especially surgeons assumed their responsibilities and "spared no pains or expense to contribute to the comfort of their inmates of the institution." A hospital band played daily, often from a flat area atop the two-story administration building called the observatory. They were mostly German and performed every afternoon from 2 to 4 p.m., in dress parades and dirges for the dead.

Dealing just with the behavior of thousands of young men was a full-time job for Dr. Hayes. Many of his orders concerned an attempt to keep this asylum under a modicum of discipline. His second order issued in 1862 was that "no patient allowed to leave hospital without permission from surgeon in charge." He would control passes for all hospital attendants, druggists, clerks, engineers, carpenters, ward masters, cooks, nurses, and laborers. The medical officer of each ward submitted a list of up to ten passes for any one day for those orderly and well behaved

Getting, keeping and circumventing the pass system seemed to occupy many otherwise idle minds. Green, yellow and red tickets were issued for specific locations and time limits, some permanent or just Sundays. Forgeries flourished. There were two roll calls daily, 7 a.m. and 7 p.m. By 8 p.m. names of those absent without leave were submitted to the executive officer. Patients who violated their liberty or returned intoxicated or disorderly were placed on the Black List. Those AWOL beyond 48 hours could be charged with desertion.

Rules for ward conduct were posted. All took a bath on admission and washed face and hands every morning. Those physically unable would be assisted. All patients were to be at bedside for rounds and standing if possible with no passes between 9 and 11 a.m.

Convalescent pass, Lincoln U.S. General Hospital, Washington, D.C. August 1861 (author's collection).

No spirituous liquors of any kind could be had without permission of the medical officer. No smoking, spitting, loud noises, slops or rubbish on floors, including storerooms and hallways, was permitted. Beds were to be made every morning by attendant, and those able to do so would make their own. No patient occupied his bed without undressing or with shoes on. No clothing or other articles were allowed under beds or mattresses.[15]

Hospital stewards determined and obtained whatever clothing was necessary for patients and attendants, dispersing goods every 15 days. The government would not replace "article for article" but only clothing lost as a casualty of war. Laundry days were Mondays and Saturdays; officers were charged $2.00 and cadets and stewards $1.50 per month for the benefit of hospital fund.

The executive officer and lieutenant of the guard would see that no person was admitted to hospital grounds without a pass except new patients, officers, chaplain, cadets, and stewards. Visitors were permitted Monday, Wednesday and Friday from 2–5 p.m. and must leave by 6. Those passes were good for a month.

Only the utmost care and attention would be acceptable for the benevolent citizens bringing contributions for the sick and wounded. Guards and sentries were expected to be courteous, polite and civil to all. Hayes expected continued praise from visiting foreigners, the Surgeon General, army generals, and government officials concerning the excellence of their military discipline.

There were armed, uniformed sentinels at both inner and outer gates who could be relieved only by an NCO or officer. They were not to quit their post or have conversation with any person unless obligated by the job. Officers were to be saluted. Rifles and bayonets were secured indoors only in rain and absence of sentry box. Every half-hour at night they shouted "all's well" and "fire" if necessary. There was no pass for bundles, all of whom were examined by the sergeant of the guard for contraband, liquor or stolen items. If an inmate left the hospital grounds without permission or if the sentinel was found conniving, both would be court martialed. Those capable of light duty were assigned guard duty by the ward surgeon because "property of government is much exposed and many articles have already been stolen."[16]

By the summer of 1863, a 14-foot fence surrounded the 16-acre complex. A guard barracks held 177 men including five musicians, seven orderlies, and clerks, with the rest guards with bayonets and rifles providing 25 sentries at a time. They were stationed in and around the hospital to warn off "*night-thieves* and other *strollers*" and to keep them a respectful military distance from the hospital in addition to discouraging deserters, bounty jumpers and importers of illicit booze.[17]

Exposing the worst truants to peer pressure may have been why the following was posted: "Private James Lamphere, Bed 48 Ward U having been placed in confinement for striking Sister Mary is at the earnest request of Sister Mary and Sister Superior released from confinement and all other punishment and will return to his ward."[18]

Another notice "published for information for inmates in this hospital" concerned the court martial in June 1863 of Private Kilpatrick of the 23rd Pennsylvania Volunteers, who was AWOL from March 2–10 and sentenced $5 from monthly pay for one month and deprived of all leaves of absence for passes for two months. Private Samuel Crumb of the 89th New York Volunteers was found guilty of forgery of descriptive lists, fraudulently drawing pay, desertion, and conduct prejudicial to good order and military discipline. He was sentenced to "be shot to death with musketry at such time and place as the commanding general may direct." Two-thirds of the court members concurred.[19]

A unique feature of this burgeoning community was the Printing Department, publishing the first hospital newspaper of the Civil War, *West Philadelphia Hospital Register*, from February 16, 1863, through June 24, 1865. It was a paper whose "contributions are as a general thing from the pens of soldiers." It was initially superintended by Hadley Lamborne, a soldier and experienced printer. Type and press-work were by convalescent patients disabled from service in the field. The two compositors and three pressmen were listed by name and unit: three from Massachusetts, one New York and one Pennsylvania. Being composed of convalescents meant the staff was transitory; a year later there were four from Pennsylvania, one from New Hampshire and three from Massachusetts. One clerk ran an office with two small presses that did printing duties for other military departments as well. A new issue of the *Register* appeared every Saturday, handsomely produced and four pages long. Initially a standard small sheet, in a year it became large format (11 by 16 inches) or "two open hands long and a hand and thumb wide." A surgeon in the field could use it as a tablecloth.[20]

In January 1864, the logo was changed from an Oriental styled physician applying leeches to an overview of the hospital. A free copy of a lithograph was given to subscribers of the *Register* and offered for sale to others.

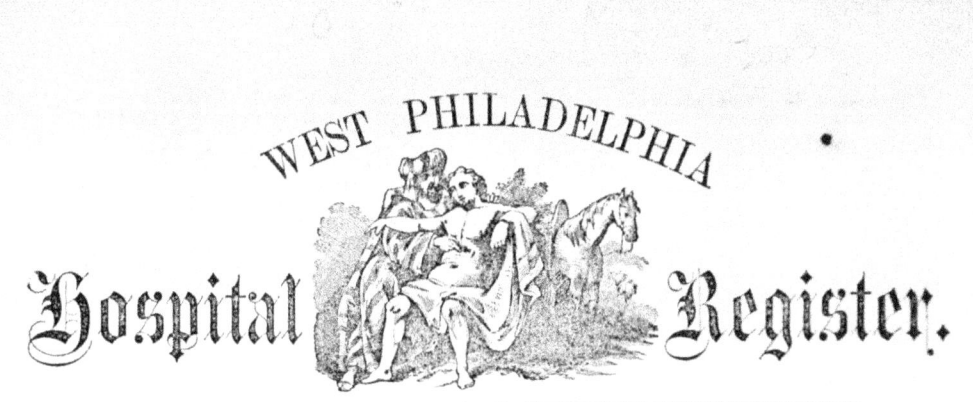

Masthead of *West Philadelphia Hospital Register,* May 9, 1963 (author's collection).

The first issue of *West Philadelphia Hospital Register* declared its origin: "Printed and published at U.S. Army General Hospital, West Philadelphia. Read o'er this: and after, this: and then to breakfast with what appetite you have." Its purpose was to support an elaborate library and reading room and solicit reports of the war and experiences of soldiers. "Jot down adventures and personal occurrences while in the field and place in the contribution box." Friends of the hospital should contribute. "Nothing of a partisan character can find a place in this paper. Soldiers who have been tried in fire of battle and found not wanting can never recognize but one people, one flag and one country. Neither will discussion in regard to merits or demerits of individuals such as generals or politicians find a place in our columns." Any article or item of news from soldiers in the camp or at any other hospital and others with an interest in entertainment and instruction of the soldiers would be welcome.[21]

Each person who contributed to the paper got five free copies. A one-year subscription was initially $1, raised to $2 in 1864 or five cents a copy for non-soldiers. The reading room was given 400 copies. Because of many donations, it was provided gratis "to some extent for hospital patients as we want every man to have it." There would be a short summary of military activities and short stories both moral and uplifting. In a plea for more subscribers, it was noted that "all visiting surgeons subscribed without hesitation and all resident surgeons with three exceptions." Some ladies donated up to $30, and several benevolent men in this city subscribed for five copies but request just one, noting "can they not give the soldiers too poor to purchase the paper the rest?"

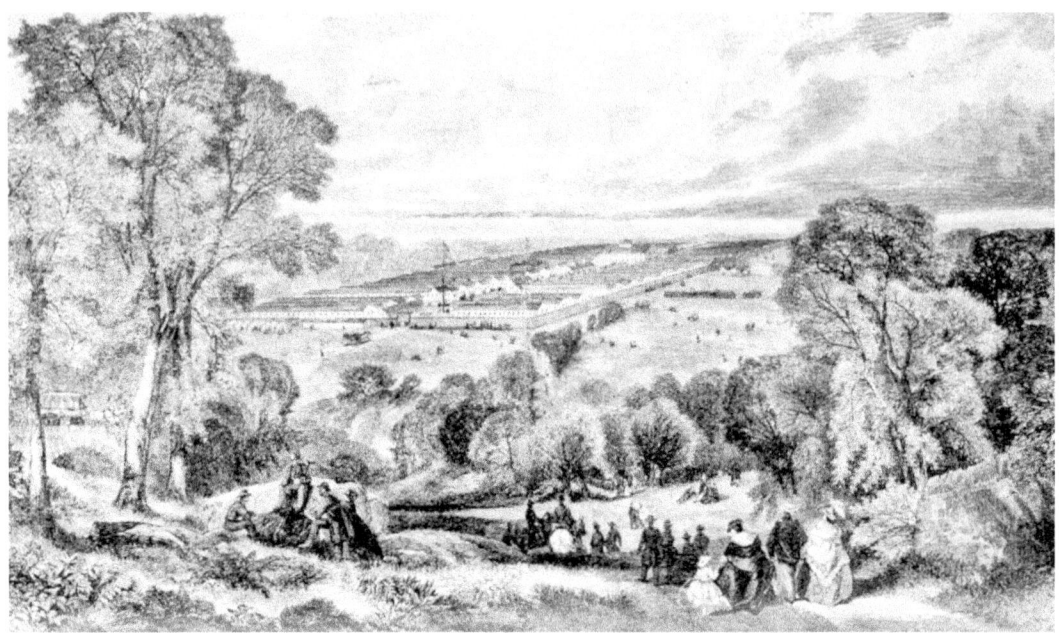

Lithograph of a new logo for *Hospital Register*, engraved by Mr. Snyder of Van Ingen & Snyder of Philadelphia (Library of Congress).

It was stressed that the paper was published strictly for the "benefit of the soldiers and not private interest." Surplus funds were for the benefit of those maimed by bullets or diseased from exposure and fatigue. A few hundred copies of "our little sheet [were] sent to the citizens of Philadelphia, hoping they will subscribe." The presses made forms for other military functions including written orders from the Surgeon in Chief and officers in other departments.

Initially there was great enthusiasm and a great quantity of material to choose from. "Scribble on, your turn will come." A weekly feature was *The Canvas Backed Chair*, a high-brow literary column concerned with the likes of Aristophanes, Plato, Cicero, Virgil, Socrates, Hercules, Faust of Goethe, Don Quixote, Virgil, Byron, and Greek and Roman commentaries. These topics were not foremost on the mind of the average enlisted man and provided literary discussions a doctoral candidate might have trouble following. Modesty and the study of antiquity were not to be slighted. "This is the most wonderful and original literary production which has made its appearance in our times and although our modesty is so great we cannot help adding that the hospital which has given birth to this prodigy is in itself a marvel of excellence and completeness." There were 500 subscribers by the summer of 1863.

Getting quality material was difficult. In May 1864 another call went out: "Attention soldiers—we want communications. Write articles, experiences in field, camp or in hospital setting that are treasured up in your mind that will be interesting. Send to the Hospital Register, Philadelphia." The one absolute restriction was "no politics as long as the present regime continues. We are pleased to print patriotism to any extent but neither Democratic nor Republican, nor Copperhead nor abolitionist, find any place in our columns."[22] Other papers did allow political discourse, making for livelier reading. The call went unheeded, as reported in August 1864.

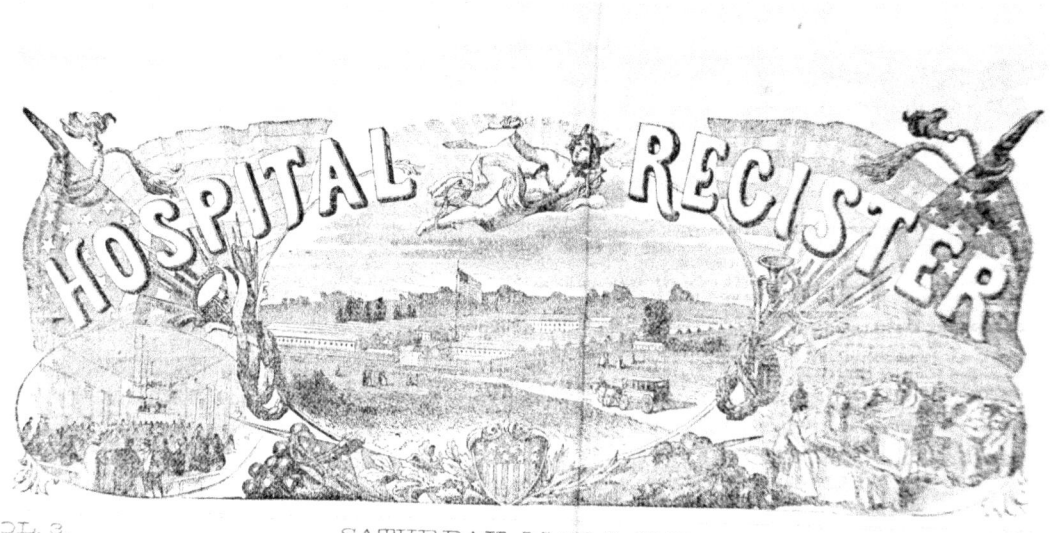

New logo, *Hospital Register*, August 29, 1863 (author's collection).

We are obliged to acknowledge that our efforts to obtain articles and communications from the soldiers have proved fruitless. There is no doubt of the ability of many soldiers to give interesting articles for their paper but there seems to be an indifference or apathy prevalent among them which they cannot or will not try to overcome. The columns of the register will be enlivened by original articles of some kind each week and a more thorough record kept of the sick and wounded arriving in this department.

In March 1865, appeals continued; "we desire contributions from our correspondents and readers who find it convenient to write. Make your articles concise with all readable brevity and suggest you select as subjects something of every day interest, including home incidents of ordinary occurrence."

One source of literary insight was the city street cars moving large numbers of humanity in wet, dusty and crowded circumstances.

Sketches in the cars explore riding home amongst travelers while nodding into slumber-land. A small sitting space opens enticing a hulk of a man to force himself in, exclaiming as if monarch of all he surveyed, "there is always room for one more." The man of size and his friends discuss the diversity in size and shape of individuals of the same race with saloon humor. The conductor shouts "41st Street," and the correspondent leaves the corpulent speaker and his motley crew. He concludes, "the most intolerable nuisance in the world is a man who sits cross-legged in the street cars and spits out the window."[23]

Each issue had a listing of ten puzzling questions put forth to amuse and stimulate, "Things Wise and Otherwise—Conundrums." Stimulating the funny bone was always good medicine.

> What is the difference between a surgeon and a dress-maker?
> One cuts dresses and the other dresses cuts.
>
> Why is a gentleman walking between two ladies a most singular sandwich?
> Because the tongue is all on the outside.
>
> Why do women never have whiskers?
> They cannot hold their tongues long enough to be shaved.
>
> What is the difference between a Northerner and a Southerner?
> One blacks his boots and the other boots his blacks.

Political satire had its appeal whether written by a convalescent or nationally renowned humorist.

> The tone of this paper needs to be radically changed. Suggested topics for study at $150 each include: how to get real pepper, what about hospital visitors, is an army without discipline all that bad, a geological study of the hospital site including its paleontology, the locations of adjacent grog shops from the hospital, and how to cheat doctors in convalescents camps. For a moral poem $150. For discussion on financial gains from descriptive lists and paymasters, the aesthetics of desertion, or a poem in blank verse $175. An epic on the war showing how it may be terminated in a manner universally satisfactory to all parties will collect $10,000.[24]

The editor exalts the Printer as the "adjutant of thought." Author and printer are engineers united in self-serving purpose, the truth givers come down from Mount Sinai.

> His missiles bombard for the ages and not just a recent battle. He stands at the base and marshals into line the force armed for truth and clothed in English for the Anglo-Saxon race. His goal is to win victory from death with his work. The printer is a laborer whose work a sublime rite flinging a worded truth grander than any missile, into the bottom of an age yet unborn. The place he stands is holy ground from whence he sends a little song like a wounded bird from the Ark that had preserved it and flies into the future with the olive branch of peace and melody, the dawning of a spring morning.[25]

The many problems of the hard-working editor were enumerated for the reader's edification and amusement.

> If there is too much political matter people won't have it, if too little they won't have it.
> If type is large it doesn't contain enough reading matter, if type small they can't read it.
> If I have a few jokes, it is rattle head, if omitted we are an old fossil.
> If complementary to a man, we are censured for being partial.
> If not complementary to a man, we are a greedy hog.
> If we speak well of any act of the President, folks say we dare not do otherwise. If we censure they call as a traitor.
> If stay in office and attend business we are too proud to mingle with fellows, if we go out we never attend to business.[26]

According to the *Register*, the first soldier newspaper was printed early in 1862 by the 19th Pennsylvania Volunteers for three months, called *National Guard* and leaving no copies. The 11th Pennsylvania Cavalry at Yorktown published another early paper called the *Cavalier*. In October 1862, a Massachusetts regiment in the Army of the Potomac briefly issued a paper, leaving no records. The first introduction of a press at a hospital was at Satterlee, in October 1862, publishing its first issue February 14, 1863.

It was common practice for hospitals to exchange newspapers. One consequence of this was cross pollination so that jokes, anecdotes, and fictional stories were sometimes republished with the origins becoming obscure. *The Cartridge Box* of York, Pennsylvania, was praised as a "very spicy little sheet. We trust it will never want for plenty of good ammunition to keep its *pockets full and strong* and loving hands to keep its *brasses bright*." The short-lived *Caduceus* was "an interesting little paper just born into the work devoted to the interests of hospital steward. It is very spicy and full of courage."

Advertisements

An extensive military directory took up most of one page. The commanding officers of the Department of Pennsylvania were listed by name, rank, title and address. Included were the Judge Advocate, Paymaster, Quartermaster, Arsenal, Mustering and Disbursing office, Provost Marshall, and Commissary Department. The latter was concerned with issuing of subsistence and supplies and payment of commutation of
rations. This was followed by the Medical Department listings, including the Medical Purveyor office and the U.S. Laboratory that made drugs. Satterlee's staff was listed in detail including all wards with their respective surgeons and medical cadets by name. Also listed were the executive officer, guard commander, pathologist, chaplains, hospital stewards, postmaster, baggage master and chiefs of ward masters, clerks, Sisters of Charity nurses, printers, carpenters and engineers. Visiting days posted were Monday, Wednesday and Friday from 2 to 5 p.m. Special passes for other hours of visitation could be procured from the executive officer, if approved by the surgeon in charge. There were ten other military hospitals in Philadelphia also listed with their staff.

Numerous advertisements took up the last page, with a cornucopia of services and products. Jay Cooke, a notorious financier, placed an ad for U.S. Treasury notes issued June 1865, bearing 7.3 percent interest per annum, known as seven-thirty loans, payable in three years. They were convertible at 6 percent to gold bearing bonds and were exempt from state and municipal taxes. Collectors of ephemera might frequent the shop of A. C. Klines on Walnut Street, whose "wanted" ad for Confederate notes, postage stamps, coins, medals, and autographs was a *Register* feature.

More relevant was the notice "for relief of families of soldiers who have fallen in battle." To apply for benefits required an application asking the name of the widow, her address, children by age, and the husband's name, regiment and company. In what battle was he killed, how much money was obtained from the regiment since his death, and what other aid was received? To apply for benefits for sick and disabled, the same information was needed including whether employed and character references. The U.S. Sanitary Commission, Christian Commission, and Women's Relief Corps were among those organizations that either provided aid or directed families to government departments who did, and at no charge.

A committee representing relief associations visited the hospital each Thursday. Soldiers could contact them by leaving their name and bed number with their ward master or directly at their headquarters on Chestnut Street.

The *Hospital Register* business directory listed four hotels, a restaurant and an ice cream parlor. For those soldiers suffering from hospital food fatigue this ad must have been appealing. "A Good Meal for Twenty-Five Cents at Ford's Restaurant. Have your choice of poultry, beef, lamb, veal or oyster pie and for 10 cents more apple dumplings, pie and milk, or ice cream." Three blocks down on 11th street in Farmers Market, it offered "Great Dinners in North End" for the same price, touting patriotism in its ad: "Wrong is weak, Right is strong, Union right, Treason wrong."

Numerous photography galleries offered portraits for loved ones back home as carte de visit, ambrotype, melannotype, ferrotype, water color, pastels, crayon or oil. There were dealers of cigars and chewing tobacco, merchant tailors, Army and Navy clothing, military goods including water proof gators, shirts, boots and shoes, envelopes and paper, blank books, paper and stationery, trunks and carpet bags, watches and fine jewelry, gentlemen's furnishings, billiard saloons, choice brandies and wines for medicinal purposes, flour and country produce from dairy farms, butchers selling beef, mutton, lamb, chicken or fish, and the ubiquitous Sutler department with "ice cream, lemonade, sarsaparilla, peaches, apples and all the best fruits of the season at the lowest prices along with new military music." Music and musical instruments were for sale "cheap." Sewing machines were "the cheapest, the best and the most beautiful does interlock stitching with all kinds of thread and sews leather and finest muslin."

Surgeon Dentist J. Lubielski had an office in the headquarters building promoting "cleansing, extracting and filling teeth." "Bad teeth make bad breath" unless prevented by tooth powder of his own manufacture. "Sets of teeth made to order on reasonable terms." Druggists and chemists filled prescriptions "most carefully compounded." J. Medhurst was an undertaker and embalmer who promised "all orders promptly attended to." On Market Street were agents seeking substitutes for those drafted and volunteers for the "highest bounty."

In May 1865, with the war just over, an ad from clothier Wanamaker and Brown guaranteed the lowest prices while castigating the fleeing ex-president of the Confederacy. Linking the Darth Vader of that period's evil empire with the steadfastness and determination of a haberdasher might seem a stretch. Patriotism sold soap, deodorant and men's clothing.

> Jefferson Davis has come to grief.
> He scampers away like a frightened thief,
> Making his specie up in a pack,
> Taking the bundle along on his back,
> Sneaking and hiding out of sight,
> Traveling as hard as he can by night.
>
> But the great Oak Hall stands up like a man,
>   Selling its goods as fast as it can;
> Selling so rapidly selling now so cheap
>   Now and hereafter determined to keep
> The best and finest goods on hand,
> Just the things to meet the demand.[27]

Library

Chaplain Nathaniel West, 68 years old, was present at the hospital's birth and first anniversary, which he commemorated by writing its biography.[28] His responsibilities included the library and reading room. The chapel was without equal for a military hospital. It was next to headquarters, having expanded from 100 to 400 seats. Subscriptions from private citizens enabled cushioning all chairs. Pulpit books, pulpit chairs, and window shades were paid for by private sources encouraged by a "contribution box." Gifted was the profile of George Washington, a photograph of General Andrew Jackson, and a large, eight-day clock. Typical was the donation of 80 copies of *The Accepted Time* by the

Reverend L. H. Christian, pastor of the North Presbyterian Church of Philadelphia, whose work allegedly "garnered precious food for the soul whose wants are too often neglected and forgotten amidst the exciting scenes through which we are now passing." Additional donations came from the Presbyterian Board of Publications: 550 books, 22,000 religious tracts, 100 devotional poetries, and 300 soldier's pocket book bibles. Numerous other pamphlets and books of a religious nature from Bible societies and individual citizens included such weekly newspapers as *The Christian Advocate, the Presbyterian, The American Presbyterian, The New York Observer* and *The Standard.*

West published a catalogue of the library's contents one year after opening, providing a glimpse of the administration's interests and ideals.[29] Almost half the books (390 out of 910) were religious in content and included: encyclopedias of biblical literature, memoirs of many reverends, Christian tracts, the *Doctrine of Scripture,* the *Life of John Calvin, Imitation of Christ, The Pilgrim's Progress, Holy War, The Christian Contemplated, Hadassah or the Adopted Child,* the *Converted Jew, What I must do to be saved,* the *Words of Jesus,* the *Angel over the Right Shoulder, Christ Knocking at the Door, The Worlds of Jubilee, The Little Episcopalian, Man and Woman, The Young Christian's Pocket Book, Sermons on Christianity, The Power of Prayer,* and *The Testimony of God against Slavery.*

Fiction made up the next largest selection including Charles Dickens, Harriet Beecher Stowe, James Fenimore Cooper, Edgar Allan Poe, Shakespeare, and Daniel Defoe's *Robinson Crusoe.* The small collections of poetry included Cowper, Shakespeare, various British poets, Milton and especially Longfellow. Travel was represented by a number on the Northwest Passage, John Fremont, *Life in China, Journey to Iceland, The Sultan and His People, What I Saw in California, Arctic Exploration, Russia, American in Paris,* and *Discoveries in Africa.*

Out of 910 books, 69 were in German, 22 in French and three in Spanish. There were many nationalities represented in this patient base, all of whom were encouraged to seek out books, magazines and newspapers. One hundred seventy-four books on history included 11 copies of the writings of George Washington, the *Lives of the Signers of the Declaration of Independence,* the *Life of Benjamin Franklin, Heroes of the American Revolution,* the *Mexican war, History of England, Napoleon and his Marshals, Life of Napoleon Bonaparte, History of Queen Elizabeth, History of the Jews,* and *The Pioneer Boy-Life of Abraham Lincoln* (six copies).

The miscellaneous category was the third largest and contained encyclopedias, the *Letters of Horace Walpole,* journals on health, physiology, zoology, gardening, chemistry, natural history, inventions, phrenology, electromagnetism, salads, and chess playing, Webster's dictionary, botany, zoology, *The Conspiracy Revealed or the Horrors of Secession,* and *Irish Eloquence.* There were ten other newspapers including *Harper's Weekly and Monthly, Leslie's Illustrated,* and *Illustrated London News.*

In September 1863, the *Register* enunciated the importance of the Reading Room as:

> an attempt to facilitate more physical and mechanical remedies of the physician. Frequently the diseases of the body proceed from the soul, since the power of unassisted thought could carry a man according to Plato. One of the principal predisposing causes of death is *weariness,* an apathetic condition induced by constant and unvarying duties and positions. Reading material detracts from morbid tendency of boredom and inactivity ... and will bring temporary self-forgetfulness and abnegation of their own maladies and sufferings.

Sound mind, sound body. For those disinterested in religious life, there was a fine spinet piano and 15 different games to play: backgammon, dominoes, solitaire, six chess sets, 28 checkers sets, 48 stereoscopic views and three viewers, numerous puzzle boards, and several chromolithographs.

The *Register* had solid grounds to claim the reading facility "detracts from morbid tendency of boredom, weakness, and depression of disease or injury." It was "cool and quiet" with lots to occupy the restless mind. The planned library door motto was "Medicine for the mind." It was administered by 12 members of the Ladies Society who were sympathetic listeners to soldier's complaints. The Library Association and the private collection of Dr. Hayes contributed, growing from 625 volumes to 4,500. He initiated a lecture series in the Reading Room on Tuesday afternoons with his experiences in the Arctic, "Glaciers," presented with magic lantern and poetry readings.

The first visiting lecture was by the Reverend Richards of West Philadelphia on "A day in the Hills of New Hampshire," with a reading of Tennyson's *Light Brigade* that "gave patriotism its due." Acting assistant surgeon W. C. Bonsall spoke on "Follies of the age." Signed passes were required, one show admitting 475.

By May 1863, the Reading Room was 20 by 200 feet with a billiard room and a separate "large smoking room in which the weed may be indulged to an unregulated extent. The narcotic clouds which float about in the atmosphere of this room proceed mainly from the bowls of pipes." Opposition to tobacco by smoke or chew came from the temperance organizations and confirmed in the *Register*. Smoking was forbidden on the wards, storerooms, kitchens or bathrooms.

The *Canvas Backed Chair* editors praised improvement of hospital grounds with gravel walks, grass plots, water fountains and flower beds. They stressed high-brow literary features, running a series on painting and sculpture. One episode was called "Phantasm" and another "Of Verisimilitude," which discussed the artificiality of modern art. The literary and debating society took up the question "what has caused the most misery, intemperance or the war?" The response was less than enthusiastic, leaving the editors to conclude that there was "decimation of the literary spirit among soldiers and regret that the number of visitors of the reading room has fallen off." The average soldier might have preferred the "narcotic clouds" coming from his pipe. A request was made for personal narratives of those who were wounded to increase reader interest.

In February 1864, a second anniversary of the Reading Room was celebrated with a 17-piece band concert and refreshments. With an eye towards rehabilitation, Dr. Hayes instituted night school and vocational training such as bookkeeping and general education taught with "fundamental branches of an English education." Preparing veterans for post-war life would be an essential hospital function.

On September 17, 1864, the *Register* announced the death of Chaplain West at age 70, noting "he was stern in manner but with much affection and kindness." Putting together this library was his achievement. A cautionary tale came from the hospital newspaper *Convalescent*, published in Baltimore, that "got folks to send books from their attics and closets thus ridding them of garbage to help build a library." They received calendars from 1823, public documents from 1826, a list of the royal navy from 1829, sermons from 1836, and annual reports from the Home of Aged Women from 1848. "Send us boxes of books not boxes of junk," pleaded the *Register*.

Specific rules were posted for the privilege of using the Reading Room and library. It was open from 8 a.m. to retreat. Ward surgeons sent a list of those deserving approval to the surgeon in chief. Those unruly, intoxicated or showing bad behavior were placed on the "reading room black list," meaning banishment.[30]

Chaplain Crane became the new director with the duties of keeping inventory, maintaining discipline, listing donations, and ensuring the facility was used just for reading and lectures without illicit libations. Ladies of Philadelphia and Directress Miss Mary McHenry dispensed books and answered only to Crane. The job of administration was transferred to the executive officer to improve discipline, control passes and provide statements for funds on hand. Many unauthorized passes had been dispatched, requiring re-registering all passes. Only neat, enlisted soldiers with proper uniforms could play billiards. Officers were excluded during daytime hours.

Sermons

The military chaplain, like the surgeon, served more than one master. He represented the soldier, the bible and the government. Religious services were held at 2 p.m. on Sunday, prayer meetings on Monday, lectures on Wednesday, and bible class on Friday. Private consultations were offered in the chaplain's office 9 to 11 a.m. From Monday to Saturday, each of the three chaplains—West, McLeod and Crane—made daily visits to six wards so that each ward saw a chaplain three days a week.

At a typical Monday prayer meeting, nine soldiers poured out their souls and in most fervent manner blessed the President and Cabinet, offering "prayers for salvation of our common country from a merciless rebellion. I fully believe He will in his own time overthrow the rebellion, cleanse a nation from her crying sins and raise her in the eyes of the whole world more glorious than ever."[31]

If all the religious tracts, pamphlets and texts were insufficient to quench the spiritual soul, there was the column Canvas Backed Chair and later the Chaplain's Corner, dispensing wisdom for the faithful and those seeking renewal and encouragement. They carried the baggage of literary snobbism in that Herodotus, Confucius, Socrates, Euclid, Aristotle, and Descartes were unknown to the average volunteer. The appeal to the reader was: "Cease your doubts and if you believe anything at all, state to this chair what it is. For ourselves, we make it a rule to believe everything we don't understand."[32] Cant, whining and hypocritical chatter were considered harmful and untruthful.

> I doubt patriotic testimony. Shakespeare and Bacon had no confidence in human veracity since the world is given to lying. In the good old times men settled their differences of opinion by the dungeon, the battle axe and the stake without regard for their commercial interests—there was no room for cant. Mankind does not calmly and deliberately listen to reason. Cant is a fungus of civilization that never fights but threatens, never defies but abuses, never resents but whimpers and scolds. It is a cowardly narrow minded feeling and now almost as popular as whiskey. Cant is empty declamations and hypocritical protestations now respectable. In the press it is called patriotism.[33]

Believing sometimes demands faith rather than a scientific understanding that exceeds the grasp of common man.

> *Believing but not understanding:*
> "I will not believe anything but that I understand," said a self-confident young man.
> "Nor will I," said another.
> A Gentleman replied "do I understand you that you will not believe anything that you don't understand?"

"We will not," said each.
The stranger replied, "In my ride this morning I saw some geese eating grass, do you believe that?"
"Certainly," said the unbelievers.
"I also saw pigs eating grass, do you believe that?"
"Of course, we do!"
"And I saw sheep and cows eating grass, do you believe that?"
"Of course, again!"
"Grass they had eaten had turned to feather on the geese, bristles on the backs of swine, wool on the sheep and hair on the cows; do you believe that gentlemen?"
"Certainly," they replied.
"Yes, you believe it but do you understand it?"
They were confounded, silent and ashamed.[34]

What is the meaning and value of *the true life*? The four grand elements of moral worth and cardinal virtues are justice, prudence, temperance and fortitude. Knowledge, truth, love, beauty, goodness and faith give spice and vitality. Prayer and the hardship of struggle provide nourishment of our natural being along with laughter, tears and music.[35] Knowledge is the universal language, allowing a man to stand before kings as he stands before ordinary men.

"Religion is an inestimable boon to all, but especially for the soldier. The life of both soldier and civilian are equally in God's hands." The bible brings unity, freshness and success. "One cannot avoid the bible; it always triumphs over scrutiny thus separating the false from the true religion. It is a true friend whose value like sound health is seldom known until lost. It is the patriot's book; societies lacking religion ultimately fail."[36]

The soldier was told he must face personal responsibility because "life is cheap now." In a war that seemed endless, patience became even more virtuous.

"You can do anything if you only have patience," said an old uncle who had made a fortune to a nephew who had nearly spent one.
"Water may be carried in a sieve if you only wait."
"How long?" asked the petulant spendthrift who was impatient for the old man's obituary.
His uncle coolly replied, "Till it freezes!"[37]

Self-sacrifice was critical to success in sports, family life and the battlefield. The Chaplain encouraged action and return to duty: "all you have suffered incident to the state of war, pray to God to pardon and heal you and when recovered go back again to the field and renew your compliments to the enemies of our blessed country!"[38] Like the military surgeon, his job included keeping soldiers in the battlefield.

In the book of Job, every kernel in his cob of life was destroyed, testing his faith as "changes and war are against me." Spiritual and material calamities oppressed and overwhelmed an afflicted nation. "In a fearful fratricidal war be prepared to meet your last great enemy which is death. Be cheered by the knowledge we were fighting a just and holy cause. The future is in His hands who have faithfully promised to be a father to the fatherless and maintain the cause of the widow."[39]

A visiting Reverend Adams spoke on "Enlisting: Who will go for us?"

God calls for volunteers from man who is born in blood; as is liberty, good government, and redemption of souls. He wants the best but will take the weak he will make strong. Enlistment is for life. If you fall in service, He will lift you up and if you suffer with Him you shall be glorified with Him, and if you overcome will sit with Him on the great eternal throne. In this glorious war his soldiers shall conquer though they die.[40]

A medical cadet penned a satiric tale about a "patriotic" volunteer with a dislike for work. His father, discovering bills labeled washerwoman were actually for cigars, cocktails and brandy smashes, evicted his son, forcing him to earn a living. He was approached by friend Major Sniggins, recruiting for the 90th Massachusetts Volunteers, and agreed to join but only as colonel. His friend challenged: "Do you go for filthy lucre or let some patriot fill your place who will carve with his sword a way to immortality?" He enlisted as a private, asking, "Do soldiers work?" Sniggins replied, "work—no! No mere drudgery, no plebian toil. A soldier's life is a life of honor and glory, and hardships far above mere mercenary labor. Plant the banner amid showers of shot and shell on the battlements of the enemy and sweep them out returning with honorable scars and laurel wreath of the Goddess of Liberty." Though his father was pleased with this patriotic fervor, he felt swindled by Sniggins, "a contemptible liar who took me in to mostly hold his horse." He slipped and fell in a cellar in Baltimore from a brick to the head and was nursed for a week by "an old darky woman." Upon reaching his regiment, he was declared a deserter and given a spade to dig Virginia soil. The only shot he fired was at a donkey he mistook for a Secesh and missed. The only shot fired at him occurred as he was stooping over a brook to drink, wounding his rear end, mistaken for a sheep.

> I went expecting glory, honor, and grateful smiles of my country and instead for twenty months dug with spade and pickaxe as a waiter for officers. An aspirant for literary fame not content to carve his way to immortality with a scalpel in his hand and a green sash around his waist put me in the *Register*. Lying on a cot with rear-end up, I have to endure listening to surgeons moralizing on fatigue and billiards, quoting Greek mythology, and appealing to the women of America for evening studies.[41]

A series on "Reflections" helped crystallize why they were fighting and the unholy hopelessness of rebellion. There could be no war without God's permission as there was sin on both sides. "I reared children and brought them up, and they have rebelled against me!" [Isaiah 1:2]. "If you refuse and rebel, you shall be devoured by the sword-for the Eternal One has spoken." [Isaiah 1:20].

The worst evil was committed by those who secretly prepared and then thrust their country into a rebellious war. Be faithful to your country and the President. "Rebellion is like the sin of witchcraft." [Samuel 15:23]. In this world sin, death and the devil had to be subdued as well as the rebellion in the South, whose secession violated the bible. Its remedy: "if thy right eye offends thee pluck it out for it is profitable for thee that one of thy members should perish and not that thy whole body should be cast into hell." [Matthew 5:29]. Both sides quoted the same passages of the bible to support their side.[42]

The chaplain recounted Moses' call for a draft amongst the 12 tribes of Israelites after exiting Egypt. All those over 20 must fight without exception. None was considered too feeble, too edentulous or stiff jointed when they left Egypt. Their light camp had no commissariat, no sutler, no purveyor, no clothing department, and no surgeons. Jehovah fed them, gave drink, provided one shirt and a pair of sandals that lasted a march of forty years. So Union volunteers; do not complain! [Deut. 29:3].

Atrocities were being committed by Southern demons rather than true men. Men and women were hunted by bloodhounds, hanged, shot and burned alive. Men boasted of being gentlemen, and their women, young and beautiful, spurred them on to rebel barbarities.

> The little child is accustomed to see men and women treated like animals and are taught to regard them as such. They see them sold, beaten, branded and driven like cattle with all decency obliterated. They have become tyrants with uncontrolled passions never opposed. Why should not men who flay

their slaves sometimes to death, burn them alive, take their women at will be expected to treat the same, men and women against whom they feel a savage hatred and whose destruction they thirst.[43]

This was a holy war; the rebels were criminals who must be brought to justice so that righteous men could achieve their full measure of salvation and enter heaven.

The Reverend West stressed that none valued obedience to orders more than soldiers. God is the greatest authority and commands repentance of sins. "Be loyal to your country, the fate of the African race is among us." At an official ceremony, the chaplain provided the hospital a new flag 36 by 20 feet. Surgeon James Williams, who was the assistant executive officer, addressed assembled troops. "Citizens can gaze with pride and admiration on this glorious banner the emblem of liberty floating in triumph over many hotly contested fields. You have just come to us mutilated, wounded and invalided from the fields of savage war where you have been nobly battling in our country's cause in the suppression of a wicked rebellion. Let us have three glorious cheers for this beautiful flag!"

On June 11, 1863, the contracts of two-thirds of the visiting surgical staff were cancelled. Dr. Hayes expressed "sincere regrets that necessities of service require a reduction of the medical staff but was authorized to state that if vacancies occur they will be first offered." This was three weeks before the greatest battle of the war, with 52,000 casualties in three days of fighting. In the first week of July 1863, there were 704 hospital admissions from Gettysburg, and many more to follow.

Christmas of 1864 celebrated the fall of Atlanta and Lincoln's re-election by majority vote. Mrs. E. T. Egbert donated $5,000 for a magnificent repast for all patients. "We cannot do enough for them. I have one dear brother in the field but where I cannot tell. How happy it would make me to give him a Christmas dinner." Two thousand copies of the *Register* were sent to family members. A half a mile of halls and corridors were decorated with wreaths of evergreen. American flags hung from the ceiling along with pictures and likenesses of Lincoln and Washington and placards such as "God bless our brave boys in the army." The names of each ward's surgeon hung in the rafters along with Generals Grant, Sherman and Sheridan.

Over the post office door was a carved American eagle made by a Union refugee with only a pen knife. A sign over the main entrance said "Our thanks to Mrs. E. T. Egbert." In the printing office, pictures of Benjamin Franklin were framed in evergreen. Christmas Dinner was served at 3 p.m. The main course was turkey, roast beef, and roast chicken with sides of apple, plum, or mince pies. The usual potatoes, greens, cakes, cookies and appropriate beverages made the menu complete. Cheers went up for Lincoln, Grant and Egbert.

Santa Claus Dead was published on January 7, 1865, after the good cheer had worn off and cold reality settled in.

> "Mama, who told you Santa Claus was dead? Did they kill him when they killed papa?" A well-dressed gentleman with rosy cheeks entered and gave with pride some toys to a little boy. Another child cast a forlorn look with longing at the dancing Sambo and the prancing humming top and when he reached the platform a plaintive voice cried out, "Mama that little boy's Santa Claus isn't dead; why is my Santa Claus dead?" Alas, Santa Claus was dead to many a child on Christmas day and the kind hands that were want to fill the little stockings and deck the tree are cold beneath the fields where our countrymen are seeking love and concord in earth covered with blood.

Temperance

There were hundreds of Sons of Temperance societies across the United States. Some organizations demanded total prohibition, others not. The clergy devoted much time and space for this issue. Assistant surgeon James Wilson addressed the society on July 23, 1864. "Employers do not want to hire young men who smoke cigars and drink. Job prospects dim if you do and are excellent if you don't."

For some, intemperance brought more misery than the war! One of the four cardinal virtues was avoiding excesses of food and drink. "The drunkard shames his nature, drowns his reasons, prostitutes his chastity and murders his conscience. He has the body of a swine, throat of a fish, and the head of an ass. Drunkenness is worse than plague, famine, war and all these calamities together. The drunkard's cups kill more than the cannon and rob heaven of more souls than war. What they do is criminal!"[44] True happiness is the absence of alcohol.

A short tale, *The Power of Religion*, by the Reverend Alfred Nevins, appeared in the *Chaplain's Corner*. A distinguished New York City lawyer only two weeks before was a hopeless drunkard, a poor, lost man. Friends tried to reclaim him but without effect. He tried with many tears to break away from drink's cruel bondage, but resolutions and vows failed. Suicidal, he went down to a river and saw a young man fishing. The stranger turned down his flask of liquor, saying, "I never drink intoxicating drink. I asked the Lord to help me never to touch it and yes I am a Christian." The lawyer went home that night and while on his knees confessed being a poor, miserable wretch, struggling against a raging appetite for liquor. He appealed to the Lord to remove it and promised to serve and love Him forever. He had not had a drop since or any desire to taste it. He frequented temperance meetings to help others reform.[45]

Aristotle declared that "man being reasonable must get drunk," and the "practice a duty to the Gods." Intemperance among literary men was common. The most powerful intellects were unable to escape the fines, bailiffs and indignities of debtorship. "A Scottish poet, near the close of his melancholy life walked alone with feeble step and downcast eye, a woe-wasted bard ignored by his partying former friends. Read his despondent letters and penitential poems on the prospect of death and follow his darkening decent to the grave in the very prime of life."[46]

Drunkards were often jovial, noting drink is encouraged in the bible. *Autobiography of a bottle of whiskey* tells of a quart bottle made in a kiln filled over time with wine, oil, candle sticks, vinegar, bitters, gunpowder, black pepper, ink, and molasses. "I was first used as a whiskey bottle by a liquor merchant who bought me from an Israelite of old iron and glassware persuasion." He was filled with "tangle foot" and purchased by an elderly lady from a boy for a pittance and then brought to the hospital and placed under a pillow. "During the night several soldier patients took part in emptying the bottle in a joyful enterprise. Bottoms up! All are happy!"[47]

Excess brings biblical doom for "Those who chase liquor from early in the morning until late in the evening, never give a thought to the plan of the Lord, and take no note of what he is designing. Assuredly my people will suffer exile for not giving heed." [Isaiah 5:11, 13].

The *Evening Telegraph* called drunken soldiers a nuisance needing corrective attention, describing several hundred hospital convalescents fit for active service who ought to be in the field. "They spend their time in the city in dissipation, get to taverns and get drunk, become boisterous and profane, quarrel, fight and disturb the public peace." The *Register* rejected the notion as an "impudent lie," insisting drunkenness was minimal. Soldiers preferred not being in the hospital, and Doctors wanted them moved out as soon as they were well.

Anecdotes and short stories illustrated the same points more effectively than sermons.

> A bright eyed little boy watched as an inebriate staggered down the street. "Mother, did God make that man?"
> "Yes, my child."
> After a moment of thoughtfulness the little fellow said: "Well I wouldn't."

> I am an old man, wealthy and respectable. But I do not know except by memories long past what joy is. I am not unhappy. I look forward to seeing my angel again and remember her love in the dim past and see her love in the dim future. When young and alone in the world, I was well educated and versed in books and men. I spent the years of early manhood in prison, lost my money, as a slovenly and vile drunkard, despised by others. I met a saint-like lady who came to my store with veil on, a well-known woman of great wealth, daughter of rich merchant. She gave him wealth, love and pride infused in a new life. She died, he mourns.

The lot of the clergy was never easy, dealing with trials and tribulations of their parishioners. The following conversation concerns a cynical and foolish English merchant matching wit with a clergyman on a railroad car.

> "Does your reverence know the difference between a priest and an ass?"
> "No, I do not."
> "Why, one carries a cross on his breast and the other a cross on his back."
> "Do you know the difference between a conceited young man and an ass?" inquired the clergy.
> "No, I do not."
> "Neither do I."[48]

Mail

Most of the soldiers had no experience away from home, especially for an extended period. War changed that, producing an ailment that had no cure in the pharmacopeia. Homesickness, sometimes called nostalgia in severe form, afflicted young and old. "Many a gallant fellow in the ranks of the Union army dies of it, but shows no wound. He is dying to go home. The cause is often home neglect and its remedy costs three cents a week, a letter from home."[49]

Absence of funds and loneliness were among the typical patient concerns. An officer recovering in a Philadelphia hospital wrote to his family in Maryland, November 1864: "I received both of your letters, one containing 50 cents and 4 stamps and the other containing 50 cents and one newspaper. Am very much obliged and am tired of asking you to send money. We are looking for the paymaster every day and when we get paid will send money home so you can come see me. Ask mother and father to write."[50] Soldiers in the field often had no stamps and used envelopes embossed with "soldier's letter" or the name of the hospital, indicating payment would be made by the letter's recipient.

Private Erastus Bugbey of New York was a patient in a Philadelphia hospital writing a friend in hopes of getting money for a trip home. "I wish you cood send me some money for if I had some money now I cood come home.to see the foakes, so I wish you wood send me some soon. Send it by Express or by a letter. If you can't send me enny tell me wat the resan is. Write soon and don't faile me. From your friend."[51]

The Post Office was located next to headquarters; mail arrived at 8:45 a.m. and 3 p.m. The master of the post office was hospital steward D.W. Martin, assisted by the chaplain, six clerks, one orderly and one messenger. Mail carriers delivered directly to the wards accompanied by armed guards. A crush of eager convalescents might remove cash-laden letters not theirs jammed in a box called the Sentinel. Ward masters were ordered to keep patients at the bedside until mail was distributed. Families were urged to include ward and bed number on the envelope, and for those letters sent with money to be registered for ten cents to avoid theft or at least guarantee the money. Money orders alleviated this problem. The *Register* published *List of Letters*, indicating those remaining in the post office in alphabetical order and those with postage due. After a week they were sent to the general post office in Philadelphia and forwarded to respective regiments. Those rejoining regiments, on furlough or dead had letters forwarded to them or next of kin to avoid the finality of the dead letter depot.[52]

From August 1862 through October 1863, they delivered 125,950 letters, 19,512 newspapers and 1,443 packages. Most of the letters were stamped rather than franked (8,841). For the year 1864, there were 174,219 letters, 33,100 newspapers, and 1,478 packages. Largest mail in one day was 1,777 letters, 590 newspapers, and 99 packages.[53]

Blacks

Mid-nineteenth century America had stereotyped views on women, race, ethnicity, and religion. All men were equal if white, Anglo-Saxon and Protestant. Phrenology and other "science" allegedly demonstrated that the brain size of a white Englishman was largest and the American Indian smallest. Caliper measurements of skull size, width of nose or calf were considered evidence of intelligence. Darky, sable, bondsman, slave, colored, and Sambo were among the adjectives applied to blacks.

Why should the funeral of a colored man not take place in winter? Because it is not the time for black berrying (burying).

On picket duty with calves head and pluck
Raiding rebels led to increased picket line duty looking out for marauders and were warned not to forage, rob or maraud themselves. Nobody passed without the countersign. After midnight Sambo and comrade on picket heard a step near them. "Halt. Who go dar." There was no answer.

"Halt. Vance an' give de countersign." The visitor was a fine yearling calf gone astray. Two bayonets were passed through his lungs and he became Sambo's prize. The officers and men had a nice veal breakfast and the black cook made the "calf's head and pluck" as the daintiest dish ever put too.

"Where did you get this veal?" demanded the officer of Sambo.

"Ober dere, cap'n; in de picket line where you dun sent me in de swamp, Cap'n."

"Did I forbid your foraging strictly."

"Yes you did. But you tole us nuffin nor nobidy muss be 'lowed to pass the lines' cept they give de counter sign. Dis feller wouldn't answer when we call him halt and so we jess run him thru with baynets, dat's all."

"How you like dem culets cap'n?"

"Very good, very good! Sam."[54]

The *Register* answered a letter to the editor in *Camp Stool* concerning the question "Will these blacks fight?"

Abraham Stoefield had the dark skin of the "despised and degraded race." An ex-slave, sullen and slow about his work, with back scarred by the lash wondered "is God dead?" Putting on the blue uniform gave a new outlook on life. At the assault at Port Hudson he bore himself with the same stubborn and undaunted courage as the whites. A dozen balls struck him and he fell dead. These heroic deeds proved them worthy of a higher sphere than our countrymen have awarded them.[55]

In February 1865, the Street Railway companies of Philadelphia took a poll of their patrons as to whether "colored persons" should be allowed to ride on their cars. The *Canvas Back* editor replied.

This we consider a perfect farce and an insult. The decision is not about your character or skin color but do you have 7 cents. Many will object to sitting next to them but not if they stand in front of their loved ones on the battle field. Our friend Mack was asked the other day how he would like to take a nice young lady in the cars and have a big nigger sit down beside her. "Well." said Mack "I wouldn't be afraid of the nigger cutting me out—I guess not."[56]

Irish

Ads for servants often specified "Protestants preferred" or "Irish need not apply." The drunk found dead at the town bridge was always Irish, never Protestant.

What animal does an Irishman carry away from a fair? A bat over his head.

An Irish colonel was escorted at night through the woods where fighting was fierce. Burial units were just finishing their work. Trees were full of bullets. Even a dead squirrel could not escape the rain of Minnie balls. The bodies were buried shallow not more than two feet deep and scantily covered with earth and debris. These dead were not defined by "privilege," as all got same burial.

"Colonel your honor, them bois 'ill niver stand aginst' the Irish Brigade again. If they'd ha' known it was us, sir, begorra!; they'd ha' brought coffins wid 'em."

"No niver! They got their ticket for soup! We kiferfed them first, will inough!" shouted the other grave digger.

"Do ye belave, Colonel," said the first speaker again, "that thim Ribals 'ill lave us a chance to catch them? By me sowl! I'm just wishin to warm me hands wid rifle-practice."

The presence of death seemed to have added no fear of it to these people; having tasted blood, they now thirsted for it and I asked myself forebodingly if a return to civil life would find them less ferocious.[57]

An officer inspecting his company spied a private whose shirt was begrimed.
"Patrick O'Flynn."
"Here your honor!"
"How long do you wear a shirt?" thundered the officer.
"Twenty-eight inches, sir."

Germans

Many of the soldiers from Pennsylvania were German, bringing their own set of customs and willingness to serve. The same was true of other minorities facing status as the latest newcomer.

Our soldiers—Along with the hardy yeomen of our country have come forth in its hour of danger and need those who have forsaken the worn-out and crumbling system of old world life to broaden and deepen the free air of democratic America. The foreign born citizens who have sprung to arms the call of their adopted country have been urged on and inspired by a thorough appreciation of the freedom for which they fought, the benevolence of that Union in which they have found liberty unknown elsewhere. They have fought side by side with our own gallant countrymen in the desolate battle field, their mingled remains lie in eternal brotherhood. They fear losing liberty for themselves and their peaceful homes.[58]

A new kind of officer is the German soldier with little English. An officer appeared at the picket line at 2 a.m. but the sentinel did not understand the countersign, "Officer with the countersign" and let him through. "Vat did he means officer with the countersign?" The German wasn't the dumbest man in the world.

*Story about **German** immigrant and soldier.*

The secesh and the German are both patients in a hospital. The secesh soldier who was very sick but now doing better was a crabby customer. His surliness increased as he got well. In the same ward was a Union soldier from the land of the kraut. The confederate led with: "Go to ----,"

"Du vat?"

"Go to ----,"

"Ah! Mine frent, you ish to kind. I cannot go to dat place."

"Why not?"

"It is now full. It ish very crowded dere. Sigel, he filt it with dead rebels. Even ter faitful has to shleep out o'doors.[59]

Romance and Marriage

Contributions by the fair sex were far-reaching. A fair for the sick and wounded soldiers was held at Concert Hall Philadelphia for two weeks in June 1863. Contributions of flowers, fancy articles, cakes, jellies, fruits were requisitioned by the *Register* for a West Philadelphia Table. It was organized and run by the Patriotic Ladies of West Philadelphia for the benefit of the hospital. They participated the following summer in the "Great Central Fair," asking Satterlee Hospital soldiers to donate "chains, rings, carvings in bone and wood, canes, paper lampshades, drawings, puzzles, pipes, pictures, picture frames, rebel relics, bullets or memorials of their battle field of any sort."

Man does not live by bread alone. The aspirations of soldiers about love, romance, the promise of marriage and family were matters of greater interest than why the Roman Empire fell or the evils of alcohol. The poem *Love's power* examined unrequited love as a ship tossed in a turbulent sea that provided heavenly thrill and heart-warming cheer otherwise unobtainable.[60]

> More welcome from the assassin's steel,
> Or keenest pang the heart can feel—
> A wound no earthly power can heal
>   Is unrequited love.

Finding the appropriate mate might involve more luck than common sense. Experience, wisdom and a sense of humor trumped the most devious machinations.

"Cut out." It was many years since I fell in love with Jerusha Jane Skreggs, the handsomest country gal that ever went on legs. We walked in moonlight that shone on our meeting lips. She meant all to me with honest double love for whom I would roam the land for the choicest flowers. A city chap came along dressed in store clothes with shiny hat and vest and moustache under his nose. She left me for a singing school in the city on the new chap's arm. My fervent love that none could drive away left a desolate heart. She married the city chap and my heart was sick and sore. Then it struck me that just as good fish remained in the sea. I went to church one night and saw a dark brown curl under a gypsy hat and soon we were married. Many years passed and I realize my gain and often bless the fancy chap that stole my Jerusha Jane.[61]

The maiden's confession. With pale cheek flushing, he whispered in my ear and took my hand and pressed it in his own. He watched my crimson cheek and brushed away a tear. My pulse was wild and thrilling. I gently said, "I love thee" forgetting some might hear.

To marry a rake, in the hope of reforming him, and to hire a highway man in the hope of reclaiming him are two dangerous experiments. Yet I know a lady who fancies she has succeeded in the one and the world knows a divine who has succeeded in the other.

What is the difference between a mischievous mouse and a beautiful young lady? One harms the cheese and the other charms the he's.

Pleasure is to women what the sun is to the flower. If moderately enjoyed, it beautifies, refreshes, and improves. If immoderately it withers, deteriorates and destroys. But the duties of domestic life, exercised as they must be in retirement, and calling forth all the sensibilities of the female, are perhaps as necessary to the full development of her charms, as the shade and the shower are to the rose, confirming its beauty, and increasing its fragrance.

A woman is always at the bottom of trouble. You remember the story of the Shah of Persia. When he learned that a workman had fallen from a ladder, he called out:

"Who is she?"

"Please your majesty, 'tis a he."

"Nonsense!" exclaimed the Shah, "there is never an accident without a woman, who is she?"

The Shah was right. The man had fallen from his ladder because he was looking at a woman in the window opposite. Many a man does this in countries other than Persia.

This was the Victorian age where women wore long skirts and blouses that encircled the neck and arms to the wrist. Dorothy Dix organized a women's nursing corps with absolute requirements being plain looking, unmarried, preferably not especially attractive gals with no perfume or jewelry and in black or brown dresses.

The poem *Mistress* let steam out of the teapot, exploring a white-hot romance where "honey lips" made for an immortal kiss and unsurpassed joy while "reposing on thy bosom" surrounded by loving arms. Fifty years passed, leaving "trenches on cheeks, eyes dull without fire, lips shriveled and withered from age." The searing passion evolved into cold darkness and despair. Love and beauty succumbed to age. The smiles were long gone from a love perhaps deceitful and vain. And now she was deaf too! A few weeks later an angry letter by a 70-year-old woman married for 50 years demanded censorship of such foolscap. "Do not allow such things to get into your newspaper again. Think of the feelings of poor old women like me who have to read them."[62]

> To drink the honey of thy lips,
> I would dare all but die for one poor kiss,
> And then rest within thy arms,
> Where joy surpassing aught beneath the sun, reposing on thy bosom.
>
> Think what havoc change will make with you and me in fifty years,
> Trenches on your cheeks, eyes now dull without fire,
> The voice that made my blood jump madly,
> The ear a worn out toy, and full of discord,
> Lips shriveled and shrunken, withered by age.
>
> To mutual loathing and the transient blaze of passion dies away,
> Cold darkness, mistress a long farewell,
> No hope that love and sympathy can live longer than beauty
> As terrible despair closes over me.
>
> Love is very foolish, tis most vain,
> And kisses of unstinted worship rain upon a feeble thing,
> Whose fleeting charms, vanish more swiftly than most war's alarms.
> The smiles of revelers then full swoon.
> When love and beauty perish mid-life's storms,

When noisome death shall seize for his own being,
Deceitful love farewell, all's vain beneath the moon.

Short stories dissected the battle of the sexes and provided a manual on bad-tempered wives, slovenly or penny-pinching husbands, and the hopelessness of bachelorhood.

How David Price cured his wife's bad temper. He hired a doctor to make a powder out of various plants and things then make a house call telling his wife the powder is for female complaints, uneven temper, and headaches. Outraged, she beats the doctor with a stick till he is forced to leave, powder in hand. "Oh Missus Price, have ye gone Mad," cried out the practitioner. From that day on Mrs. Price has been wholly cured of her scolding habits. David has only to look her in the face and say "I'll get a box of liniment and there be an end to the matter." He honorably paid the doctor to forget the pummeling.[63]

The effects of marriage. Men who marry late lose their little oddities after marriage, they being pruned away. Once shabbily and carelessly dressed with frayed shirt collar, they become a pattern of neatness. Hair and whiskers look like other humans. Long beards and snuff are gone as a wife is a grand wielder of the moral pruning knife. The little corners are rounded off; the little shoots are pruned away in married men. Wives generally have much more sense than their husbands especially when the husbands are clever men. The wives advice is the ballast that keeps the ship steady. They are the wholesome though painful shears, snipping off little growths of self-conceit and folly.[64]

An old curmudgeon of a husband gets off a volley on damsels' nature. "As soon as calico is scarce and expensive the ladies wish to wear it: and were there to be a sudden dearth in the sackcloth and ashes market no doubt the dear creatures would insist on clothing themselves in that scriptural but at present not prevalent style of garment."

An ounce of prevention might be *bachelorhood.* Some poor souls despite the best intentions are destined for a life without romance, family or children. They are called bachelors.

One old bachelor we know was so coldly correct in every transaction in life that when he died he left no one behind him to lament his loss—not even a creditor.

The lost found, or the proposal. By Mrs. S. Stephens. I have a great deal of charity for old bachelors— that is for genuine nice single old gentleman of fifty who have not been disappointed in affairs of the heart more than half a dozen times and who have neither taken to eating, drinking or shaving notes as a substitute for love. Bachelors are the more philanthropic class than married men as their homage to our sex is more general and disinterested, devoid of selfishness of exclusive devotion; whereas the married are too often churlish and unsocial. Bachelors are mostly gentle, urbane, useful, so kind and gallant and not crusty ill-tempered, selfish with avarice. They are a much abused race. There was a man repeatedly losing at love, along with his hair on top of head, now single, old and hairless as well as heir less. So he bought a wig and went to Paris where he meets a widow; her daughter and dog all favorably impressed. He writes a marriage proposal which the daughter mistakenly uses for hair dressing and does not deliver to her mother. He returns to the U.S. from another failed romance and his situation unchanged.[65]

Soldiers far from home got non-judgmental affection from pets, but risks of bites and infections including rabies were a grave concern. By February 1864, there was a great number of mongrel curs that Dr. Hayes felt "infect the limits of this hospital having become a nuisance are no longer tolerable." Orders were given that all dogs within camp must wear a collar with the owner's name or other designation. Those without went to the dog pound, and if unclaimed in two days were terminated.

Health Care

The *Prose of Battle* contained a serialized description of medical care on the battlefield. Mass casualties, painful ambulance evacuations, broken soldiers and hard-working but realistic surgeons sorted out and treated masses of pulsating sick and wounded.

Ward 1 was under the care of Dr. A. A. Smith, who had served previously as medical cadet in the same hospital where he was described as "ever attentive to duty, obedient to his superiors and constant in his attention to the suffering soldier." The ward gave him a presentation sword which was promptly stolen. He was given an even better replacement in a ceremony where the assistant executive officer, Dr. James Williams, spoke about the "responsibility of the true physician's life and the anxiety he feels for those patients under his care." Speechless and overwhelmed, Dr. Smith could just say "thank you."

The *Register* noted the affection hospital wards had for their surgeons, bestowing gifts and Christmas cheer, "We tender to our brethren of the quill or scalpel our affectionate greetings," decorating that issue with tease and humor.

> A surgeon in the army was making rounds seeing a patient struck by a bullet in the left chest right over the region of the heart. The doctor's surprise at the narrow escape said "Why my man, where in name of goodness could your heart have been?" "I guess it must have been in my mouth just then doctor," replied the poor fellow with a faint and sickly smile.[66]

The term *Saw-bones* was first applied to surgeons employed in a conflict where 35,000 amputations were done on the Union side alone. The mortality rate for open fractures of the shin-bone in peacetime was 25 percent, and the thigh 50–75 percent. Lister's seminal work on antisepsis was first published in 1866 and not accepted world-wide for over 20 years. The dilemma was to avoid deadly infection in an era absent antibiotics and sterile techniques. To avoid infection, extremism in the form of surgery was no vice. Sacrifice a limb to save a life, but never sacrifice a life to save a limb.

The *canvas backed chair* related the hard facts of war to an audience well versed. "Those who live at a distance from the state of actual warfare can never know or appreciate the real horror of war. The list of casualties of battle is but one page of many in the history of war's desolation where lands are laid waste, homes destroyed and deaths met without glory." A soldier shot above the ankle fracturing both bones pleads to try and save his leg willing to endure painful daily dressing changes. His parents arrive in despair. The elderly father in tears is consoled by his son now febrile and rapidly declining. Amputation was in part designed to avoid infection, the "scourge of military hospitals." The wounded man insisted he was not going to die inspiring false hope in both father and mother despite the surgeon's unfavorable prognosis. He finally succumbs after smoking his final "cegar." Parents take their only child home, crushed and in despair. Days later, the father died suddenly of a broken heart. "The once happy home is now desolate with despair."[67] Such was the fate of so many families.

There is often a wide gulf between the writers and the readers of war literature. Here the witness wrote narratives simple and honest, encouraging empathy in active participants or those far from the battlefields.

> A soldier is stationed near a heap of human limbs. The bare armed surgeons with bloody instruments leaned over rigid and insensible figures while comrades of the subject look on in horror. "The grating of the murderous saw drove me into the open air. In the second hospital I visited a wounded man who had just expired and encountered his body being carried out. Lanterns were hanging and they thought me the doctor. Men with arms in slings were restlessly moving about, some sweltering with fever. Those with wounded lower extremities, body or head lay on their backs tossing even in sleep. Some with wounds still containing metal balls shouted periodically "Doctor!" or "Help!" or "God! or "O!" with loud spasmodic cry and continuing the same word till it died away in sighs. The act of calling seemed to lull the pain. Many were unconscious or lethargic, moving their fingers and lips mechanically but never moved or opened their eyes, ready to go through the valley of death from unutterable agony of the mortally wounded to mercifully leave this earth. Perhaps to soothe dying

groans, the next day a band played as full ambulances kept coming and the red flag of the hospitals floated in the dark of midnight.[68]

After the battle of Fair Oaks Virginia a house was commandeered for surgical headquarters and the wounded lay in the yard and lane under the shade waiting their turns to be hacked and maimed. Some curious people were peeping through the windows at the operations. As processions of freshly wounded went by the poor fellows lying on their backs, looked mutely at me and their great eyes smote my heart. The house was filled with thirty wounded Federals lying in their blankets on the floor: pale, helpless, and hollow–eyed making low moans at every breath as flies reveled upon their gashes. Several had only stumps for legs. They were but fragments of men, to limp forever through a painful life. Such wrecks of power I never beheld. Broad, brawny and buoyant a few hours before, the nervous shock, the loss of blood drained them to the last drop. Faces white as the ceiling, whining like babes, only rolling eyes distinguished them from mutilated corpses. Some were broken in spirit. One wept noticing his fate with pitiful glances towards a missing leg. The cow shed had seven corpses in a row. They were scarcely cold and had no history: and people call such deaths glorious! One federal was shot in his foot and howled at any attempt to remove his boot. The leather shoe was removed in pieces, cut with a knife. Among confederate wounded were fine vigorous fellows, one married just three days before: "Doctor I feel very cold. Do you think this is death? It seems to be creeping to my heart. I have no feeling in my feet and my thighs are benumbed."

An Irish federal soldier, a jovial fellow came along with a bucket of soup and proceeded to fill canteens and plates. "Come pardner, drink yer sup. Now old boy this 'ill warm ye; sock it down, and ye'll see yer sweetheart soon. You dead, Allybammy? Go 'way now! You'll live a hundred years, you will; that's wot you'll do, won't he lad? What! Not any? Get out! You'll be slap on your legs next week, and hev another shot at me the week a'ter that. You with the butternut trousers! Sa-ay! Wake up, and take some o'this. Halloo, lad! Pardner, wake up!" That man was stiff and very dead.[69]

A boon for humanity was the discovery of general anesthesia. In Edinburgh, Scotland, obstetrician George Simpson used chloroform with great success. It was cheap, easily made, had few side effects in surgeries lasting but minutes, and especially important was not flammable, a great virtue if working by candle light. Ether, when first demonstrated at Harvard, was hailed immediately as "no humbug." Its negatives were higher complications, expense and being flammable.

A two-part series detailed experiences with *ether anesthesia*. It was providentially true that ether made a person insensible to pain.

After a deep breath he saw New York from a height then out to sea and then woke up. With more ether he became a space traveler at great velocity, seeing vivid colors, followed by a voyage to the regions of the damned where he was warned "behold your doom" not returning to life to which he responded with "torrent of abuse and his entire stock of hard words. The trip around earth ended with an awakening and chill."[70]

A soldier with a gunshot wound to his shoulder has an ether dream with a nightmarish turn. The surgeon says, "well my friend we will have to perform an operation on your arm before you can get well. We will have to take out those pieces of bone that are causing so much mischief. The operation had better be done tonight. It is too hot in the day and the evenings are long and cool. What do you say?"

"As you think best, doctor."

"Tonight then at eight. Don't eat anything in the meantime." And on he passed to others of the brotherhood of suffering humanity.

"I felt a total indifference as to the result with passive carelessness about the operation. I mentally reveled in my helplessness. The wound purchased me a respite from the labors of the camp and picket duty, all wants are provided without an effort on my part." He was moved to ward's end, screened by curtains until his turn came, surgery by candle light.

Bed 26 was called and two nurses carried him to a curtained room with Sister of Charity holding lamps. A sponge with ether was held over his mouth and was told to take a good long breath. "I took a short breath. The odor was sweet and pleasant as perfume of orange blossom. A deeper breath and then another. It made me strong and I was aglow, my blood danced, my head was a vast hive with bees singing a wild melodious chant, an orchestra shrill and cadenced, slow and faster, then hushed. I was alone, all alone, my body was below. That frame was mine but was not I. I was sailing in space and seized with visions of eternal immunity from all earthly relationships. But the droning world returned and exquisite and unalterable pain raked my whole system. Incidents of years gone by seemed to occur again." They were more than memories as flames flew around him, becoming a scorching hiss. "I tried to scream but could not: my tongue was swollen and choked me. I struggled wildly, every muscle tried to free me from my fiery enemy." He faced a stone wall which stopped him cold. The flames chased after him and then subsided as he sank into unconsciousness and loss of all memory. "The next morning I was told my deep breathing had scattered the vapor of ether so that it had caught fire from a lamp held injudiciously nearby and that as the surgeon engaged to extinguish the flames my struggling had caused me to roll of the table and fall upon the floor."[71]

[Twenty-first century medicine requires that before each surgery, all members of the surgical team confer briefly about medications, allergies, site of surgery and fire risk assessment. Is the procedure above the end of sternum or within twelve inches of an oxygen source, and will laser, cautery or alcohol-based skin preparation be used? Last year there were over 600 operating room fires in the U.S.]

On Christian street was the Hospital for the Maimed under chief surgeon Dr. Levis. Their specialty was soldiers with amputations or deformities of limbs from battle wounds. They applied prosthetics and had patients share their experiences with other amputees. Vocational training was instituted including telegraph operating, bookkeeping, penmanship and other "practical matters" of business. The goal was to bring public attention to the disabled soldier to gain favor and jobs. "Influential persons" assured that large number of these men would receive employment. The mayor employed many in the Police and Fire departments. In their first weeks of operation, 300 maimed were received for training. The *Register* appealed to the public to supply them with books, instruments, and other donations.

Specialization in hospitals produced medical advancement. In Philadelphia, the hospital at 16th and Filbert Streets was assigned patients with "chronic rheumatism, chronic affection of the heart, organic or functional hitherto resisting treatment, impaired locomotion or action of a limb consequent upon cicatrices, or lesions of nerves or muscles from gunshot wounds or other injuries, and all cases of suspected malingering." Turner's Lane Hospital, inspired by William Hammond, was the first facility to specialize in neurological disorders such as head and spinal cord injuries, peripheral nerve injuries, seizures and psychiatric disease. This was staffed by Silas Muir Mitchell, one of the first American neurologists.

The chaplain of a New York Cavalry regiment visited the hospital and was impressed with the courtesy of officers and men and the neatness of rooms, though access in muddy seasons was "somewhat forbidding." Soldiers were well cared for and housed from "tumult and waste of war. Institutions like this assuage the horrors of war."[72] He stayed the night and shared the comforts of sick and wounded. He had a favorable impression of the self-sacrificing Sisters of Charity and conveyed the heartfelt thanks of a grateful country.

Letters to Chaplain West from mothers mirrored the same sentiments. "The few weeks in Philadelphia left many pleasant reminiscences. I really feel that the poor sick soldier has much cause for gratitude to your hospital. The sentiment you penned in my notebook 'read much, studies more, but pray most of all' has been heartfelt by my son and I," Mrs. Reed of Binghamton, New York, wrote about her son Elwin: "he was but a mere frame when he left the hospital but now weighs 130 pounds. I feel quite sure you would not know him. The five weeks I spent in Philadelphia are ever present with me; the long wards, the patient faces of the poor sufferers, the calm sisters, and the kindness I received. I am certain the kindness of the people of Philadelphia cannot be surpassed."[73]

Surgeons listed those who would benefit from furlough for 20 or 30 days, or if unfit for service for 60 days, to be placed in the Invalid Corps. The most efficient could be doing guard duty or serve in some capacity, including amputees. A letter to the editor claimed the disabled were forced to serve. The *Register* denied this, replying they were confined to garrison, hospital nursing, and guarding deserters and conscripts. It was considered a "great honor" to be attached to this corps, and they had not heard of anyone forced to take that position. An order of April 1863 listed employment opportunities as clerks, cooks, nurses and attendants for "any convalescent wounded or feeble men who can perform such duties" instead of giving them discharges.

Some viewed the hospital as an oasis from a turbulent world, finding the cover of bed and blanket preferable to the cacophony of the battlefield. The following two poems illustrated the dilemma of who shall serve, who are disabled and who takes their place.

I'm too sic to go bak to the war
O the doctor he sez I am wel;
   but ill nevr be well eny mawr,
Its the rummytiz sure I kin tel—
   im too sic to go bak to the war
Im afrade ive a spine in mi bak
   un my hart is awl gawn at the core;
I am sure I cant march with a pak—
   im too sic to go bak to the war
There's a mizzery, too, in mi bed
   An mi legs they kin scarce reche the door:
Im shure id be beter in bed—
   im to sic to go bak to the war
Im a blacksmith bi trade, an if ev
   er I git to go home enny mawr,
I wil hamer an slave, but i'll nev
   Er be sic az I am uv the war.[74]

On the excruciating torture of chronic rheumatism, malignant type.
Mi bak is stif and sore
   Mi legs are thin and weke
And when I tri to wak about
   I here mi ne pans kreke.
And I want to be discharged
   And get mi pai whats du
And ill give a green-back kwik
   If I cud get put thru[75]

No event was more momentous than the discharge of soldiers unfit for service. Dr. Hayes was unequivocal.

> Numbers of discharges are too high. Each soldier costs thousands and every man is needed in the field. The number of discharges sent out daily from this Hospital is very great and bears entirely too large a proportion to the number of patients in hospital. Men will practice every deception possible to avoid returning to the field. A gunshot wound through the muscles does not furnish sufficient disability for discharge. Debility resulting from remittent or continued fever is not sufficient cause of discharge. Discharge for chronic rheumatism is forbidden.[76]

Patient evaluations needed state the cause of discharge, be it lameness, loss of use of arm, gunshot wound, paralysis, inability to march or carry knapsack, general debility, tuberculosis, fever or dyspnea.

Hospital patients needed to come to terms with their new universe and prepare for the future. Getting out of bed and taking that first step is always the hardest. Inertia must be overcome.

> *The convalescent.* The hospital patient has a nervous fever. He has a sick man's dreams. He is a king on his throne of pillows only to change sides faster than a politician. Within the four curtains surrounding his bed he is absolute, supreme selfishness is thrust upon him as his only duty. He wears his crown, the pillow king, wrapped in calico. He has put on the stone armor of sickness, wrapped in the callous hide of suffering, keeps his sympathy, and conceives himself as the sick man.[77]

Two dreaded complications after amputation surgery were infection and secondary, life-threatening hemorrhage. A medical cadet described such an incident concerning Private George Dash of New York, who sustained a mortar wound to the shoulder, tearing off his left arm at Chancellorsville. The surgeon removed the head of the remaining bone, thus excising the fracture, and applied cold water dressing. The wound became infected and sloughed necrotic tissue. The patient now thin and pale developed bed sores. Tonics iron and quinine along with poultices failed. The gangrenous tissue continued to slough and then bleed. A styptic was applied to the mangled stump without success. A proximal incision to tie off a feeding artery failed. Pressure was applied round the clock by a team of 14 medical cadets alternating every 30 minutes, and that failed. The infected, foul-smelling wound grew to three by three inches. He re-bled 48 hours later, the exact source uncertain. He was still and deathly pale, mumbling, "the next time I bleed I shall die." A Sister of Charity sat next to his bed for three days, helping as she could. "Poor Dash, don't you wish you were in Heaven?" He feebly replied, "yes." The pressure of the cadet's fingers could not stem the tide and save his life. "At 6 a.m. dark blood welled up then dripping in little puddles on the floor. A handkerchief hastily snatched and crammed into the orifice was all that could be done but Dash went the way hundreds go who die of their wounds."[78]

A sorrowful bride came from afar to visit Captain Wallace of Ohio, mortally wounded at Fredericksburg. His fiancée was in Washington the morning his limb was amputated. A marriage ceremony was performed post-operatively. She left for a boarding house to regain composure for the next day's nursing care but was urgently summoned back, only to find him dead. During the night the nurse in attendance noted the bloody dressing. The wounded limb began bleeding profusely, which could not be stopped with a handkerchief.

The most calamitous infection was tetanus, which afflicts the nervous system, causing seizures and lockjaw with 100 percent mortality. A case was published in the *Camp Stool* of a private from Maine who survived eight battles including Gettysburg and sustained what seemed a slight wound of the hand. Infection set in. Surgical consultants recommended dressing changes only, as surgery would likely prove fatal. Two weeks later he was described thusly:

> In extremis, distorted by terrible spasm, bent bow shaped with only head and heels on the bed. You might have passed a large pillow under his back, muscles were corded into hard knots, stiffened as of carved out of a block of stone. He did not groan or utter complaint; jaws clenched with a choking and peculiar cough. He was conscious to the last, tortured thus for six days. He died unknown and unwept for, except by those who saw him pass away after suffering long weary marches and many battles by one of most appalling of all deaths.[79]

Another case of tetanus occurred in a soldier sent home on furlough with hopes of recovery. At Gettysburg, an Ohio sergeant sustained a gunshot wound to the right shoulder, entering above the clavicle and passing backward, a lump of lead removed from the lower neck. Gangrene converted healthy flesh into "masses of loathsome putrescence, eating away slowly but surely. The shadow of pyemia hung like a pall over this chosen victim. A deluge of hemorrhage caused a feeble cry for help. Tetanus went wild with agonizing pain and grunt of despair. He reeled and rolled from this revengeful merciless monster, bent and twisted into inhuman forms. Paroxysm after paroxysm of agony, the wretch prayed for death ultimately granted from this punishment of hell." Having failed to return from his two-week furlough, he was listed as deserter. The government eventually corrected the records, which gave solace to the family but did little for the deceased.[80]

A recurrent theme was the notion that love conquers all and the faithful wife could heal that which the doctor could not. The patient was written off as hopeless by surgeon and nurse, only to be rescued from raging fever and desperate wound by an angel in the form of invincible love: the fiancé, wife or mother, arriving just in time. Will she still have me deformed with empty sleeve? She cheerfully proclaims, "I will be your right arm."[81]

A poem commemorated the loss of a hand at Gettysburg. "I have no right hand to wave, our flag above the dead lying all silent smeared with gore, but countless tear I shed." He awoke in the West Philadelphia hospital, surrounded by others suffering a similar fate, and was welcomed. "They brought cold water to my lips that scarce had strength to open and kindly whispered hope. Our chaplain was so tender and offered a library full of books to read. I'll toss in the air my cap tattered and torn, to see and give one shout for the Union and the next for Satterlee!"[82]

> "My dear, said a returning volunteer to his wife, "have you noticed any difference in my height since I left for the war?"
> "No, what do you mean?"
> "O, nothing," holding up his injured limb, "only I am shorter one foot!"[83]

Dr. James, the namesake of the "celebrated powder," was asked the difference between a doctor and an apothecary. His analogy was about a monkey residing in a gentleman's house that watched the butler go into the cellar and take the spigot out of the barrel, draw a jug of ale and return it. When the butler left, the primate Jacko wishing to imitate but, lacking the capacity of the original, drew the spigot out of the barrel, but not knowing how to return it let the beer run all about the place while he frisked up and down the stairs in the greatest fright and confusion imaginable.[84] [Competition and jealousy between health care providers is common in any era.]

The laissez-faire attitude concerning government regulations allowed patent medications free rein, enjoying great popularity with the public. Effective ingredients were alcohol, cocaine, opium or quinine. The *Register* published peer review and patient outcome studies in a unique and satiric way.

> *Patent Medicines.* Ramrod's tincture of Gridiron has "subtle invigorating fluid allied to nervous systems or magnetic fluid of the body and becomes a specific and infallible remedy for almost every complaint of mind and body which human nature has been subject since the flood. It gives relief against accidents, and quickens circulation and muscular exertions.
> "Walking near the machine of a mill I was a caught and carried between two cog-wheels and every bone in my body broken to pieces. A phial of Ramrod tincture of Gridiron being thrown in the mill-pond I found myself restored and as whole and as sound as a roach. Dick Whirligig."

"Riding out the other day I accidentally fell into a ditch and broke my legs, my arms and neck. On taking a little of the Tincture of Gridiron I instantly recovered and have never been near a ditch since, nor felt a desire to approach one." Tom Tumble.[85]

Battlefield Experiences

The *Register* asked, "Why is a cowardly soldier like butter? When exposed to a fire they run." What separated bravery from cowardice could be a thin line determined more by illusion and context than character and deed. European military experts believed that issues of modern warfare depended on scientific strategic combinations in which the individual soldier was just a mathematical unit. The days of mace, axes and sword were over. No forbidding castle or building could resist the pounding of artillery. The battle field was no longer just a mass of struggling men with steel rods. The opposing forces were spread out by rifles and cannons. Personal prowess, zeal, and intelligence availed little in the "big picture." Brute force was replaced by strategy and maneuvers.[86] Napoleon's army fired the notoriously inaccurate round ball and thus required massing of troops to increase efficiency. The Minnie ball was twice the size and velocity and very accurate and destructive at a few hundred yards. If you could see it, you could hit it.

How much lead it takes to kill a man explored this issue. "The real cause of bravery is the apparent security of one's own safety after volley upon volley from the enemy fails to hit you."[87] General Rosencrantz reported that out of 20,000 rounds of artillery fired at Murfreesboro, 728 hit the enemy. Out of two million rounds of musketry, 13,832 were effectual.

A New Hampshire volunteer on Ward M wrote the *Register* about the horrors at the Battle of Williamsburg. After heavy marching, hard fighting, and dodging falling shots, the dogs of war were weary. "Why should we be melancholy whose business it is to die? Grape, canister, shrapnel, shot and shell pour holy upon us." Nine thousand blue coats were allegedly against 40,000. "The shattered remnants of our divisions fell back with rain pouring down. Our ranks sadly shattered and decimated rested upon their arms."[88]

More fearsome was the *thunder barrel* filled with sulfa layered with 12-pound spherical case shot until the barrel was full. "They burst and roared as if ten thousand devils had broken loose upon earth, scattering and shattering into atoms everything within a circle of fifty yards. In the distance came cries of twenty men in agony. The next morning torn, burned and horribly disfigured cold corpses illustrated the practical effect of a thunder barrel."[89]

Rebel shelling struck and blew up a caisson, tearing the horses to pieces and whirling an artillery gunner into the clouds. The ammunition wagon exploded, filling the air with fragments of wood, iron and flesh.

> A boy stood at one of the fires combing out his matted hair. Suddenly his head flew off, spattering the brains; and the shell, which I could not see, exploded in a piece of woods, mutilating the trees. The effect upon the people around me was instantaneous and appalling. Some were partially dressed, and ran on their heels. In a twinkling our camps were deserted and the fields and woods alive with fugitives pushing, swearing, falling and trampling while fierce bolts fell among them making havoc at every rod. The confederates sent an infantry wave into the mass of dying. Union infantry failed to stop them until an assist from artillery drove them back.[90]

The bloody footprints of Antietam, the largest one-day total of American casualties ever, was described by Sergeant S. H. Sloan of the 95th Pennsylvania Volunteers.

> At an early hour the enemy sent in a flag of truce asking permission to gather up their dead and bury them. But they had been engaged in that occupation while they were retreating across the river into Virginia. Of all the spectacles I have ever seen nothing equals this field of carnage. The greater portion of our dead had been removed while the enemy's dead still remained where they had fallen. The ground had lately been ploughed and we could see by their dead where their lines of battle had been. Some were horribly mangled by cannon shot, heads arms or legs being carried away. It was awful. Some lay with their faces turned to the ground, some in heaps of three or four with faces turned up toward the sky. Scores lay in rows as they had fallen, pierced by grape and canister as they advanced to meet us. Covered with mud and dust they rotted in the sun as parties were engaged in burying them as rapidly as possible.[91]

A hospital patient who experienced over 20 battles put his memory to pen in *delusions of soldiering*. He marched to war in step of fife and drum before cheering crowds "that made me maniacal, similar to the effect produced by a private conversation with a pretty girl." He returned home a renowned hero, slightly wounded, and became the "object of interest and admiration to all especially the feminine portion of society. I was insane and enlisted to prove myself to be so." A handsome blue uniform attracted commiseration and respect of all citizens and predictions of an easy and quick victory mainly by those not participating in the actual fighting. Bull Run showed that newspapers and politicians made deadly mistakes and deceitful false statements such as

> the soldier becomes inured to grape shot, canister, shell or cavalry and is no longer terrified, astonished or stampeded by it. I am convinced that soldiering is to the vast majority of mankind a delusion and a snare, entering into it self-deceived. Warfare is not pleasant by any means and men do not achieve the rewards bestowed upon gallantry because they are careless of life, despise the horrors of a battle field and become overly excited of the scene or desire glory enough to overcome the instinct of self-preservation. Do not ask returning soldiers about the propriety of war because they lie and do not ask mothers for their views as if it was their fault. The truth will not be found in speeches, posters, bounties or advertisements.

Humming religious tracts about the hereafter or pining about a lady love back home was "sentimental, vain and unsubstantial" and "won't keep the rain out of your blankets or the gnawing tooth of hunger out of your vitals. So take the advice of an old soldier my fine young recruits, and prepare for the worst."[92]

Sacrifice and Patriotism

Replacing ever-declining numbers of volunteers lost from sickness or wounds required a draft, not especially popular with those likely to be called. As the *Register* jested, "What brings on an illness, cures it, and pays the doctor, a draft!" A satiric letter to the editor expounded on how to dodge service.

> I am neither coward nor copperhead. How to avoid the draft is what I want to know. It is a dark cloud. I am unfortunately neither halt, lame nor blind. I am perfect in my frame, have all my teeth and am not at present in the service of the government. Not a confirmed drunkard, Quaker or clergyman: all exempted. I might without difficulty become either but it's of no use. I am likely to be drafted and likely to be shot. Is there any way I can avoid from being torn from home about the first of July by a Provost Marshal and forced to do what my soul revolts at? I am not iron-clad; I have a serious objection to being shot, something almost inevitable if I rally with that crowd who shout the

Battle-Cry of Freedom. Resolve in your mind Mr. Editor and in mercy tell me if there is no way for me to avoid becoming an unwilling justifiable homicide.[93]

The stories about the volunteer getting girl and glory while showered with honor and respect did not fill the ranks. Private Robert Yew of a Pennsylvania regiment wrote to a Satterlee hospital patient after Gettysburg about sacrifices made by private citizens and soldiers in *Tide of Victory*. The enemy was driven to the wall as the blue coats worked like "Trojans and suffered like martyrs." He found an old house with a chicken that he unsuccessfully chased with fixed bayonet. The owner, an elderly woman, asked him to leave it as the rebels took her cow, calf, and chicks. "Now I aint got nothing but this one chickin." "I understand that every one of the brave sons of Pennsylvania who have turned out in this trying hour to protect the invaded hearthstones of the Commonwealth is to be presented with an appropriate medal. It will testify in future years to the sacrifices made and the dangers passed through in this trying hour."[94] For parents and wives whose only "chickin" was the volunteer, the price of victory was steep.

All of society needed to support the war effort for it to succeed. "Treason stalks, fraud deletes the treasury and currency depreciates to an alarming extent. We need unity and confidence. Public feeling is the aggregate of individual feeling and public expression the aggregate of individual expression. Do not be despondent."[95]

The term "copperhead," originally referring to the brass cap of the coin figurine of the muse "liberty," was used in derogatory fashion, describing the Democratic Party and opposition to continuation of war. It referred to a treacherous, deceitful, venomous viper hiding in the weeds to be avoided if convenient and eradicated if necessary. The snake rewards evil for good, kills more than it can eat, coils around its victim and squeezes them to death. As in the bible, the serpent is the devil to be feared, avoided and destroyed. Opposing this obstinate enemy of good is the policy of Christianity and nation-saving patriotism.

While the *Register* declared abstinence concerning politics, they were vigorously pro-administration. With the renomination of Lincoln, the cause received a final blessing and dedication.

> Copperheads have been assaulted, defeated and rests beneath the heel of liberty. The loyal people demand the country be cleansed of this blot on her fair frame and we trust its death warrant decrees our chief magistrate the first choice of the people. We should pity our enemy had he not insulted the nation and humanity by his atrocious acts committed on our prisoners. They will be avenged, and the instruments of such wanton cruelty, violence and cowardice, extirpated from the land.[96]

The re-election of Lincoln meant that the war continued until the goals stated in the Republican Convention were met, the end of slavery with union. The nation had laid at the President's feet all the resources in men and money needed to put down the rebellion.

There was never a shortage of critics. The *London Times* issued a guarded prognosis as to the future prospects of the republic. "The Americans have already sacrificed their liberty to the Union. The constitution is violated and the old system of government lost." the *Register* replied with some deception,

> That is nonsense. In the South both state and individual rights have been trampled. People hurried into war against their wishes and without an opportunity to be heard. Conscription and taxation was carried to a tyrannical and oppressive extent in the extreme. Anarchy replaced good government, robbers in the garb of soldiers plunder their own citizens and neither life nor property is secure. When they parted from the union they parted with their liberties. For the North the war is the

people's war. Conscription has been cheerfully acceded to and unusually heavy burden of taxes have been borne without complaint. In suppressing the rebellion the people lose nothing of their rights and privileges and maintain their liberties. The Constitution secures freedom to all men living under it of whatever condition or color.[97]

Generals

News items on key generals and the war's progress was monitored weekly. William Tecumseh Sherman, with no love for the second estate, was described by the *Register* as "the successful and great man." "I am popular as long as I am successful. Not only the American press, but the London papers praise me as the general of the age. Why? Because I have crossed much of this country by long and perilous march and have caused an important city to fall into our hands. But if I fail in the ensuing campaigns, every laurel I have won, everything I have done would be forgotten. There is not a tree high enough to hang me upon."[98] By March of 1865, the North had *Cheering Prospects*. Sherman was portrayed as an invincible conqueror, "all is right and doing finely." He was destroying immense quantity of rebel property and stores, capturing cannons and hundreds of barrels of powder.

Stonewall Jackson was a celebrated and cherished hero of the south, but was considered "killed at the right time" from the northern perspective. If his achievements had begun to ebb, he would have exited this earth with few regrets and fewer tears. "We care not for antecedents, family position or West Point training as long as we are led on to victory in a righteous cause."[99] [As a future five-star general would proclaim, "there is no substitute for victory."]

Another favorite was steady and aggressive "Little Phil Sheridan," on his black charger with attractive qualities for a general: speed, dash, brilliancy, and a spice of caution and energy. In spite of mud and flood, he pushed rapidly on to surprise the opposition. At the pinnacle was U. S. Grant, "long lives our little Hercules." His name and portrait often hung from the ward rafters, on banners and placards. Like Napoleon, he led in person and planned the movements of his forces. "He was modest without any apparent personal ambition and impervious to flattery without sign of show or ostentation. Plain and unassuming he made no triumphal entry into Richmond and required no pompous surrender of Lee's army."[100]

Lincoln

On April 8, 1865, a glorious headline trumpeted, "Richmond has fallen!" The hospital was ablaze with excitement. "Fire bells rang and firemen scampered pell-mell thinking a fire existed. The steam whistle screamed and shrieked, snorted and puffed as pandemonium broke loose. Patients crowded, huddled, jammed and jostled some on crutches, others with canes and all with a broad grin as the band played *Hail Columbia,* the *Star Spangled Banner* and *Yankee Doodle*." They cheered for Lincoln, Grant, Sherman and themselves.

The issue of April 22, 1865, was framed in black in consecration of the assassination. A national calamity and the pain of martyrdom transformed great jubilation and hearts filled with brotherly love into a demand for revenge and justice.

A black pall of mourning enveloped the entire land. Lincoln was about to enjoy the sweet and richly earned fruit of his patriotic and unflinching devotion to the cause of his country. Never was a ruler more humane whose heart overflowed with milk of human kindness. He never forgot charity and forgiveness, but dealt too leniently with incorrigible traitors. He extended the hand of friendship and pardon. Their response was blood more blood; and blood they shall have. Every vile traitor shall be quickly swept from the land.

Lincoln's genius as complex figure of frontier origins became bigger than life and other-worldly. "His temper was soft, gentle and yielding, reluctant to refuse anything presented to him as act of kindness, loving to ease, with a melancholic temperament and deep and fixed seriousness." Under Lincoln amnesty for rebels was expected, but under Andrew Johnson the same was impeachable. With the end of the rebellion came a demand that its authors suffer extreme penalty for a terrible deed and for the high crime of treason.

Intramural games between hospitals and regiments brought out combative spirits not fully spent on the battlefields. On June 3, 1865, Satterlee Hospital's baseball team took on the Mercantile Hospital Warriors with a final score of 34–28. The West Philadelphia home team had access to the largest population of players, but fielding a team at war's end was difficult as the best got well and went home.

By June 1865, the fighting was done and soldiers were eager to leave, awaiting bonus, disability and pension status to be resolved. In one week, 700 convalescent patients were discharged home. The *Register* had published no issue in three weeks because all but one of their staff were mustered out.

Two

Armory Square Hospital Gazette

The Department of Washington was the largest, with 25 hospitals: 17 in the capital city, five in or near Alexandria, one at Point Lookout, Maryland, and one in Fairfax, Virginia. The bed capacity was 21,426, which by December 17, 1864, had 13,805 occupants. (See Appendix II).

Armory Square U.S. Army General Hospital, with 1,000 beds, was located at the intersection of major thoroughfares with ready access to wharf and railroad. In the summer of 1862, construction began at Seventh Street opposite the grounds of the Smithsonian Institute between A and B Streets, now the site of the Air and Space Museum. Adjacent a foul sewer and open canal requiring cleanup, it served as triage center for the Army of the Potomac.

Serious cases unable to travel further were brought here, accounting for an average mortality rate of 12.7 percent, the highest of all hospitals. Some admissions were actually dead on arrival.[1] Other hospitals far from the battle field averaged 2 percent mortality or less. The type of patients determined this discrepancy and not the healthfulness of its site or the skill and efficiency of its surgeons. Their pride was justifiably offended, offering this response in an *Armory Gazette* piece, *Great Mortality*. "There is a report in Northern papers that mortality in this hospital has reached sixty a day. This is a mistake. Although some die on the way here from the front they are often brought to Armory Square Hospital for burial. Yesterday thirteen were dead on arrival. Our greatest mortality in any one day has been twenty-one and the largest number brought here in any day is twenty-seven, making a total of dead in one day forty-eight."[2] In a later issue, they reiterated the high number of acute cases other hospitals did not see. "All those who die on transports on the way and those about to die are brought here. Often we have men who died before being removed from the stretcher on which they have been brought."[3]

Witnessing so many fatal casualties had an adverse effect on staff and convalescents alike. As one hospital patient put it, "three men died in this ward since I came. One from my regiment was here and another in the next ward. He also belonged to my company. There is no more notice taken after a man's dying here than killing a fly at home or not much more."[4] For the year 1864, admissions were 4,647, return to duty 1,413, discharged 259, furloughed 1,724, transferred 1,497, deserted 197, and died 668 [14.4 percent], dead on arrival 187.[5]

The hospital design was 11 parallel buildings separated by the width of a building. Pavilions were 149 by 25 feet long and 13 feet high, holding 50 beds each, which could be increased simply by adding another row. The rear end of each ward was used as the dining room, and sometimes lodging for female nurses until better quarters were created.

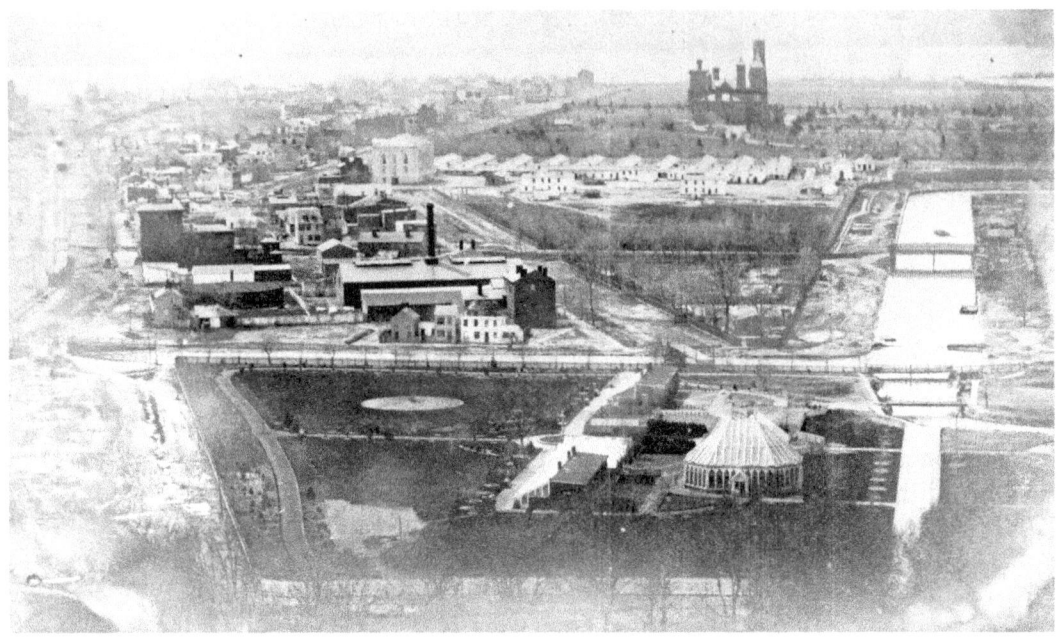

View of Washington D.C. from Capitol looking west-southwest. Armory building to left, Hospital in front of Smithsonian Castle in rear, Potomac River in background, Botanic garden in foreground, Washington Canal to right (Library of Congress).

The other end was either a bathroom or water closet. Ventilation was by ceiling ridge shafts and floor inlets as per the custom of this period. Administration took the center building with five separate wards on either side. Each structure was interconnected with a covered walkway at the rear and transversely in the middle. Connected directly in back was the general kitchen, 105 by 25 feet, a laundry 47 by 17 feet, and a bakery 36 by 16 feet. Offices for the surgeon in charge, dispensary, general offices, linen room, post office, store room, officers' quarters and mess room were included in administration headquarters. Separate units held a coal house and ice house. Later construction on the right flank, near the stable and knapsack room, added the chapel, chaplain's quarters, rooms for female nurses, and a dead house. Behind the kitchen and laundry and between them and the guard house were two barrack buildings erected to house contrabands [blacks] and guards. On the left side was the Columbian Arsenal, a three-story brick building, 102 by 57 feet, that was converted for additional wards. Tents were available for mass casualties.[6]

There was steady improvement over its two and a half years of existence. Spring cleaning meant bringing in the "white washers" who renovated with white and blue. Ward A was given a "pretty roof of blue covering with white rafters making the patients think that was the sky of heaven if he pleased." By October 1864, there were "extensive repairs for the comfort of our brave men in this hospital," all roofs shingled and rooms plastered. The central administrative building was entirely remodeled along with medical offices, surgical rooms and linen and dining rooms, making it "beautiful and convenient. New floors of good material were installed." At the end of renovation there were 700 occupied beds.[7]

Soldiers' private quarters tended towards disheveled and disorderly as ward masters varied in ability to discipline. Foggy Bottom tends to be a haven for roaches and vermin even in modern times. The hospital barracks were inundated with rats despite the usual

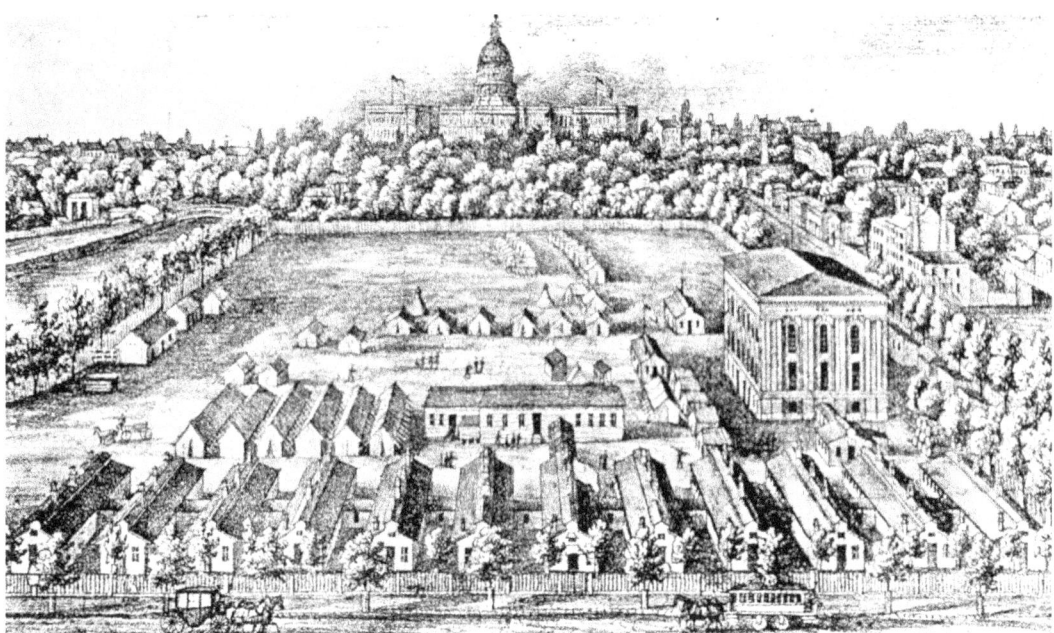

Armory Square Hospital, Independence Avenue and 7th Street, SW. Building on right is the Armory. U.S. Capital building in back. Current site of Smithsonian's National Air and Space Museum (U.S. National Library of Medicine).

counter-measures. A letter to the Editor came to the rat's defense. "Let the rats alone. Why do you want to get rid of them? They are useful. They are scavengers, and carry off the filth nothing else reaches."[8]

A clean water supply was critical. Water you could see through was considered potable. This was referenced in a brief anecdote. "Easterners have a way of giving an encouraging pat on the shoulder to the witty. One friend was in great danger of a broken shoulder when on drawing the water which supplies the city and hospital remarked that it was evidently not 'all quiet on the Potomac.'"

The chief surgeon was Brevet Colonel D. W. Bliss, who entered service with the 3rd Michigan Regiment Volunteers in May 1861. By September he was promoted to brigade surgeon. He served in the Peninsula campaign and was then appointed medical director. Due to illness, he was removed from the field and placed in charge of the Armory Square Hospital, where he performed numerous surgeries. The Gazette described him as "kind to patients, approachable to subordinates, courteous to strangers and gentlemanly to all. Being a thorough disciplinarian he governs well without use of red tape and favors election of Lincoln."[9] Handling the fatal gunshot wound of President Garfield earned the charge "ignorance was Bliss."

The medical staff initially included nine and ultimately 15 assistant surgeons. Doctors become ill just like their patients. Dr. William Butler was sent home to Buffalo, where he died after a "lingering illness of several months from tuberculosis," leaving wife and family. Dr. E. H. Horsey was summoned one evening for a medical emergency, only to be surprised with a reward in gratitude for kindness to his patients, a gold watch and chain. Six weeks later he was dead, another casualty of disease.

Patient gratitude was extended to Dr. Stearns, mustered out April 1864, to his home in Massachusetts. A grateful patient wrote, "I should never have lived through my sickness if I had not had such a good surgeon to take care of me." Soldiers under his care planned to present him a memento, but he declined.

A small room at the rear of Ward A was the office of Dr. Alcan, a French practitioner of electricity for the relief of wounded and disabled soldiers. He had an award from Emperor Louis Philippe on the successful treatment of cholera by electricity, along with other medals. He came from New York City to help, served on the front for two years without pay, and was now a hospital steward. The *Gazette* was baffled by his work and foreign accent.

There were five hospital stewards, one medical cadet, and 13 clerks: chief clerk, carpenter clerk, furlough and discharge clerk, statistical and post return clerk, postal clerk, assistant postal clerk, descriptive list clerk, register clerk, burial clerk, commissary clerk (2), linen room clerk, and muster out office clerk (2).

Army chow did not typically rate high on the culinary scale, though here it allegedly excelled compared to field level cuisine. One hospital patient who "brought up the sick men's supper and gave it to them" had a different assessment, advising his friend back home, "would you like the kind of rations we get? Hardly, I think."[10]

The head cook of the officers' kitchen was surprised with a ceremony and gift of silvery gratitude: "two very handsome long handled spoons and a pair of pancake printers." Getting meals to large numbers of patients required mass transportation. A railway with covered cars was installed "along the rear of the wards to supply soldiers with hot food." The newly arrived men of the 3rd Iowa Regiment registered thanks for their treatment in letters to the editor. "We wish to express our thanks to the staff of this hospital for the troubles that we have been to them. When we arrived here we had nothing to eat or cook with but soon found that men who had been to the front and endured hardship and privation had plenty of friends at the Armory Square."

D. W. Lefebvre of Ward K in this hospital wrote home as a convalescent working as cook, on February 2, 1864.

> I have got pretty well again. I am second cook for 130 sick men. We have not had any cold weather here this winter and the streets are so dusty you can hardly see at all. I would like you to call around and see me some evening. There are a great many sick and wounded in the hospital. I do not know how long I will stay here. I was examined this morning to return to duty so I suppose I will go before long. I was in Congress and the Senate. They had a good time discussing the $300 clause. I think they will not get it thrown out. Give my love to all. Write soon.[11] [The $300 commutation fee allowed paying another to take your place in the draft.]

A lady nurse was preferred over the more common male as they tended to exude kindness and sympathy. "The nurse on this ward is a nice, lively woman-always having some fun going on and the boys are all such lively fellows and we have some good times." Many left comfortable homes to help suffering soldiers, mostly unrelated. They reminded each soldier of family, offering heartfelt thanks for their "faithful devotion" while "honoring and cherishing their pleasant faces." The *Gazette* honored by name the 11 single women each assigned to a ward whose "laboriousness and responsibility" in dispensing medicines and stimulants, supervising the distribution of special diet, made wards cheerful and home-like and the duties of medical officers lighter and more pleasant. A surgeon remarked to one Lady Nurse, "You ought to have your name and rank published in the *Gazette*." She replied, "No need of it, if you please sir! Our rank is that of private. Since we are privates, our names should remain private." She received affectionate encouragement from her friends, the other nurses, and a complimentary newspaper. They were much praised for self-sacrifice and devotion, women whose gentle presence and kindly acts made them "ministering angels."[12]

There were many distinguished visitors, including nationally known religious, political, military and temperance leaders, and Mrs. Lincoln. Hospital visits were encouraged but regulated. City residents provided music with guitar, violin and song, drawing patients involuntarily into cotillion or waltz. The wife and daughter of the Vice President brought turkey dinner and "won golden opinions from the soldiers for the great interest manifested in their cheer." President Lincoln was a frequent guest, receiving copies of the *Gazette*. Limits on visitation were necessary because of theft, security matters, smuggling alcohol, and sight seekers. "There has been a great desire to visit our hospital recently from high and low. It became a necessity to limit visits; the men most imploringly call for it. Congress has instructed the committee on the conduct of war to see why hospitals are closed to visitors. When they investigate the matter it will be understood."[13]

Beware of impostors warned inpatients to give articles of value only to those with specific hospital responsibility. "Yesterday a dying man sent me to inquire about his wallet given to a stranger for safekeeping. I returned without finding that person. As I entered his door the poor man was being carried out a lifeless corpse. The villain who would rob a sick soldier will meet his due punishment hereafter. Let our soldiers beware!"[14]

There would be no freak show, visible piles of removed limbs, or need of "dreadful gloom" in any hospital and especially at Armory Square. A New Hampshire state agent wrote to the *New Hampshire Journal* that their state's hospital was the best managed, lacking gloom and doom that others displayed. The *Gazette* editor thought the statement "ridiculous and presumptuous," and "calculated to discourage enlistments and give erroneous impressions of our hospital system to those at a distance."[15] He would find none of that despair in Armory Square Hospital, where the surgeon in charge was the truest friend of even the humblest soldier.

Writing to the soldier was considered a priority. Friends and relatives were encouraged to write frequently. Those dismembered with ghastly wounds and "the fever" might ease their troubles with hope and cheer from family and hometown news. The hospital post office was open twice daily, centrally located in the administration building, and secured prompt and safe delivery of mail to hospital inmates. Every letter was registered, both received and sent. In one month over 14,000 letters were so posted.

The *Armory Square Hospital Gazette* was a four-page sheet with the motto "Ask nothing of Society but the liberty to do it good." The editors were a string of chaplains whose influences were manifest in sermonizing, with emphasis on the temperance movement and full support of the war. It was published every Monday from January 6, 1864, through August 21, 1865. A one-year subscription, initially $.50, was increased in 1865 to $1. Delivery outside the hospital in Washington was $0.50 extra. Advertisements cost $.10 a line. The printers were convalescents who at home earned $18 a *week*, not the enlisted man rate of $13 a *month*. The printing office of the *Gazette* also made cards, circulars, bill heads and envelope addresses.

The goals of the *Gazette* were definitively stated in the salutatory address:

> To the support of the government and to the distraction of copperheads and traitors, we fervently pledge ourselves. No peace through submission to armed rebellion is our motto. We are soldiers and believe in meeting the enemy by hard blows, and not by supplications for peace and feel this is shared by all who will read this soldier paper. This hospital is an episode in a soldier's life—sometimes a

Armory Square 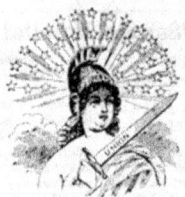 Hospital Gazette.

"Ask nothing of Society but the liberty to do it good."—F. H. HEDGE.

VOL. 1.   ARMORY SQUARE, WASHINGTON, D. C., OCTOBER 22, 1864.   NO. 39.

The Song of the Light Artillery.

FROM U. S. SERVICE MAGAZINE.

On the sustained sward of a gentle slope,
Full of valor and full of hope,
The Infantry sways like a coming sea,
Why Bugles the Light Artillery?

Action, front!
Whistling the Parrots like children's toys,
The horses strain to the rushing noise;
To right and to left, so fast and free,
They carry the light artillery.

Drive on!
The gunner cries, with a tug and a jerk,
The limbers fly, and we bend to our work;
The 'hand-spike' in, and the 'implements' out,
We wait for the word, and it comes with a shout—

Load!
The foes pour on their billowy line;
Can nothing check their bold design?
With yells and oaths of fiendish glee,
They rush for the light artillery.

Commence firing!
Hurrah! Hurrah! our bull dogs bark,
And their triple line is a glorious mark;
Moodfronds fall like grain on the lea,
Mowed down by the light artillery.

'Fire!' and 'Load!' are the only cries
Which are thundered and roared to the vaulted skies;
Aha! they falter, they halt, they flee,
From the hail of the light artillery.

Cease firing?
The battle is over, the victory won,
See the dew is dried by the rising sun;
While the sunset bursts on, hip a full-volleyed sea,
Three cheers for the Light Artillery!

Naval Action in Mobile Bay.

The following clear account of the naval fight in Mobile Bay, is by a young man who was on board of the fleet. We extract it from a letter in Zion's Herald:

"As soon as the last pair of vessels were past the forts and out of range, there were three such cheers went up from the fleet as are not often heard. Each vessel then cut adrift from her consort and stood by for a fight with the rebel fleet. As soon as the smoke cleared away, we could see the rebel gunboats, Morgan and Gaines, and the ram Tennessee, close under the fort, and the gunboat Selma steaming up the bay as fast as she could go. The Metacomet being the nearest, immediately gave chase, and soon coming within range gave her the blows as fast as she could fire. The Selma returned pretty lively, but the Metacomet was too much for her, and after about a quarter of an hour of close fighting, she surrendered. As soon as she hauled down her flag, we sent up three more rousing cheers from the entire fleet. The Admiral then signalized for us to come to anchor, which we did with fifteen fathoms of chain, and our shipping gear on, and it was lucky for us we did so; for the ram Tennessee, seeing the Selma surrender, and hearing our cheers, steamed out from the fort and came slowly towards the fleet. We did not think she meant to fight us, but was only reconnoitering, but we stood by to slip our cable in case she meant fight. She worked slowly and gradually, yet almost imperceptibly, nearer to us. When all at once she put on a full head of steam and made directly for the Seminole, at the same time firing her bow gun. The shell went over us and burst about a dozen yards from us. We were then lying broadside to her. I stood by the chain to slip, and when the shot came, the first lieutenant cried out 'Slip,' and with one blow from my hammer we were clear of our anchor, and making tracks with full power, giving the Tennessee the contents of our battery as fast as we could fire, but apparently with no more effect than flinging beans at a barrel. The monitors and the rest of the fleet came promptly to our relief, which drew his attention from us; and then ensued one of the most grand and magnificent combats that man ever beheld. All three of our monitors ranged close up along side of him, and all firing at once, but as the ram could steam a third faster than any of our vessels, he would keep breaking away from them, but we were so many, some one of us would head him off and hold him at bay till the others came up, and while thus engaged, the Lackawanna bore down upon him and gave him a butt fair amidships, with full speed, knocking her bow all to pieces, and hardly jarring the ram, both firing as long as they could bring their guns to bear.

The Monongahela then butted him, but got all the damage, her bow being shattered, while the ram was apparently uninjured. The Hartford and Brooklyn then closed on him, giving him the most terrific broadsides, and he, keeping as clear of our monitors as he could, tried all his force to sink our wooden vessels by trying to butt them, but he did not succeed, though he gave some dreadful close shaves, and every shot he fired went through and through the Hartford and Brooklyn, until they hauled off and left the whole affair to the monitors and at it they went in earnest too. At this time the ram appeared in as good order as ever, and so did our monitors; but in a few minutes one of the monitors shot away his flag staff, and soon another took away his smoke stack close down, and then went out the deafening cheers from our fleet, and there seemed to be no end to our cheering, for hardly had the smoke stack fallen, ere a shot went into one of his port holes and cut both his wheel ropes, and now he was at our mercy, and he did the best thing he could do, which was to surrender; and then there was such a shout as never before came from our throats. This closed the fight, making three hours of as hard fighting as I wish to see. We then went and picked up our anchor, spread awnings and took some rest, while the ram Tennessee lies within thirty yards of us, with the American flag flying over her, and the gunboat Selma ditto."

Vices of Genius.

Coleridge was such a slave to liquor that he had to be kept an unwitting prisoner, by Christopher North, on an occasion when some literary performance had to be completed by a certain time, and on that very day, without even taking leave of any member of the family, he ran off at full speed down the avenue at Ellerary, and was soon hidden, not in the groves of the valley, but in some obscene den, where, drinking among low companions, his magnificent mind was soon brought to a level with the vilest of the vile. When his spree was over he would return to the society of decent men."

De Quincy was such a slave to the use of opium, that his daily allowance was of more importance than eating. 'An ounce of laudanum a day prostrated animal life during the forenoon. It was no infrequent sight to see him asleep on the rug before the fire in his own room, his head on a book, his arm crossed on his breast. When this torpor from the opium had passed away, he was ready for company about daylight. In order to show him off, his friends had to arrange their supper parties so that, sitting until three or four in the morning, he might be brought to that point at which in charm and power of conversation, he was so truly wonderful."

Burns was not less a drunkard than Coleridge. It was the weakness of Charles Lamb. And who can remember the last day of Poe without an irrepressible regret? He was on his way to marry a confiding woman, stopped in Baltimore, and was found by a gentleman who knew him, in a state of beastly intoxication, unconscious as a log, and died in the ravings of delirium tremens. Douglas Jerrold was a devotee of gin. Byron was a tippler, and his vile Don Juan was written under the inspiration of rum.

Steele the brilliant author of the Christian Hero, was a beastly drunkard. Men wrote of him that very often he would dress himself, kiss his wife and children, tell them a lie about his pressing engagements, heel it over to a groggery called "The Store," and have a revel with his bottle companions. Rollin says of Alexander the Great, that the true poison which brought him to his end, was wine. The Empress Elizabeth, of Russia, was completely brutified with strong liquors. She was often in such a state of baccacle ecstacy during the day, that she could not be dressed in the morning, and her attendants would loosely attach some robes, which a few clips of the scissors would disengage in the evening.

Hail, Maryland!

No merely partisan triumph could awaken the joy wherewith we announce the accession of MARYLAND to the sisterhood of Free States, increasing their number to twenty, and carrying their southern boundary down to the Potomac. Delaware, thus isolated from the slave region, must soon assimilate her institutions with those of her immediate neighbors; her remnant of Slavery having for years been retained by means of an apportionment which gives to once-half of her freemen living in the anti-slavery county of Newcastle but one-third of the representation in either branch of her Legislature. Every one in Delaware has long known that she ought to be a Free State; but Slavery is here one bond of affiliation with the Democratic Party, so the Democratic Party has insisted on keeping her a Slave State. We trust she is about to be delivered of her incubus. The redemption of MARYLAND will powerfully hasten this consummation.

Had the anti-Slavery men of Maryland but known that they were to be stubbornly resisted, they might have largely increased their vote in Baltimore and the Western and upper Counties. But how could they suspect it? The Convention prescribed that only loyal citizens should vote—nay, that every voter should take an oath that he had never aided nor sympathized with the Rebellion—and this debarred from voting at least two-thirds of the white males of St. Mary's and Prince George's, with half those of Talbot, Somerset, Anne Arundel, Caroline and Worcester. In fact, not half the men who have just voted against the New Constitution can truthfully swear that they are not Rebels at heart. But Reverdy Johnson—who last Winter voted to abolish Slavery throughout the Union by Constitutional amendment, declaring that he had been anti-Slavery these forty years—suddenly came out for McClellan, and of course became an upholder of Slavery. On the eve of the election, he publicly advised the pro-Slavery men to take the oath and vote, saying it was unconstitutional, therefore of no validity. They have generally taken his advice; or rather, we presume, they have defied the requirement of the convention, and, in the Counties and precincts under their control, have refused to administer the oath, and voted everything that wears suspenders, law or no law. They have thus rolled up enormous majorities in the lower Counties—majorities which evince the serfdom which the poor whites are held by the slaveholders rather than their untrammeled convictions. The pro-Slavery party have polled a great vote in all their strongholds—a vote which embodies their wrath, their hatred, and their desperation. It is a burning shame that Baltimore, Frederick, Alleghany, &c. &c., had not been polled out as thoroughly. But thousands doubtless hold off because, having all their lives voted what was commended as the Democratic ticket, which was always pro-Slavery, they did not choose now to vote so as to preclude the possibility of their old party's triumph through M'Clellan's election. They wished Slavery dead, yet hated to throw the stone that must kill it. This is lamentable, but, happily, not fatal. THE NEW CONSTITUTION IS ADOPTED; MARYLAND IS HENCEFORTH A FREE STATE; and the Rebellion is finally driven from her borders. Let us thank God and take courage, for the end visibly approaches.

Unionists everywhere! give a welcoming cheer to Free Maryland.

Armory Square Hospital Gazette. Armory Square U.S. Army General Hospital. Washington D.C. (Library of Congress).

painful termination of it, and has many an event worthy of chronicle. To friends far away, we shall record the last hours of their dear ones dying here, and provide a brighter page about returning well with sound limb, ready to do the work which shall yet save this country and events which transpired in this large family now home to many whose distant homes are lonely without them. To all the dislodged classes whose interests touch so closely upon our own—we are sure this little and inexpensive paper will be welcomed.[16]

The printing press was owned by the surgeon in charge, the press-work and printing done by invalid soldiers. Mistakes were made and jealousies festered. In March 1864, the harbor froze along with the boxes of type and was the reason why there were "no papers recently." The previous printers and editors had left to work at another newspaper and failed to warn the newcomers.

Paper cost one cent a sheet so that the initial yearly price of $.50 was rock bottom. Two columns would be devoted exclusively to communications of soldiers in the hospital. The first editor was Mrs. H. C. Ingersoll from Maine, formally a nurse in the hospital. She was replaced by the Reverend E. W. Jackson, the hospital chaplain, reflecting an emphasis on more religious themes. Overall command remained with Dr. Bliss, "who is responsible for all articles published in the *Gazette*." Communications from all friends of the soldiers were welcome; the expected audience was 500 or 600 soldier patients. "We ask for a generous and fore bearing public to overlook imperfections in the outset."

It was common practice for newspapers to exchange with each other. Sick and wounded soldiers were eager to read local news in papers from their own state. "From some of the largest states from which we have the most men, we never receive a single paper. For this reason if no other we put ourselves on the exchange list." *The Crutch* and the *Reveille* were described as "larger and better looking than our own." *The Cripple*, "a sprightly little sheet" from Alexandria, Virginia, was $1 yearly. "We welcome the new sheet and say with all our heart, 'go it cripple.'"[17]

Submissions of poems outnumbered prose three to one. In the Union army, the sword and the lyre seemed hand-in-hand, "the minstrel boy, to the war hath gone!" The *Gazette* solicited financial and literary support for brave, patriotic and loyal men of the army. "Items of interest and short pithy articles are wanted from soldiers and friends. To make it interesting we must have contributions from officers and nurses. We solicit them. Please give us a helping hand."

An official directory was included in each issue, including hospital staff, the 22 hospitals in its department, medical inspector general and director general, acting medical purveyor, pay officers for discharged volunteer and regular soldiers, transportation office and Provost marshal. Posted each issue were the names of patients admitted to the hospital, including rank and company, returned to duty, furloughed, transferred to other hospital, deserted, discharge or died. In one week in June 1864, over 400 admissions were recorded, covering two pages; 41 died and 17 were dead on arrival.

The Hospital Fund covered conveniences and extras beyond the regular ration. Varieties of food such as milk, eggs, butter, vegetables, and fruit were often difficult to obtain and cost extra. Purchasing power depended on sale of the *Gazette* and embalming profits. The cost of running the paper was $5 a week, with the rest going into this fund. "We ask every friend of the soldier, every patriot and every Christian to become a subscriber, at only $1 a year."

The need for more subscribers and funding was unending. Two agents were sent to adjoining states to gain new readers, who in turn would get others to join. Postage was to be paid quarterly in advance. In December 1865, the paper was enlarged and the third page devoted entirely to the Temperance movement. Articles entitled *it must pay* estimated a need for 400 more subscribers to fund this overhaul. The fourth page contained ads, which despite low rates often went unpaid. "We must charge something; we need to make it pay to create revenue for the Hospital Fund for our suffering men. We will remove every word from our fourth page which is not paid. Businessmen will take notice and govern themselves accordingly."[18] Their publisher, Benjamin B. Russell, supplied a "beautiful picture" of the bishops of the Methodist Church, thinking it "should have a place at least in every family of that church." The price was $1.50 and few were sold.

Temperance

By 1864 the seating in the one-story chapel with thatched roof was expanded to 300, containing a room for a library and another for a printing office. It was oiled, varnished and then dedicated in a formal ceremony by the Reverend E. Marks with assistance from "the kind ladies of the city who provided excellent music, anthems and hymns." The Temperance Society met Monday and Wednesday evenings; bible study and lectures by the staff and visitors took up the rest of the week. Religious services were held twice on the Sabbath, mornings for enlisted men and afternoons for non-commissioned officers. Short services were held on each ward. Preaching in the Chapel occurred on Sunday, Tuesday and Friday at 7:30 p.m.

Over the life of this hospital, 800 men joined the Sons of Temperance. It was not considered flattering that there were no officers beside the chaplain. This was a total abstinence society, the first originated in a U.S. hospital. Strong drink was the "soldier's worst enemy and the curse of the American army both among officers and men. Every patriot and Christian should spare no effort to save these men from the curse of king alcohol." The proposed model was moral suasion for the poor and unfortunate drinker and legal suasion for the vile trafficker.

A new excise duty on whiskey brought high prices for fine wines and spirits and was thought just the remedy to decrease consumption. It did not. A "temperance alliance" was formed by another group of young men. They pledged no alcohol between 8 a.m. and 5 p.m. but no restrictions between 5 p.m. to 8 a.m. and a $10 fine for violation per glass consumed.

The national convention of the temperance movement was held in Connecticut in 1865. Its president, Dr. Charles Jewett, and Governor Buckingham did not support the imposition of total abstinence. The local chapters in Washington regretted that position but were in favor of open organizations that would still "promote the glorious cause." It was common to see members of Congress tripping the streets of Washington under the influence of spirits amidst the malarial airs of the Potomac. Was there no way to reach such poor, unfortunate men? "Teetotalers in Congress should become acquainted with each other and organize a society and win them over to the cause."[19] On this as well as most other things, Congress was hopelessly divided.

Even men of genius succumbed to the lure of the grape, so what could be expected of ordinary, mortal men. "Alexander the Great was poisoned by wine, Coleridge an unwitting slave and prisoner to liquor, and Byron a tippler." General Grant's predisposition was well known and his alleged first general order offered effective ammunition for the movement. "The use of intoxicating liquors by any persons on duty in the military railway service is positively forbidden and if detected using liquors or carrying them on any military road will be dismissed from the service."[20]

The chaplain, in his *Temperance Drawer* column, admitted many a church and ministry had no interest on the subject of abstinence in view of the ever-present goblet of wine and the Holy Eucharist. Hospital temperance meetings seemed well attended. The Chaplain of the 19th Maine Regiment, a graduate of Wesleyan University, spoke on how to avoid drink, the Reverend Parker on total abstinence and the dangers and miseries of drunkenness, and the Reverend Pierce of California on the physiologic effects of alcohol on the human system, and prohibitory laws.

At the hospital opening, the surgeon in charge ordered "the chaplain shall do all the profane swearing and all the getting drunk done on the premises. We utter our solemn protest against any infringement of these rights is contrary to military discipline and good order and earnestly request that all concerned take notice and cover themselves accordingly." Good morals demanded that the Chaplain report monthly to the Secretary of War on vices of swearing, drunkenness, and gambling. He then jested, "there is little of either here."[21]

Lectures on temperance were given every day except Sunday in at least one of the 17 Washington hospitals. Much of the newspaper was devoted to this subject by sermons, short stories, poems, anecdotes, and letters to the editor. A 35-year-old lawyer with wife, daughter and promising career became destitute, crumpled up on the floor of a dingy bar in his usual state of drunkenness and ruin. Soldiers marching down the streets of Philadelphia were offered a pitcher of ale. One big fellow declared, "What you need is a good stimulant!" A soldier placed his hand in his pocket, bringing out a Bible, and said, "that's my stimulant, Sir!"[22]

The lady nurse of Ward A told a sad story, a warning to those who did not resist the "enemy within the camp," death-dealing liquor! She picked up a man in the street so emaciated and haggard he was all but unrecognizable as a patient from her ward. He had chronic diarrhea which caused delirium, leading to his wandering off without food or water. The surgeon thought he might have been saved if liquor had not destroyed him, as he died in the arms of his brother in Armory Hospital.

Temperance will save your life! One well conversant with a soldier's life noted, "the sick and wounded cold water man always withstood diseases, wounds and operations better than those who drank liquor. Diseases of the camp, wounds, and amputations were but death warrants for drunkards."

A widow had two sons. The 19-year-old was tall with fair skin, dark eyes and hair. He bid her farewell with "don't worry mother, God will spare me to return. I have faith that he will." He became an exchange prisoner. Her other son was not a soldier and worse was a drunkard! "I would rather my boy perish on the battlefield or die in prison than be like that." She went to Annapolis, searching for her soldier son. The surgeon thought he had been mortally wounded but she did not believe it. "Oh no, he is coming back," pleaded the little lady in black. She eventually found her son whole except for his absent right hand, but manlier than ever and not like the skeletons of other prisoners that had been released. He was still bronzed, brave, strong and alive.[23]

The *Temperance Drawer*, now the entire third page of the paper, described a drunken soldier carried back to the hospital by the Sons of Temperance through the streets of Washington to the central guardhouse "to be punished as criminals instead of being cared for as heroes." [The 6,000-page MSHWR devotes two short paragraphs to the problems of alcoholism and delirium tremens. Alcoholism was considered an administrative problem and moral issue, not a disease.]

A temperance poem *Come sign the pledge*, asks the sinner to support the cause, sign temperance laws, and drink no more, and the ladies would be there to assist. As for the dreaded D.T.'s, with its hallucinations, delusions and a mortality rate of 25 percent, a cautionary tale was told.

> *A snake in the grass—the horrors of delirium tremens*[24]
> He trembles with fear,
> And acts very queer
> Hubby shivers and shakes.
> When he wakes and raves
> About great hard snakes!
> Though no one can see the Viper
>   But bear to hear the poor lunatic ball,
>   How they crawl all over the floor and wall!"
> Next morning he took to his bed,
>   And he never got up
> To dine or to sup.
> Though properly physicked and bled.
>   Next day the poor fellow was dead.
>   You've heard of the snakes in the grass my lad,
>
> Of the Viper concealed in the grass.
> But now you must know,
> Man's deadliest foe
> Is a snake of a different class:
> Alas: *Tis the Viper that lurks in the glass*!

Sermons

A New Year's sermon predicted that 1865 would be "the year of victory." Slavery was dead, the oppressors broken and millions in bondage would soon be free. Great moral victories came as fathers sacrificed sons, and wives husbands, to save their country. "The rich have poured out their wealth; the poor gave their time and strength, and gentlewomen rose with ministers and teachers to comfort the wounded and support the dying. The Lord has been on our side when men rose up against us. What enemies are left: profanity and intemperance?" Armies are by definition profane, and changing that nature is equal to removing stripes from zebras. But clergy persist as this short missive indicates. "How shall I stop swearing," said a poor wounded and dying man. "I want to seek God but find it hard to keep from profane words in these sufferings. I have been committing this sin my whole life. Oh! The power of habit would that we all take warning from the testimony of this dying soldier."[25]

Another habit on the religious hit parade was use of tobacco, smoke or smokeless.

> Tobacco chewing seems to be an inveterate habit among soldiers. As for smoking, I cannot in the limits of this article, even touch; there are so many arguments for and against it as a disinfectant in-hospital life. But what can be said for chewing? It is something to do when a man has nothing else. I think a man must be brainless or a copperhead to have done so.[26]

Sermons delivered on Sunday included tracts on temperance, the religious character of George Washington, the practice of Christianity, and heroism. Titles included "outrages upon a soldier's widow," "Sin and misery are not lovers, but they walk hand-in-hand just as if they are," "never sulk," and "the refining power of religion—it expands the mind of the possessor and purifies his taste."

Being *too fond of pleasure and not enough earnest* was not bad luck but lack of hard work. A handsome and intelligent college man failed because his socializing, carousing and billiards play drew him away from books and classes. A job opening in engineering had two applicants. One was not as smart as the college man but hard-working and honest. The college man could be counted on going hunting, fishing and other places." His life seemed plagued with self-delusion of "ill luck" and "things go against me."[27]

Dr. Sunderland [minister and publisher] spoke to soldiers with "thrilling eloquence," making religion and patriotism inseparable: "It is I and my children, and my children's children that you have saved." Others echoed the notion of "my country, right or wrong." "Every loyal patriotic citizen of the United States should support the government in these ominous and portentous hours of trial. Sustain the administration in a vigorous prosecution of this war and after victory we shall perch our banners and peace pervade our land. There will be ample time to adjust all wrongs."[28]

Visiting clergy spoke to full houses. The Reverend Ward Beecher seemed wordy, long-winded and too high-brow for some. There were many eulogies for the many deaths. By 1865 an end was in sight, making the lesson "to forgive and forget" appropriate. The Reverend Garnet warned: "Let us not be like the Bourbons who never forgot anything and never learned anything."[29]

The biblical story of Joseph and his brothers served as backdrop for the *Sentinel*, a tale about a volunteer falling asleep on picket duty, then getting pardoned by Lincoln. He rejoined his peers in battle, only to die of wounds, saying at his end, "God bless the President." A *day of fasting, humiliation and prayer* was initiated by the President in the summer of 1864. "Let us humble ourselves under the hand of him who has sent the affliction wrought upon his country, on account of our impiety and transgressions and for individual and national obligations to him." Along with that was a call for 300,000 new volunteers.

On Christmas 1864, the *Gazette* appealed to those who could to leave gifts for those fallen. "Many wives mourn their losses. Many children have been made orphans. There are fewer in the family circles this Christmas day. We would do well to remember the afflicted." Santa arrived late, the first week in January 1865. Each soldier's bed received a bundle containing diary, comforter, fruit and other small articles such as made the soldier think he was "a child again just for one night."

Romance and Marriage

The shadow we cast was a sermon concerning the relationship of young married couples and how their souls grappled for love in the search for happiness. In another vignette a young man and a woman were caught in an icy river but survived the buffeting of rapids with luck, faith and hard work. "I hope that our voyage down the river of life may be more pleasant than was our excursion down the St. Lawrence."[30]

There were numerous observations on the female condition:

"The railings of a cross woman are like the railing of a garden: they keep people at a distance."

"Never trust a secret to a married man who loves his wife; for he will tell her and she will tell her sister, and her sister will tell everybody."

"It is no misfortune for a nice young lady to lose her good name if a nice young gentleman gives her a better."

An advertisement was placed for a wife, requiring applicant to submit her carte de visit. One correspondent replied: "I did not enclose my card, for though there is some authority for putting the cart before the horse, I know of none for putting one before an ass."[31]

Local fairs brought in donations of goods and cash. The *Gazette* reported that in the South it was said that women refused to dance with men who had neither enlisted nor offered gifts to sustain the Army. Confederate papers intentionally distorted the news in hopes of keeping morale high by publishing propaganda rather than the truth, hoping to demoralize the enemy. [Both sides practiced such deception.]

Patriotic appeal was made for and by the women of America. "Stop buying foreign goods! We cannot help in battle but our hearts are filled with intense longing to serve. We pledge ourselves to purge imported goods where American can be substituted. This will check the immense debt we are incurring."[32] In one day the receipts of duties in New York alone were two million in gold where business was booming.

A recurrent theme was the heartbroken mother or widow touched with bitter grief but always a willing donor to the Union cause. The son died alone or survived fever and amputation thanks to a mother's loving care, returning home to cheers and a happy and rewarding new life.

Costly sacrifices were made by unheralded women who received no medals or cheers from the crowds. A just-married man in his twenties bade farewell to his beautiful wife. He was the only son of a wealthy farmer but was tanned with callused hands. His father could have gotten him a commission but he preferred being a private. A year later, in a federal hospital in Alexandria, the same young lady was six months a nurse and much praised by the surgeon. Just a month after departure, her new husband was shot while on picket duty. "She is only one of many, an *every-day heroine*!" said the surgeon. The pale faced young widow, going about her daily rounds amongst the wounded, was more truly noble-hearted than Joan of Arc, whose words and deeds fired inspiration. "She does this for the sake of her own dead husband soldier."[33]

Another tale of womanly devotion concerned the noble Mary Fails, niece of Judge Weston, who was in love with Private Harry Sanford of a Maine Regiment though her hand was promised to a man of higher station. Harry pleaded, "will you write often, so often that I shall have no chance to think or fear that I am quite forgotten?" Mary tearfully replied, "Oh, Harry as if I could forget you, the only friend I have in this wide world." He was wounded at Antietam, becoming delirious with fever for which the doctors offered no hope. Mary found him and cried out, "I am here dear Harry. I will never leave nor forsake you again." The magic power of love! Who can withstand it? What life is worthy without it? Harry, pale as marble though outwardly calm, sensed his end was near. In the bed next to him was Colonel Graham, who promised Harry to take care of the lovely Mary if he failed to survive. Back home in Maine a year later, the colonel said to her, "can you learn to love me, Mary?" She replied, "There is no need that I should learn such a lesson. I loved you once for dear Harry's sake. I love you now for your own." It was Christmas Eve, and they watched the star of Bethlehem in the heavens, giving them a benediction.[34]

A women's rights activist, Miss Amy E. Dickenson, spoke to a large and somewhat hostile crowd who hurled "offensive missiles" at this petite defender of women's rights, who stood her ground eloquently with "wit, pathos and a sweet voice." Hers was the "voice of God" according to the *Gazette* review, a triumph for women and for freedom. She vindicated the right of women to speak for the repeal of unjust laws, women's right to property and to vote, her wages, her children, and herself. An editor responded.

> We have small room for controversy only saying that we also believe that woman is not half as strong as man! We think too that she has a great many imperfections! Our dearest wish is that she should *improve* rapidly. In sober sadness we fear that neither woman nor the nation can be saved until both the big and little jealousies are put away and magnanimity and cooperation take their place.[35]

Library and Donations

The Armory Square Library was open daily except Sunday from 9 to 12 a.m. and from 1 to 4 p.m. The chief librarian was a soldier from the Invalid Corps. Books were all hand-picked for suitability and contributed by friends of the institution, often clergy. By 1864 there were over 1,500 books, with newly donated bookcases to accommodate them.

Donations of all sorts were received from widespread civilian sources. Ninety-six single ladies from Wheeling, West Virginia, gave $60 to Ward A to purchase rocking chairs and foot stools. A northern Maine girls' school sent a barrel filled with rags for bandages. Massachusetts sent 14 pairs of slippers, 50 fans and pure liquors for "medicinal purposes" only. Mrs. A. Fogg of Maine sent a "loaner gift" of a quilt flag in red, white and blue to aid a soldier on Ward F who "cheerfully putting his best foot forward" was wounded and "declined any special title of valor or patriotism." The white stripes had patriotic sentences and lines of poetry. The editor requested more quilts to be shared by other such brave volunteers. Fifty pairs of calfskin shoes and 50 pounds in cash from an Englishwoman were received and appropriately distributed.

Embalming

Twelve percent of the Union army died from disease or injury, some interred under Southern soil and the rest back home. National federal cemeteries were established where one in three casualties were unidentified. The Treasury Department posted a directive on how to apply for financial aid and for claims on deceased or discharged soldiers: a plain written letter with company, regiment and state, date of death or discharge, and if a city resident, both street address and number.

Dr. Bliss took great pride in providing the cheapest embalming in the Union army. "Every soldier who dies at this hospital is embalmed requested or not." The ordinary cost was $25–30 each. He charged $3 for materials and $10 for the "embalming package and encasing the body." Those who could afford paid, and those who could not did not. Those requiring disinterment were charged $15, less than half of city rates, profits going to the Hospital Fund. Family and friends of deceased soldiers were immediately notified by telegram. If they desired the remains to be forwarded, a telegraph with an address was sent. All expenses could be paid on delivery or money could be sent through express mail and telegraph.[36] This service was provided on the account of the hospital and in the name of the surgeon in charge.

The Christian Commission and state agencies sent the deceased from other hospitals for "treatment" to be sent home. "For two years we have been saving them unreasonable annoyance and expense charged by others practicing in the city." Mrs. James Cray wrote: "the body arrived home one week ago today looking perfectly natural. It was a great consolation to me." "Our prices are so low that the poor as well as the rich can have the precious dust of their own. Persons in distant states having sick or deceased friends need only telegraph us *send home, expenses follow* and it will be done."[37]

In April 1864, the newspaper notified *friends of the deceased* that the government prohibited further exhuming of bodies before October 1. "We shall continue our fixed practice of embalming those who die at this hospital to assist friends and save them expense."

January 1865, was a traditionally cold month in Washington, where being "frozen stiff" was not uncommon.

> The Armory Square Hospital is as careful in having a proper temperature in our dead house as in our office. We recently received a body of a good and brave man from a nearby hospital to be embalmed and sent to his wife and found it so frozen it could not be embalmed until the next day. It would be cruel to have the wife, sister or mothers come to look upon their precious dead and find them frozen as though they were of no account. We believe it matters how one cares for and buries properly. Our precious dead should receive more attention.[38]

Ceremonials for the deceased were processed by official protocol. "Funerals of all who die in this hospital are attended in the chapel at 2 p.m. Bugles will sound 10 minutes before service commences." Prepared bodies were taken from the room they were placed after death by military escort to the Chapel. The American flag was then placed upon the coffin. "Funeral services and appropriate scriptures are read, prayers offered and appropriate remarks made in the manner of bearing our dead." Mrs. Lincoln, a frequent hospital visitor, "left choice seeds for our flower garden. We have been under obligation to this excellent woman for contributions of flowers to be placed in the coffin of our soldiers sent home for burial."

A *Gazette* advertisement was placed by Dr. Holmes from nearby 451 Pennsylvania Avenue. He claimed to be "the first embalmer of the dead in the United States, the first in Washington City and in the Union Army." He listed the names and dates of his prominent customers since the commencement of war. Included were one major general, four brigadier generals, 15 colonels, one lieutenant colonel, ten majors, and four doctors.[39] Getting formal testimonials from his dead clients must have been difficult.

Advertisements

Another unique addition was the "first class hospital sutler" who provided hard-to-get items desired by soldiers: Segar's [cigars], smoking or chewing tobacco, oysters raw and stewed, apples, cakes, pies, cheese, nuts, oranges, lemons, stationary, beer, cider, soda, and sarsaparilla.

The state agents for Massachusetts, New Hampshire, Indiana and Connecticut placed notices for their respective soldiers to get aid for transportation home, rations, and back pay. There was a directory of the Sons of Temperance and ads for military boots and shoes, military goods, hats and caps, merchant tailors, fashionable clothiers, booksellers, wall paper hanging and window shades, hardware, house furnishings, drugs and medicines, watches, jewelry, restaurants, and gold filling to save teeth! Photographic portraits, especially carts de visit, were popular and inexpensive. Attorneys and solicitors for demands and claims against the government, including pensions and pay stoppages, were ever present.

Overlapping soldier relief associations duplicated distribution of supplies. The hospital provided all clothing gratis. This prompted an editorial about "a serious and growing evil" on the distribution of supplies, irresponsible manner of hospital visitors, agents of state and other aid societies indiscriminately issuing food and clothing.

> Send your supplies to the front, not to this hospital, which is supplied in abundance. Send clothing and food to the thousands of our emaciated and half naked paroled prisoners arriving at Annapolis from Andersonville. Why not unite all our charities in one common depository? This is especially true of the Christian commission who are duplicating the work of the Sanitary Commission who has given comfort to thousands and given material not otherwise available. Local aid societies, state societies, and others should be combined.

The Sanitary Commission did yeoman work but was wrongfully credited with activities of the medical department such as providing "tables, food and other material for soldiers in Washington at a recent event on 6th Street."[40]

Politics

The *Gazette* encouraged the exchange of political ideas while rigidly maintaining its unassailable point of view. "We believe in the honesty of Lincoln, the ability of Chase, the firmness of Stanton, the hopefulness of Seward, the bravery of our Army and Navy, the downfall of the rebellion, in the pluck and patriotism of the Yankees and the holiness of our mission in establishing universal freedom in America."[41] As for the notion of compromise or working together for a common goal, time stood still. "Universal distrust is the *rule* in Washington. If there is a man here, who believes that his next door neighbor is an honest man, we wish he would step forward for inspection!"[42]

An opinion piece, *A few plain truths*, outlined one version of political warfare.

> Some argue the government is waging an unjust war against the rights of the southern rebels. Is a combination of traitors entitled to any other than the right to a fair trial? When they arose in arms they forfeited all right to property and government protection. Alexander Stephens, vice president of the claptrap slave-holders government in his speech declared slavery is the cornerstone of the southern Confederacy! Our government has had a great amount of forbearance. In Europe insurrectionists are hanged or beheaded and leaders suffer extreme penalty. Our government magnanimously offers pardons to those who return to their allegiance. History furnishes no such parallel of leniency to traitors.[43]

Accusations of disloyalty and treason were directed at members of the Democratic Party living in the North who opposed administration policies. A Union soldier wrote the editor, "There are very few copperheads in the Army. I never saw but one and he was a coward. The fact is a soldier cannot be a copperhead, since it is only another name for traitor and it is not in the nature of soldiers to be either."[44] Fernando Wood, a Democrat from New York, was a leader of the opposition declared disloyal by Republicans. "His speech exhorted the rebels not to succumb and hold out till next fall when the chances of a copperhead triumph in the presidential election will give them peace on their own terms."

A soldier from Ward C protested the constant denunciation of the opposition and their definition of copperhead. "If you mean traitors then say traitors. I am inclined to think you mean Democrats. I am a Democrat and pride myself in being a loyal man and deny any imputation of disloyalty. You might say 'there are several kinds of Democrats; what kind are you?' I am a war Democrat, a McClellan Democrat. I don't expect you will publish this but if you do, you will oblige many Democrats of Ward C."[45]

The editor replied that copperhead meant "traitor." The term was reserved for Northerners who

> discourage enlistments, oppose government in its efforts to put down the rebellion and urges Congress to make peace on any terms without compelling rebels to submission. These men are mean, groveling and sneaky, would go down on their knees to the South, restoring slavery and every concession possible if they would come back with us. Don't you think the term very descriptive and appropriate? We can't believe such a snaky skin fits any soldier here and should no more think of a copperhead when thinking of our brave soldiers.[46]

With the Presidential election of 1864, the rhetoric and passions reached a crescendo on both sides. The Democratic Convention met in Chicago; a pithy summary of their voices was offered by the *Gazette*.[47]

> The leading democrat proposed; "let us demand of the convention, above everything else that they give us peace."
>
> I have done nothing to help the war that I could avoid. It will only bring destruction to the people, collapse our finances and send desolation and death through all our homes. Has not that been the result?
>
> War Democrats are not Democrats they are abolitionists. This fall we will bury them in the same grave as the abolitionists and damn them to eternal infamy.
>
> Those who support the war are a Judas and should be cast out as an enemy to humanity and to God.
>
> The Democratic government must be raised to power, and Lincoln with his cabinet of rogues, thieves and spies be driven to destruction. "What shall we do with him?" "Send him here and I'll make a coffin for him, damn him." "Yes," continued the speaker. "Damn him and his miserable followers."

There was not a word against the rebellion, only against the government. Not a cheering word for the soldiers, only pity for their hardships. Peace against Richmond and war against Washington was their battle cry. The *Gazette* returned fire through editorials and sympathetic write-ins.[48]

> Who commenced the war? Has Lincoln said one word, directly or indirectly against the administration of Jefferson Davis? Has he said one word against men endeavoring to kill your brothers and sons on southern battlefields? Stand by the administration because it is engaged in a struggle against a gigantic rebellion, attacked by enemies sworn to destroy our union. Millions will be sacrificed if we fail and the rights of man and human liberty will be blotted out forever. The world is watching how we deal with the principles of despotism and tyranny. The happiness, peace and liberty of our children could be sacrificed and millions yet unborn will curse our memories, if we fail. In this contest there can be but two parties, patriots and traitors. McClellan wants to cease hostilities with those who offer no concessions, no words of repentance and no acknowledgments of wrong.

A great Union demonstration was held three weeks before Election Day in a spacious hall next to an attached building of the hospital, festooned with flags both large and small. Bands played as a chandelier with jets of gas lit up the sky for a large, enthusiastic audience. Dr. Bliss was whole heartedly supporting the Baltimore Convention of the Republican Party and re-election of Lincoln and chaired the meeting with a stable of eloquent civilians and officers from several other hospitals. They resolved, that

> the Chicago Convention and its disgraceful platform deserve the execration of every true American, of every soldier and citizen. We must defeat the champions of the Chicago convention having met the armed legions of the rebellion upon many bloody fields with the sword. We are now prepared to encounter their allies at the polls and by our ballots defeat the dark designs of the would-be assassins of our country. Ever praying for peace, we know that across the battlefield is the only pathway to an honorable and permanent peace.[49]

Informal polls showed two of three patients favored Lincoln, an electoral fact mirrored in all Union hospitals. The need for *suffrage in the field* drove Pennsylvania, Rhode Island, and Connecticut to grant this right. Other states followed suit, helping to guarantee victory for Lincoln.

M. Prevost Paradol, a liberal writer for the French paper *Journal Des Debate*, was stunned and overjoyed by America's latest experiment in democracy.

> After four years of cruel suffering were Americans willing to lay down their arms or engage themselves for another four years? It was disunion with General McClellan or Union with Lincoln. One English journal says Lincoln's reelection is the installation of a military dictator. Others see a discordant love of war. This government surrounded even in its capital by declared partisans has sent not a single one to the scaffold and has allowed them to convene in public meetings in great number, and give speeches by the press and by the ballot for the interests of the enemy. No nation of the old world has yet been subjected to such a trial; no government has yet been reduced to trying it.[50]

General McClellan was reportedly sailing for Europe with wife and child. "Goodbye George! If anyone asks you on the other side whether you ran for president tell him: 'I don't remember.'"

In December 1864, there was a call for many more men. The *Gazette* hoped for "real men, not bought men" who often fled as soon as the bounty was paid.

> Give the President all the men and money he asked for and will soon use up the rebellion. The government should stop the miserable business of accepting bounty jumpers, the off scouring of creation and the very refuse of the infernal pit as substitutes for American soldiers to disgrace the veterans already in the field. Government pays enough to secure a better class. General Grant has hung a lot of these fellows lately for desertion. If he can get hold of and hang the brokers who are instrumental in putting such worthless fellows into the service, he would be a public benefactor.[51]

A letter to the editor suggested means of accomplishing that goal with tongue in cheek.

> Blind men have a fine sense of touch and a few regiments of them could feel the position and strength of the enemy. Blind men and laymen might be drafted together, the blind carrying the lame on their backs. Call that backing your friends. Idiots could serve as generals. Draft all in the lunatic asylum. The madder men get, the better they fight. Dumb men would be serviceable soldiers as they can just say "no surrender." Those men could quickly fill up the depleted ranks of the Army. Crush the enemy with large bodies of troops. Draft all men by all means. Confirmed drunkards armed with rifle, whiskey and sustained by a battery of delirium tremens would do great execution to somebody. A brigade of old maids would be useful in repulsing the enemy. They are sometimes good in an attack. By all means draft Congressmen. They might do a little good in the Army as they are of no possible good where they are now.[52]

Vigorous debates took place on how many men were needed and how to recruit them. This anecdote bolstered the administration and the *Gazette*'s point of view.

When George Washington was president, Congress debated the establishment of the Federal Army, but limited it to 3,000 men. Washington suggested an amendment that no nation could ever invade the country with more than 1,000 soldiers. Laughter smothered the proposition.[53]

Lincoln

By 1865, "Old Abe" was 56 but with his face and heart etched for the ages. A young woman of Newburyport sent Lincoln a pair of woolen socks. "On the bottom of each is knitted the secession flag and near the top the Stars & Stripes, so that when worn by the President he will always have the flag of the rebellion under his feet."

His murder was a crushing blow. Homes, businesses and newspapers were framed in black, the nation awash in tears. The enormity of this high crime was matched in the degree of sorrow and the swath of those deeply affected. "Mr. Lincoln was a good man; one of the kindest and most generous hearted of men, doing and wishing no one any harm but laboring day and night for the good of the people. He was not only a good man but a great man; God does not make men wicked, but finding wicked men he uses them to carry out his wise designs."[54]

Blacks and Company

Some debunked the myth of *the slave instinct,* a state of mind and fact lasting as long as a whip or gun was held to their heads. "In spite of the habit of years obeying and believing their masters they will not credit what they say and prefer to cut loose forever from their associations. Sherman's expedition found itself followed by 7,000 blacks with gray hair, some in the prime of manhood, women and children."[55]

Most Americans did not believe in equality of races on any level and felt that slave mentality was irreversible. The anti-abolitionists argued that freeing the slaves would be criminal because simple-minded and childlike people would starve to death, being unable to care for themselves. The Reverend R. J. Toomey expressed the moderate Union point of view in his sermon *firing the peculiar institution.*

> I have observed for some time many improprieties in the behavior of a portion of the colored population of this city [Savannah]. They do not see it themselves but it is man's pest on the streets and everywhere is evidently on the increase and will if not checked grow to be a serious evil in society. There are some who wear their freedom with commendable modesty, despite their erroneous idea on equality of the white and black races. They are ignorant and should not be condemned but pitied. Legislation cannot equalize the different races solely by human enactments. Justice demands all men should have equal opportunities under the law. These men need to be instructed as to their proper places in society.[56]

At the American Anti-slavery Society meeting, a black man rose to give a portrait of Southern slavery.

> If I were a painter, I would paint a huge engine working from daylight to dark, with its iron arm crushing body and soul. Beyond would be victims destroyed in the millions for its murderous purposes. The wheels creak over the bones of innocent men, women and children. A nearby pool is filled with clotted blood with the stench to remind us of the cruelty of slavery. An entrance to a tomb in prison is littered with mangled remains. Slavery must die in the center, a heartless helot's hellish image with the scorpion staying in a hyena's heart.[57]

The *Gazette's* position echoed the Lincoln administration and experience of the army as to racial progress, though with rose-tinted glasses.

> All the important presses of the country are taking the position that slavery cannot be tolerated in any reconstruction of the union. There are two reasons for this: the success of colored people in supporting themselves and their unflinching bravery in the field. A black men doing his duty as a soldier will soon be considered just another good fellow. They forget the color of his skin, prejudice melts away like the morning dew, and they find it in their hearts to treat the despised race like men. The colored man feels happy to know that his good conduct has won respect and they fight side-by-side like brothers in a good cause. Officers now readily accept black soldiers where they did not in the past.

It was reported that colored soldiers in Gen. Burnside's core seemed not to be affected by the heat. The surgeon in charge of the fourth division hospital reported that when put in front at Petersburg, only 40 out of 4,000 Negroes were unfit for duty. They had fought well though neither white nor black troops could hold their ground. "There is no discount on colored troops in the Army of the Potomac. They will not be made the scapegoats for other men's shortcomings, nor drummed out of camp of their own."

Blacks were assigned the job of burying the fallen, which due to the large numbers meant hastily in shallow graves. In preparation for interment they found letters, photographs, medals, diaries, spare clothing, gold- and silver-cased watches, and money ranging from pocket change to $50. In a brief account *Only a Nigger*, a deceased Union officer was found on a riverbank by two Negroes, who buried him while preserving his papers, cherished photos and cash. Inquiries were made, and all the cash and documents had been preserved and sent on to the family. He had been carefully buried in a makeshift coffin because rebel guerrillas were stripping bodies of shoes, clothing and valuables. It was the blacks who performed burial duty, along with Jews depicted as usurious merchants.

> *On love of home*—the Jews when forced to leave Jerusalem in their exile forgot not its hallowed associations but prayed that the right hand might forget its cunning and the tongue cleave to the roof of the mouth as if the preferred people are not above their chief joy. Even an uninformed savage wishes to return to his home.

> *On the mule*—by Josh Billings. The mule is half hoss and half jackass and then comes to a full stop nature diskovering her mistake. They can't hear any quicker nor further than the horse and has big ears lik snow shoes but cant hear that well anyhow. You cant trust them with anyone who's life ain't worth more than the mules. They ain't got any more friends than a Chatham Street Jew [peddler stalls near Wall Street] and will live on Huckleberry Braise with an occasional chaser of Canadian thistles You cant tell their age, they get no disease that a good club wont cure, and no such thing as a dead mule.[58]

Sacrifice

While most of the deaths and hospital admissions were for sickness, gunshot wounds of every conceivable type and severity tried the skill and ingenuity of the medical staff. Just as there were mood swings on the battlefield dependent on victory or defeat, so ineffective medical treatments and the natural course of disease resulted in the joy of survival or the despair of failure and death. The overall mortality rate of 12 percent meant 88 percent survived and returned home alive.

> The soldier's heart is always turning fondly homeward, but most impatiently in the hospitals wounded and sick. Loved ones from home encourage the patient and under the wise direction of the

surgeon produce a bounty of benefits. Parents from Ohio came to see their son who lost a limb. The father grabbed the hand of the manly hero, while mother covers his face with her plain bonnet and gave him a warm kiss on his sunburned face. He was twice blessed.[59]

The chaplain described his experience on the wards to emphasize need for courage and patience but distorted and beautified that which was deformed, grotesque and painful.

> *Pluck* is another name for the heroic endurance of torturing wounds, and is so frequently seen in our wards as to occasion no remark in the want of it. It is noticed in all cases with wonder the high tone and spirit of our wounded heroes. A leg off is nothing. Men have lain three months with compound fractures, through all the heat, scarcely changing their positions, and throughout all displayed the same bravery that charges a rebel battery. A wounded man with broken leg exclaimed, "Don't pity me." I replied "poor fellow—God help you!" after which he seized my hand and kissed it, thanking me for that word.[60]

The summer of 1864 produced many casualties for Grant's army of over 60,000. An ambulance train a mile in length stopped to allow regiments to pass. Cheers went up for the wounded and three more for Grant.

> There were some horrible looking sites [sic] among the wounded; some with their arms or legs amputated already on the field, others with chest and head wounds. I have seen a number of these ambulance trains lately and I have not heard one murmur or cry of pain. All stand it manfully, and have words of encouragement for those who are taking their place in the field. A soldier is jolly under the most trying circumstances.[61] [In real life no recent amputee is jolly, no fractured leg without severe pain and the absence of complaint occurs only from those absent a pulse.]

A patient in a Washington hospital was upbeat on his experience on a cold and rainy day in 1863:

> I am tired of staying in a hospital. We enjoy ourselves here pretty well but there isn't the excitement that there is with a regiment in the field. I thought before I came here that almost any place was better than the regiment, but I have changed my mind.... I have all I want to do watching sick and dying men. There is some work but not so very pleasant. You may think that only those in the field do anything that contributes. If you come into some hospital, you would see there is something to do there as well as in the field.[62]

Society needs heroes and heroines. The wounded need hope, reassurance and encouragement. Miss Amy E. Dickenson addressed the House of Representatives on the pluses of being wounded and maimed.

> I never pass a private soldier without a feeling of the most profound respect, the deeper if possible, if missing a limb, the presence of crutch or his face *made beautiful by a scar*. The maimed heroes of the war already number in tens of thousands hold an exalted place in the affections of their fellow citizens and will inherit a peculiar glory in which those who have passed unscathed through the fiery ordeal of battle will never share. The old Romans bestowed the highest civil honors of the Republic only upon those who could exhibit to the people their wounds and scars received in the service of the state. Let therefore, the heroes of our hospital not waste a single regret upon what under some circumstances would be a misfortune, but which sanctified by such a cause, will be the brightest glory of their lives and the richest inheritance of their children.[63]

Health Care

A young doctor in a new town was asked to contribute towards enclosing and ornamenting the village cemetery. He replied that "if he fills it, he was already doing his part." The medical staff became the most experienced and knowledgeable military surgeons on earth. European military surgeons visited to learn the latest in surgical techniques and hospital construction.

The *Gazette* was sympathetic to the assistant surgeons they deemed "long overlooked and underestimated." Patient rounds started at 8 a.m., often lasting until 1 p.m., during which diet and medicines were prescribed. Three afternoons a week he served on the examining board for those seeking entrance to the Invalid Corps or discharge from the service, meetings running to 5 p.m. Evening sick call was 7 to 9 p.m. He made a casebook for all patients on his ward and assisted at operations or performed them, all at a salary of $100 a month. He could not apply for clothing at the government warehouse, was subject to the draft, and was rarely was promoted past captain. "Many left a practice or a position at home at great pecuniary sacrifice only for motives of patriotism. They rotated from medical officer of the day to ward inspector at night. They also inspected knapsack room, dead house and laundry and food at each meal 'to ascertain if it has been properly prepared and of sufficient quantities and to report in the morning to the surgeon in charge.'"

A self-described faithful surgeon with a religious background was at the battle of Fair Oaks, operating in an old tobacco warehouse.

> After a full day of surgery at 11 p.m., I fell asleep, our candles nearly gone. A man in agonizing pain had been shot through the mouth dividing a large blood vessel supplying the tongue which was terribly swollen. He was faint from blood loss and could not speak but wrote on paper he had traveled two miles and was told by a surgeon there was no help for him. I pressed my finger against the carotid artery to see if the blood came from the opposite side and as it did not told him he could be saved. The previous patient was removed from the table and the new one placed him-self ready for surgery. Two candles were not enough for light and so a tin basin was scoured with ashes to make a reflector. It took a half an hour to perform what I could do in a few minutes in the daytime. The next day the patient was walking around and returned to his regiment. He was promoted to First Sergeant and was very grateful to me.[64] [Tying off the carotid artery is rarely done as it is fraught with complications, including brain damage and death.]

Another surgical adventure concerned a volunteer with a gunshot wound to his esophagus, suffering from excruciating pain and thirst. Oral intake found its way out both sides of his neck rather than into his stomach.

> I took a long flexible tube and pushed it below the wound into the stomach. Some canned milk and water gave the poor fellow much joy and relief. "More, more," he said. Gradually we gave him toast and strained soup and when last I saw him still had the tube hanging from his mouth with the syringe he had learned to use him-self. It remained until the holes in his throat closed.[65] [Esophageal fistulas often heal if food and liquid can be diverted.]

Doctors and patients may disagree because one is wrong or another has a different perspective of the same facts. A convalescent was fed very weak beef tea for days on end; the very sight of it becoming repulsive. "I shall starve to death; give me some beefsteak, mutton chop or something to chew. It is not nourishment enough to keep a fly alive." His nurse, Niles, replied, "You are recovering from typhoid fever and could get a relapse." The patient disagreed. "I have no faith in starving a man to death and hope of curing him. My doctrine is feed a man when he's hungry." His mother, more experienced with the medical community, said, "I don't think doctors know everything, or any more now than they used to when I had a family to take care of." He shed a tear, asking for one more morsel, and was told, "the doctor knows best."[66] [Typhoid fever causes bowel inflammation and ulcerations which if perforated are fatal. Placing the gut at rest meant a very light diet in an era of no intravenous fluids.]

Amputation dates from the stone age. It was the subject of many stories and anecdotes finding their way into the arena of politics. The public saw many returning veterans with crutches and an empty sleeve or pant leg. Sermons stressed that those who sacrificed got their just rewards, ranging from society's eternal respect to the girl back home.

"I have lost one leg and would lose the other too before I would ask for any peace except by conquering the rebellion." He took hold of his stump in an affectionate way, having done its duty for country. He was sixteen months in the hospital and never complained. If Fernando Woods wants to know what the soldiers think of his peace compromise let him have conversation with these men. Does he ever enter the hospital? Let him ask men who have lost an arm or a leg what they would do, lose the other or make a peace which will prove the first sacrifice worthless.[67]

In the hospital are long rows of beds where pale white forms are stretched and patiently lie there never complaining about doing too much for their country. Some hobble around on crutches, with one leg, or carry a limp sleeve that tells the loss of an arm. Yet their eyes are not downcast and their faces are not sad when they feel that their country has been worth the price they have paid. In Congress are heard voices proposing to call all their loss and sacrifice, all their hard-won victories in vain by offering the South recognition and independence. Do not allow treason when our life and limb have been offered to put them down.[68]

Mrs. Virginia S. Ruth wrote *Lost a Limb* about a woman's devotion to a brave and valiant soldier who was desperately wounded. He received a mother's blessing anointed by her tearful eyes, praying for his welfare that she feared will be gone forever.

"Why this man is dead!" said an orderly.

"No, he still lives though feebly. Lift him carefully and place gently on our palette," replied the surgeon. The surgeon examined his patient with a gentle touch. The youthful and noble face was so bruised and mangled as not recognizable. The limbs were crushed and lying useless, broken in several parts. "This man may live, his health restored but the frame will be crippled, the restoration beyond the skill of surgical power." For three weeks he watched the young soldier wrestle with death but slowly rallied, as "God knows and marks the fall of every sparrow. God does all things well."

He sends a message to his betrothed, "I cannot let you marry a cripple." But what of her consistency and devotion to you, can you repudiate her claim upon your heart?

His betrothed answered, "I am his promised wife. He cannot break the love he has received with the sanction of God. While he lives I will follow through wounds and woe. Because his poor frame is maimed and mutilated shall I hastily yield to his request? Though crippled he may be, it does not change his noble soul. I will not be proved false or falter in my duty to him."

The soldier healed and traveled home receiving shouts of joy and cheer from his friends and neighbors who gathered from far and near to welcome back the patriotic soldier. None was as loving and tender as the devoted home-town girl who whispered, "How could you doubt me?" They married and live forever happy. Every day you see those who *lost a limb* in their country's service. Pass them reverently as they have sacrificed a limb on the altar of the Republic. Come judgment day they wear the vestments of immortality among God's chosen: those who stood nobly and courageously and sustained our country in her darkest hours.[69]

A medical cadet authored this story of a wound complication following surgery ending with a live patient and a grateful future wife. A private was in competition back home with an officer, the son of a wealthy man, and unknowingly won her heart. She arrived in the nick of time to save the broken but noble young hero. In the end the enlisted man got the girl and glory.

"You might take off the upper arm just here without asking."

"What's the use? He won't last out the day. Anyway, we might as well let him go even if we had time to waste in unnecessary operations!"

"I'm not so certain about that. Give the man a chance for his life. Where's the ether?"

"You need no ether; he is totally insensible!" The words fell meaningless on the ears of John

Carlisle as he laid just one in a multitude of wounded and dying men in a weather-beaten old shed. The busy doctor and the kindhearted young cadet made no impression on his mind. He heard what they said, as if they were talking about someone else. Life seemed ebbing away from him as the sparkling tide ebbs from under the stranded boat. All at once there was a sharp sudden pain as the surgeons [sic] keen instrument cleft the arm, and then followed insensibility.

"Ten to one, he'll die," said the surgeon indifferently as he replaced the glittering tools. "There's no use bandaging it so carefully."

But the young cadet knelt down to fasten the wrappings wondering in his secret heart if the time would come when he too should speak so carelessly of a fellow creature that God gave life. The grim old surgeon to the contrary, John Carlisle awakened days later recalling his last conversation back home with the fair town ladies.

"I am a common private and now crippled for life. They should have let me die that dismal night in the hospital when the ligature slipped off and the red life stream drained my vital sources; that night when fever throbbed in all my veins and I madly fancied I could feel Harriet's tears dropping on my cheek." He was twenty-six and already weary of his life.

His secret love Harriet arrived asking forgiveness for her heartless and cruel attitude towards him. "Indeed I loved you all the time, even when I was most willful and I love you still! If you will only let me be your little wife, I will nurse you so tenderly and care for you, so fondly. Don't send me away or I shall die."[70]

Infected wounds often spelled disaster, especially after an amputation. Necrotic tissue including artery and vein could result in irreversible bleeding and death. A medical cadet described such an event. After the second battle of Manassas, a sergeant underwent an amputation six days after injury and now had a necrotic, sloughing wound with blood trickling down to the floor off the rubber poncho across his bed. The consulting surgeon, along with other surgeons, did not think a higher amputation would be successful. His regimental Colonel delivered the verdict with the patient's sister and aunt bedside. He was sinking fast and would not survive the hour.

"Sergeant, we shall halt soon. We are not going to march any further today."

Seeing his Colonel in tears, the sergeant implored, "do you mean that I am soon to die? I am glad I am going to die. I want to rest. The marches have been long and I am weary. I am tired and want to halt." He said to his sister and aunt, "do not grieve, do not weep for I'm going to rest in heaven. Colonel, tell my comrades I died bravely for the good of the old flag."

Those were his last words, his pulse becoming feebler as blood trickled faster and faster down the bedside. The dew of death came and went and flickered for a moment over the pallid face and then he halted and rested forever. His bivouac now was in heaven.[71]

A 19-year-old was mortally wounded in the chest. The surgeon noting his condition informed the youthful martyr his time was short. Receiving the sad tidings with little emotion, he glanced at the ghastly wound, took his mother's picture and pressed it with her letters to his bosom, and gave them to the surgeon. He then called to his favorite companion, "They say I must go but before I do, let's give three cheers for our glorious old union." He then sank to the floor with a sweet smile on his bronzed features and died, or so the story went.

An Irishman from a Zouave Regiment of New York sustained a severe injury just above the ankle, requiring amputation of his foot. He was lying in an ambulance waving his hand to the passing regiments. "Tis in troth, a hard thing for a man to leave half his understanding on the field; but, by gar, it's thankful to God I am that the Johnny Rebs didn't take my raison." His companion commented, "I believe you'll die with a joke on your lips." "Well, I hope I'll have my pipe along 'wid it."[72] [Getting this past the censors could not have been easy.]

Sergeant Henry Walker of Cooperstown, New York, sustained a gunshot wound of his shoulder on May 6, 1863, at the Battle of Chancellorsville.

> We received a warm reception and got through the woods and found five lines of battle drawn up in front of us and caught in cross fire from church and a small log house. Woods were so thick that we got broken up. I can't give you any idea of the scene, it was terrible frightful and sickening. The rebs were closely following us and orders given by the colonel to retreat. We regrouped at woods edge, came to a halt and about faced "to pay their compliments to Johnny Reb.

He was transferred to a Washington hospital for a draining wound, writing home on July 24, 1863.

> It is very warm this morning and I am almost too lazy to write, but I have got tired of doing nothing. I have been waiting for the last two hours for the surgeon to come up. He is going to try and take the ball out. When I went to him Saturday eve he looked at my shoulder and said he would examine it the next morning and yesterday morning he probed it and thought he found the ball and that it could be taken out. He thought the sore was becoming fistulous and he would cut into it so that he could get his finger into it and then he could tell certainty about the ball and if it could not be taken out-could be fixed so that it would heal up. If he should be successful in getting the ball out I might have another leave while it is healing. I went to church here in Georgetown yesterday morning and heard a Reverend Dr. Stanton [a Presbyterian] preach and there were services by the chaplain here in the afternoon.... The doctor was so busy yesterday forenoon that he did not do anything to my shoulder and ditto this forenoon too but I hope he will attend to it tomorrow morning but he may not.[73]

Disabled Veteran

Matching poems follow, first the wounded warrior reluctant to be a burden, followed by his hometown love whose loyalty was absolute. No matter how deformed or disabled, she will welcome him home with open and loving arms.

A soldier's hospital letter and a true woman's answer.[74]
I'd write with a great deal of pain, dear girl;
I've not been able before since the fight;
And my brain is still so much in the whirl
That I can tell, but little tonight.
I'm wounded—'tis not very bad,
Or at least it might be worse: so I said,
When I thought of you, I'm sure she'll be glad
To know that I am only wounded—not dead
I've lost my left arm—there, now you know all!

I've had throughout the most excellent care,
And I'm doing fine, the surgeon says,
So well indeed, that the prospect is fair
For a homeward trip before many days.

You are released from the promise to be my wife;
You'll think me foolish at first: then you'll think
Of the loose, armless coat sleeve at my side:
And your proud and sensitive heart will shrink

From the thought of being a cripple's bride
'Tis a bitter struggle to give you up,
For I've loved you more than ever of late:
But down to the dregs. I drained the cup.

And I'm calm, though my heart is desolate.
I'm coming home, and of course we must meet:
My darling, this once, one boon I implore,
Let us still be friends, for that will be sweet.
Since now, alas: we can be nothing more.

From Sweet home, June[75]
My Robert, how noble and brave you are!
Too brave and too noble, I know for me.
But you've too little faith in me by far,
If you believe I want to be free.

I'm not released from my promise—no, no!
It was never so sacred to me before:
If you could but know how I've long to go
And watch by your side, you doubt me no more.

The blessed tears, by and by, came again,
   And I felt as you in your letter said,
   A feeling of gladness, amidst all my pain,
   That Robert was only wounded, not dead.

You're coming home to be happy and rest
   And I wait the moment of full bliss,
   When I shall be held to a soldier's breast,
   By a patriot hero's one strong arm and the other amiss!

    The death of Captain Charlie Wayne's father did not prevent him from joining his regiment despite the fear his mother had that he would suffer the same fate. Though severely wounded in arm and leg, pale and weak in a hospital bed, he rejoiced at his mother's presence. The assistant surgeon's assessment was guarded; "He has borne the operation much better than we feared. We shall save his legs though he may always be a little lame. His arm is off but according to present appearance; we think he will get well. His courage will go a long way. He never groaned through the whole of it." Her boy was alive and likely to survive. She reached out and touched the remnant of his left arm and neck but could not hold back sobs and tears. Her brave boy was no longer tall and strong, but maimed and halted. Secretly he wished to die rather than be helpless and disfigured, shut out by fate from manhood, work and woman's love. His mother's passion of tears did him good as she nursed him back to health. "Mother, you would rather have me as I am, then not to have me at all?" "Charlie, God is good." He resolved to live not only for himself but to be contented with life for her sake. Captain Charlie was glad he was allowed to make a costly sacrifice for his country. "My work is over now. Perhaps God thought you needed me most. This was his way of sending me back."[76]

    Not everyone is a hero, in fact few are. Most longed for the warmth of home and family, occasionally in a pathologic way. The medical community regarded extremes of "homesickness" an ailment and impediment to health. A sermon on this subject quoted *The Dying Gladiator*, by Byron. "He heard it but he heeded not, his eyes were with his heart and that was far away. He racked not of the life he lost nor prize, but where his rude hut by the Danube lay." The chaplain maintained that personal attachments and friendships that "prop and hold up a man" are not necessary to military life and cause suffering that is hard to measure. "The physician knows how a soldier's homesickness is sometimes the greatest foe to his cure. Those who suffer least are the ones kept busy along with the love of country."

Cannon Fever

There are always those who exaggerate ailments or pretend to have a condition that exists only in their minds or not at all. Some hospitals were accused of being a refuge for slackers rather than a healing zone.

> *Malingering* refers to the artifice of feigning sickness or lameness in order to procure a discharge. There are always men who are not above deception. Honest men are often jealously suspected of practicing deception by surgeons who have been imposed upon. Men under the suspicion are sometimes returned to duty which they cannot perform and so an honest man suffers for the faults of the rogue. Every good soldier should frustrate the schemes of the malingerer when he finds them out.[77]

The skeptical surgeon with some experience could usually smell out a skunk or those with incurable cannon fever.

> "Doctor, look at that poor fellow moving with such difficulty and evident pain up the ward," said the lady nurse.
> With a sly glance the doctor replied, "You don't think he is shamming! I know you don't but he has been so ever since he has been here, just look."
> "It would never do for me to look at him, he would faint away! He couldn't go a step further if I should look round," she replied while looking hurt and with the surgeon suffering somewhat in her estimation of him.
> Days later, the "cruel" surgeon administered a slight dose of chloroform. The result was an erect gate, a smart walk, and a run up-and-down the ward to the vast amusement of the boys.
> "How are you, creeper?" they shouted.
> We will not attempt to portray the down heartedness of the victim, when he came too, nor the emotion of the lady who acknowledged her being "sold!"[78]

> *The Cannon Fever*[79]
> What is the cannon fever?
> Tis a dread of that voice like thunder
> In fear it comes, those ugly bombs,
> Might tear one's limbs asunder.
> It pains the heart—it shakes the nerves,
> It causes the frame to tremble
> It makes a man forget himself,
> And meanly to dissemble.
> He leaves his regiment in the field
> Gives up his guns, his sword and shield.
> Forgets his country and her honor,
> When rebel bands are loose upon her.
> He is sick yet still his cheeks are round.
> Apparently he looks quite jolly.
> The doctors come, ah! Then he's found
> Dejected—seems quite melancholy.
> Then in a faint and hollow voice
> He tells him of some hidden pain
> Deep seated in some vital part,
> Perhaps his leg, or arm is lame,
> He limps around from room to room,
> Expects discharge and pay day soon.
> Quick as it comes he feels quite gay,
> Receives it, throws his stick away,
> Gets citizens dress and sports a beaver,
> That's what I call the Cannon fever.

The Volunteer

There was no higher or nobler example of fidelity and heroism than the Union soldier. "The countries honor was entrusted to their keeping and how well they executed their trust." Those who fought at Chickamauga were more than equal to the armies of Caesar, Napoleon or Wellington. They were as "brave and gallant" as the old revolutionary guards of America, the former "greatest generation." Comments on battle-field experience were compiled from interviews in *Chat with a Soldier*.

> "I have been in as many battles as I wish to but not as many as I expect too."
> "I am always sober going into battle."
> "Soldiers never speak to each other when they are going into the fight."
> "All is still."
> "We think of everything we ever did in our lives. It all comes up before us then."
> "We can't turn back without disgrace and shame. We must do our duty. We cheer and yell and forget everything but the fighting. I don't know why both sides cheer and yell after every volley they fire. I have come out of battle so hoarse that I could not speak when at the same time I did not know that I was hollering."[80]

The lowly private should get honor and all the rewards to which he was entitled. He marched on foot through mud, frost and snow, erected bridges over swift streams, charged deadly rifle pits against squared columns of the enemy, and confronted them face-to-face amidst showers of fatal bullets, charging with fixed bayonets. Was it a greater test lying in a crowded hospital ward with gnawing pain on slowly passing days and nights amidst stifling smells and heart-rendering sounds, where the enthusiasm of battle was absent and hope was based on faith in the gospel and justice of the cause?

"The noble suffering and dying patriots who are wounded and mangled in every conceivable manner have no regrets." Instead they told of happy homes, hard marches and deadly fields of strife. "None regret the sacrifice he had made, or thought it was too great an offering on behalf of his imperiled country. All showed a willingness to lose even life itself, that the nation might be preserved. They regret their inability to again enter the field and meet the foes of our liberties. All honor to them."[81] [The *Chaplain's Drawer* was filled with ever optimistic sermons supportive of the war effort. Any man losing an arm or leg, suffering deformity and disability for life, has regrets.]

Going Home

Soldiers returned, some to cheering parades and others for a final rest.

> *The Soldiers Last Plea*[82]
> Take me home, oh, take me home
> Ere death's shadows o'er me fall.
> Let me hear my mother's voice,
> Let me answer to her call.
> Let me say goodbye, and hear her
> Bless me, as in the days of yore—
> She will love me just as dearly
> Though I am wounded, weak and sore.
> She would press me, oh so fondly
> To her throbbing loving breast.

Gently soothe this burning fever,
Lulling me to a peaceful rest.
In my dreams I see her,
Hear again her cradle song—
Open wide my eyes to greet,
Find alas! That she is gone.

The Contrast[83]

We sit at home, not feel that they
Who fight upon the distant plain
Are falling faster, day by day
A harvest of the slain.
We lightly walk the busy street,
Where trade, and gain rolled swiftly on
They march a battlefield to greet,
And die as it is one.
The trumpet calls them in the night
To die for freedom: and the boom
Of canon from the fortress height
Still calls them to their doom.
Unmoved we read of how they fell
To shield the starry flag from shame;
Dauntless through storms of shot and shell
In the red battles flame!
They lie upon the lonely hill
On blackened plane in dreamless sleep,
Their rest eternal! Never will
They wake, like us, to weep.

Prisoners of War

Getting prisoners of war returned was a thorny issue. Lack of basic living requirements, disease and untreated injuries were known to be taking a fierce toll. General Benjamin Butler seemed adept at moving in non-governmental channels to obtain exchanges and was popular with the public. "General, the best way to relieve our prisoners is to take Richmond. If you do that you will be the next President." The General instantly replied, "That would be a very great work for very small pay."

Lieutenant Colonel Farnsworth of the 1st Connecticut Cavalry had been released from Libby prison after Governor Buckingham pleaded with Lincoln and then Stanton to intervene when eyewitness accounts revealed widespread sickness and death from lack of medical treatment and basic necessities. The Colonel noted that there were 300 New England shoemakers on Belle Island and although men were dying from starvation at the rate of 40 a day, "they all refused offers of extra rations and other privileges if they would work for the Confederacy. They would stay there and starve before they would ever draw up a stitch or drive a peg for the rebel Confederacy."[84]

Large exchanges late in 1864 shocked the nation as skeletonized prisoners came home, some dying in passage and others days and weeks later.

Barbarism[85]
by the Reverend H. N. Powers
Even love itself is fired with holy rage

By scenes that bathe the nation's heart in tears
Reading what woeful visions fill my eyes,
The loathsome prisons crammed with starving men,
And baleful swamps where 'neath the open skies
The brave, like beasts are herded in their pens!
I see their crouching forms, their vacant stare,
The hopeless look of eyes that cannot weep,
The wane pinched faces that was once so fair,
Of heroes gnawing their foul rage in sleep.
I see their bony fingers spread in vain,
For one sweet morsel to take.

There coiled in ditches through the wintry night,
To shield each other from the cold they strive,
On basing fetid chambers they pray for light
Or prone on blistering sands creep just alive.
These are thy fruits, O thou barbaric curse!
This slavery is the crown that decks thou brow,
This is the Christmas spirit thou dost nurse
These the kind deeds thy charity allow!

Valedictory Address

The final issue proclaimed: "the paper was an experiment which we flatter ourselves has been a successful one. It has afforded pleasure to many a sick and wounded soldier. The surplus income after paying for materials and printing, were used for little luxuries otherwise not obtainable." Breaking up an established institution that once held 1,300 patients was "herculean." A great deal of labor transferred hundreds of patients, removed furniture and beds, and inventoried all property on hand for return to the medical department. On August 21, 1865, the hospital closed. Over three years, 13,059 patients were admitted and 1,388 died.

On the closing of our hospital—Our hospital is nearest the wharf from which wounded from Army operations before Richmond were landed. We receive the worst cases and therefore greater mortality than other hospitals. On one occasion in July 1864 we came up from the White House with 250 badly wounded men most from the steamer on stretchers and transported here. No hospital ever afforded finer advantages to the young surgeon for improvement than this. One cannot conceive of a gunshot wound that has not been treated here. Such an opportunity for the practice of surgery, or the study of pathology in the treatment of disease, will not probably occur again soon. As for the hospital we have some regrets, learning to love its pleasant walks, its flowers, its fountains. Within its walls we have learned many a lesson of wisdom, of patients under suffering, of the keenest grief. We have seen many a gallant hero lying upon his couch during the silent hours of night suffering the keenest pain yet uttering no groans, waiting patiently for the calming of the last great victor, death. They wear the unfading wreaths of a blessed immortality, noble martyrs in a glorious cause.[86]

William A. Clark of the 17th Connecticut Volunteers saw the war's end and his return home, writing from a hospital in Washington on February 28, 1865. He was mustered out of the Veteran Reserve Corps on August 18, 1865.

I was happy to hear from you but sorry you were not all in good health. When this reaches you may you all be well again. My health has been very good most of the time and I am now enjoying my share of the blessings of life. I have been neglecting to write on account of having no stamps.... The general opinion is that the Rebellion is about played out. Prisoners are arriving daily. They said they had fought for "Jeff" long enough, there were about 40. I think by the looks they were in a dreadful state, dirty, lousy, ragged and half-starved wretches. Never did I see such a sight before. They appeared to be happy to get here where they could see a civilized people once more.... I saw the State Agent last week and he said the Connecticut soldiers were going home to vote this spring. I think I shall be one of the lucky ones. My love to all.[87]

Three

The Soldiers' Journal

Christopher Columbus Augur was born in New York and grew up in Michigan. He graduated from West Point in 1839 along with Ulysses Grant, graduating 16th out of 39, then served in the Mexican War and Indian conflicts in the west and was commandant at West Point in 1861. He received multiple wounds at the battle of Cedar Mountain in 1862, later becoming a Major General and serving in the siege of Port Hudson in Louisiana. From 1863–1866, he was commandant of the Department of Washington. It seemed appropriate to give his name to a burgeoning new hospital near Alexandria.

To accommodate thousands of new recruits, prisoners and convalescents, a large complex was established just outside Alexandria. The deluge of sick and wounded soldiers required an organized health care system in proximity to the battlefields.

> Men were coming in each day by hundreds from nearby hospitals, men who were just able to leave sick beds and were so prostrated by the exposure and fatigue that they scarcely recovered before becoming subjects of hospital again. They arrived without overcoat or blanket and often slept on the ground without straw, hoping to keep out dampness or use fire against piercing cold. I have seen a poor fellow come shivering to sick call without even a shirt unable to procure another. It was a camp made up largely of sick men which forced the government to transform its operation.[1]

Convalescent Camp Post Hospital was a tent community established on August 22, 1862. It was renamed Rendezvous of Distribution Hospital on January 14, 1864, and finally Augur General Hospital on February 7, 1864, morphing into a 668-bed unit with Surgeon G. L. Sutton as medical officer in charge.

In September 1862, on Shuster's Hill, a camp in three parts was organized. The first was for convalescents, the second for stragglers and deserters fit for duty, and the third for recruits. By October 1862, the convalescent camp held 10,000 men thought unfit for duty, living in tents without floors or heat. Three surgeons were assigned to determine those disabled enough for discharge. The second and third camps were moved five miles away. In December 1863, construction of fixed barracks with 500 beds for the Medical Department Convalescent Camp was begun, completed in February. By January 1864, there were 50 barracks holding 5,000 men, including a bakery with a capacity for 16,000 loaves a day and a kitchen serving 15,000.

The public sent gifts such as snowy linen, dressing gowns, blankets, fruit and even coffins. A soldiers' cemetery was located in the rear of the hospital, holding initially 1,000 grave sites within a fenced enclosure. Each grave had a head board with name, company and regiment. From September 1862 to December 1863, the dead numbered 266.[2]

It was the disabled of the Invalid Corps who leveled the camp grounds, removed

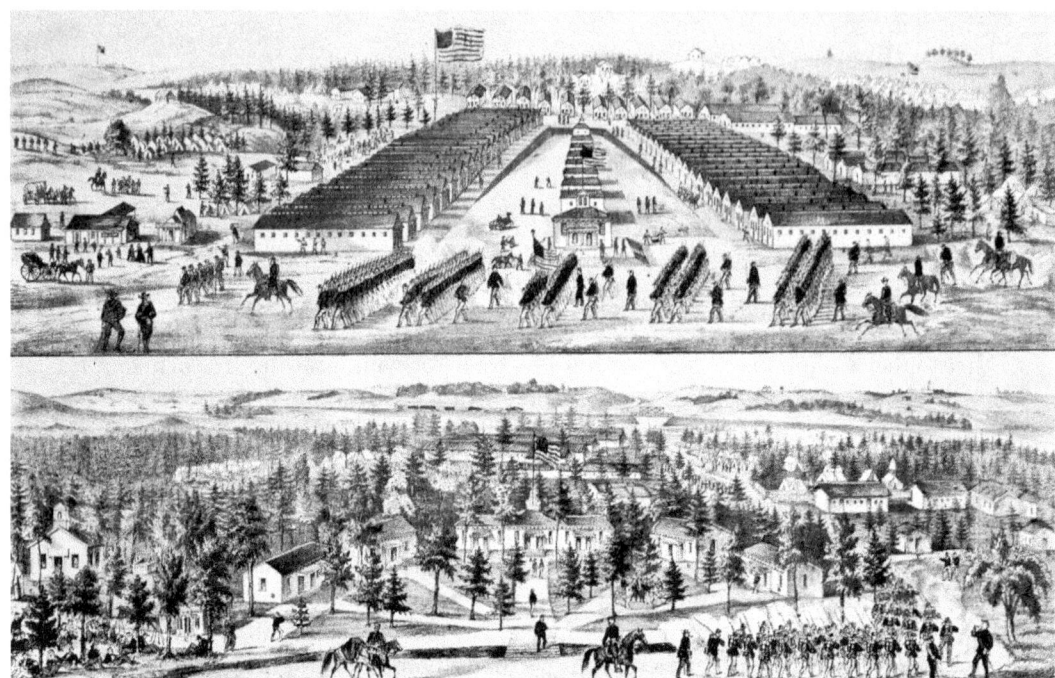

Two bird's-eye views of Camp Convalescent near Alexandria (Library of Congress).

tree stumps, and beautified hospital grounds by sodding and trimming neat walkways. A flower bed created the badges of the Army of the Potomac Corps in a garden with "geometrical accuracy." Vegetable patches were planted and edible livestock farmed though at risk of being stolen. "Fifteen young chickens were cooped in the stables, given as luxuries for the very sick in the hospital that need them far more than the scoundrels guilty of stealing them."[3]

As late as February 1864, soldiers did their own laundry. Eventually wash houses with stoves and boilers were built. At reveille, men stood in line and answered roll call, at least those who could stand and walk. Details for the day were made. Windows were opened, and blankets and bed sacks were shaken and hung out in the air for two hours. Floors were swept three times daily, bunks dusted, grounds policed, and washing stands at the rear of the barracks were cleaned nightly with soap and water. Being a "nuisance" or lounging in bunks with boots or shoes, smoking or spitting on the floor was not permitted. Dirt and rubbish went into a barrel at the rear of the ward. Haversack and canteen were to be hung up. Plates were to be kept clean with no cooking on the stove. Boards under bunks were to be left in place. There would be no cutting or defacing bunks or wards, and lights out at taps meant silence.

When the hospital was renamed for General Augur, its appearance improved inside and out. Buildings were lined with heavy quality paper, making it look like plastered walls. Ceilings were decorated with variegated tissue paper hangings artistically cut and arranged. A grouping of freshly built barracks was no match for nearby city of Washington crowded with office hunters, businessmen, pleasure seekers, porters, boot blacks, "American loafers of African descent," newsboys, soldiers and sailors all dressed in "true blue," officers of every grade and ladies of all sorts. A newsboy shouted "Philadelphia Inquirer;

another great battle; defeat of the rebels!" Newspapers put up "sensation stories" to increase sales. The "glorious news" might be an ambiguous line about a non-event or a total fabrication.

> A Washington newsboy cried "a great battle in Alabama" and sold a copy of the Star to a colonel who scanned the paper and found no battle.
> "You little rascal, I cannot see any battle here!"
> "No," answered the boy as he widened the gap between himself and the officer. "And you never will see one if you loaf around this 'ere hotel!"[4]

> Squads of rebel deserters are seen in gray and butternut, patched and dirty in most cases. Those with a good pair of shoes are considered an infallible indication that the wearer is a rebel deserter. Grant's order induced a great many to leave enhanced by a new pair of shoes. Washington has contrabands of every size and condition. These are "right smart" and will be found up to snuff in all matters of business. The city is a curiosity shop well worth a visit, at least we thought so.[5]

The Soldiers' Journal was published weekly from February 17, 1864, through June 21, 1865, by the Rendezvous of Distribution at Augur General Hospital. This was a thoroughly Union paper whose primary object was "to promote the interests of the soldier in the ranks and to keep good order in their accounts with the government." Soldiers in the hospital would learn how to procure pay and clothing, obtain furlough, and when discharged got prompt settlements without claim agents.

It was printed every Wednesday on site. A one-year subscription was $2, and single copies were five cents. All proceeds after expenses would fund orphans of soldiers who had fallen in the cause of the Union. Hospital literature would include interesting, original and selected material necessarily lively and readable.

Miss Amy M. Bradley was in charge of a relief station, a branch of the U.S. Sanitary Commission "home" in the Convalescent Camp, working with "untiring zeal and devotion for the welfare of soldiers." She brought into Washington a train of ambulances loaded with sick and discharged men who had been receiving her care. In the prior ten months, 5,000 men passed through, of whom 125 sick and wounded who received medical care in hospital tents. The esteem she was held in was demonstrated in February 1864 when, after a "half-recovery from a dangerous illness" at Augur Hospital, she was presented with a diamond, emerald and ruby watch and chain with ring.[6] She proposed a hospital newspaper to the military authorities of which she would be proprietor. The Sanitary Commission provided funds and the means to publish initially from Philadelphia. R. A. Cassidy was the editor and publisher and was fervently pro-administration.

> Southerners are guilty of the highest crime that can be committed against any nation. No sin can go unpunished. They deserve and must receive all retribution their causeless rebellion and treason brings upon them. There will be no compromise and no peace commissioners and no retreat. Unconditional submission is the only way. Publication of the reports of the U.S. Sanitary Commission will be published in this paper. We will establish a regular system of correspondence from various departments of the army.[7]

Advertisements were encouraged at ten cents per line, cash only. The importance of paying customers was emphasized. "A Western paper announcing the illness of the editor added; all good paying subscribers are requested to mention him in their prayers. The others need not, as the prayers of the wicked avail nothing; according to good authority."[8]

The paper had selling agents locally and in Maine and Massachusetts. They were

The Soldiers' Journal. Augur U.S. Army General Hospital. Outside Arlington (Library of Virginia).

"indebted" to William Ames of the 20th Connecticut Volunteers for "substantial assistance in the circulation of our paper in camp and hope that there are many more like him willing to devote a portion of their spare time to the noble cause in the interest of which our paper is published."[9]

The first edition sold 1,000 copies and the next 1,500. After ten months, the ledger book showed a profit of $546 and no debt. By June 1865 there was $1,500 earmarked for the orphans. They hoped to establish a suitable national home and school for "those worthy of aid by their martyred patriot fathers." Additional donations were solicited from the Army, various societies, and individuals.

In June 1865, hospital steward C. H. Phelps of Hammond Hospital in Point Lookout Maryland wrote Miss Bradley as owner of the paper:

> I am desired by the surgeon in charge to return you his thanks on behalf of the patients in this hospital for the thirty-five issues of your valuable paper forwarded for distribution here. They were eagerly received and read by Union boys looking anxiously for just the tidings the journal brings them, especially *mustering out* and *getting home.* May *The Soldiers' Journal* live while the Army lives! By adapting itself as it does to the *needs* of the soldier, the paper will become an indispensable companion, counselor, and friend none of which he ought to be deprived.[10]

Other papers gave praise and encouragement. The *Virginia State Journal* described them as "ably conducted, spirited and well printed. They are devoted to the interests of soldiers and receipts of which are dedicated to soldier's children and has progressed well into its second volume." The *Erie City Pennsylvania Dispatch* noted, "the main object of this enterprise is to raise funds for a home and school for soldier's orphans. We recommend it to the patriot and liberal everywhere."[11]

Anonymous literary contributions were not accepted. Author names were listed by initials or usually not at all. The printing office rules were similar to other like publications. "Enter softly, sit down quietly, do not inquire of the news, subscribe for paper and pay in advance, read news for yourself, do not touch the poker, engage in no controversy, keep six feet from table, hands off type, do not talk to compositors, and keep eyes off manuscript and proof sheets. By a strict observance of these rules you will greatly oblige the printer and need not fear the 'devil.'"[12]

Advertisements

The last page of the newspaper contained ads, chock-a-block with information concerning places to go for any contingency. Details were posted for religious services, temperance meetings, and hours of business for all government activities. The *Soldiers* directory for Washington listed lodgings, soldier homes, transportation office, commutation of rations office, discharged men transportation, adjutant general office and paymaster general office. To avoid swindlers and sharks concerning pensions and other pay matters, the Paymaster General took steps to keep soldiers' money from falling into the hands of fraudulent claim agents. Camp stationery, news depot and post office for sending money, packages or letters were listed as well. Because of the hospital's location, ads for local businesses did not exist.

There were no Red Cross, Social Service departments or Veterans Administration as we know it today. The U.S. Sanitary Commission and other private organizations assumed these roles without much support or encouragement from the Lincoln Administration. In the east and west, 48 commission offices were established. The Hospital Directory of the Sanitary Commission listed the names of soldiers in hospitals across the nation. A designated office with five clerks stored books, each with 300 names of soldiers and their most recent location across the nation. They were listed by hospital, date of admission, rank, company and status: discharged, returned to duty, furloughed, deserted, transferred or dead. If the name was not in a book, a clerk sent a letter to the regimental surgeon asking the soldier's whereabouts. A stamped envelope was sent to the field hospital for the reply.

The Sanitary Commission, as in other hospital newspapers, ran ads offering assistance on locating soldiers, receiving pay, pensions, bounty and enlistment money: all services provided without charge. At 14th and H Street in Washington were the Commission's relief offices, dealing with men from every state, some with amputation awaiting discharge papers along with pay, furloughs or passes. Meals or lodging were provided. Attached to the business office were the dining room, kitchen, sitting room, stove, lodge, comfortable beds, books and paper. They pledged to get any and all moneys due to the prisoner's wife, children, guardian or widow also without fee.

Even their supply department was listed in detail. This was organized benevolence providing soldiers with Havelocks, crutches, mattresses, bedsteads, blankets, socks, medical supplies, clothing, cordials, delicacies, condensed milk, beef stock, wine and other spirits, crackers, coffee, sugar, potatoes, cabbage, sour kraut, lemons, oranges, vegetables, and anti-scorbutic tonics.

What is the Sanitary Commission doing? Their books and work were open to the public. *Money collected by Sanitary Commission* reported that in three years, $1,000,000 was collected. Nearly 95 percent was spent for supplies and transportation, and the rest went to support its homes, lodges, hospital train care and machinery of distribution. The hospital directory, hospital and camp inspections supported 25 soldier homes or lodges where 23,000 soldiers received care daily. Claim agencies secured bounty, pension and back pay, collecting $20,000 daily. The Hospital Directory cost $20,000 a year to maintain with 60 hospital inspectors nearly constantly in the field. Their average expenditure for each battle was $3.20 per man, and $10 at Gettysburg. In July 1864, for every $100,000 worth of supplies sent by the commission, $80,000 came from available money and less from sanitary fairs. Two years prior, $90,000 came directly from the people without any cost to the Commission. Making up the difference was becoming harder.[13]

A testimonial for the Sanitary Commission described:

> an institution only asking the government for permission to live and the opportunity to work. They depend on generosity and efficiency of a free people who are honest, refined, energetic and able. Women with quick brains and hands bathe a poor grazed head with ice water, rewarded with a grateful smile from the patient parting soul. She pours a little brandy down the throats of the wounded till they can feed and clean themselves. They go groping their way at night through torrents of rain, receiving the blessings of thousands while doing noble work.[14]

The Field Relief Corps of the Sanitary Commission are prompt on the battle field reaching sufferers even before their own surgeons. Said one man, lying there badly wounded: "And what do they pay you for this? What do you get?"

"Pay! We ask nothing; only from the soldiers a God bless you!" Our beloved are taken to the hospital where science is doing its utmost on their behalf.[15]

Mail

The Camp had its own photographer and gallery. Nothing was more important for morale than mail. The post office at Rendezvous of Distribution Virginia for one week in February 1864 received 3,426 letters. Some weeks 15,000 letters were received and delivered, some containing money forwarded to families and friends of soldiers.

Unclaimed letters averaged 350 per week. For the last week in June 1865, there were 2,290 letters forwarded and 957 letters received.

The Adams Express Company handled money orders and packages in an effort to avoid losses from theft or negligence. The camp paymaster was allegedly robbed of $70,000 he stashed in a trunk kept under his bed, later found empty in the barn next door. The money and thief were never apprehended. It was recommended that soldiers enclose their letters in hospital-addressed envelopes for surer and quicker delivery, with their name, company and regiment. Printed examples were available at 30 cents per four sheets, folded once with names arranged around the U.S. shield.[16]

Library

Another means of occupying the soldier's mind was a library filled with books, newspapers and magazines.

> It is impossible for our friends to fully realize the amount of relief they afford by the contribution to soldiers libraries of books and magazines. Educate the head of the soldier and his heart will be better able to appreciate the momentous issues he is fighting to establish. The soldier should not be ignorant of the principals involved in the cause the government is battling. Political principles can be gleaned from this library. Fill up the small vacuums in boxes sent with lint, bandages and edibles with volumes from home libraries or the nearest bookstand. Historical, theological, biographical, poetical, scientific, dramatic, and miscellaneous would be welcome.[17]

The library grew rapidly from 600 volumes first gathered from Sabbath schools and Reverends of Boston donating religious tracts such as "How to spend holy time." The Augur Hospital library received 134 new volumes in the summer of 1864, with numerous magazines and newspapers from Ladies of the Bunker Hill Soldiers Aid Society, Sanitary Commission and Congressional Publications from the hospital Chaplain. "It allows our sick boys to pass time more pleasantly and avoid the tedium from recovery from serious illness."[18] The Reverend Calvin Foote, an agent of the American Tract Society, sent 21 bound volumes of religious tracts, all new and thought by the hospital chaplain "good, useful, and entertaining reading of good moral tendency."

Because of the small size of the library room, it was moved to the Chapel, undergoing a design change. A librarian was appointed and comfortable seats installed creating a quiet reading room.

The Literary Debate Society met every Saturday at 2 p.m. in the 1,000-seat chapel. All were invited at this attempt at "self-culture." Questions for debate included "Resolved that the North American Indians have greater cause for complaint than the African Slaves," and "the law of Capital Punishment should be abolished."

Religious services were held every morning at 9 a.m. with bible class every afternoon at 2 p.m. Preaching was every evening at 6 p.m. during the week except during Temperance meetings. A Divine service was held in the hospital dining room every Sunday at 2 p.m., open to all. Catholic service commenced in January 1865, in a large tent put up for that purpose and maintained weekly. A priest came from Washington for a well-attended service. The paper noted 34 generals in the Union Army who professed the Roman Catholic faith, which included Generals Meade, Rosencrantz, Sheridan, and Sickles.

Temperance

A branch of the Sons of Temperance was officially initiated at the camp on January 4, 1865, meeting every Wednesday and Saturday at 6 p.m. in the Chapel of the U.S. Christian Commission. The evil of intemperance was considered "a subject of importance to all demanding the earnest attention of everyone laboring for the good of the race. Cursed are the maddening baneful effects of intoxicating liquors. The poor wretch sink lower and lower, a foul blot upon our enlightened civilization, the acme of human degradation and guilt into a drunkard's grave." Abandon sin, control wayward appetites, commence a new life of domestic tranquility and virtuous happiness, and seek redemption. Maine's Senator Morrill addressed soldiers, first praising their patriotic devotion, privation and exposure to peril. Intemperance produced disgrace and misery best avoided by abstinence. He noted with some despair that "outdoor snow ball fights were more spirited than indoor fights against the evils of grape."[19]

Keeping busy was doing the Lord's work, idleness the work of the devil leading to drink and gambling. "Don't lend your influence to disseminate vice and increase misery in the world. Do your duty and be employed. Find a book, an intelligent companion, learn or do something, make bone rings or carved walking sticks. Don't sit down listless and inactive and thus enter a course that will make you a curse to yourself and to everybody else because Uncle Sam foots the bill and furnishes rations."[20]

The Union army consumed a river of wine, brandy and whiskey for medicinal purposes. Florence Nightingale opposed such treatment, noting, "the long cherished idea as to the necessity of ardent spirits for the British soldier is thoroughly exploded. A man who drinks tea or coffee will do more work than a dram-drinker, though he may be considered sober."

A *Great Indignation Meeting* described a dinner attended by bottles of wine meeting to discuss their future. Was the temperance movement to avoid inebriation or total prohibition, with no alcohol even for cooking or medicine? New doctors joining the division were not going "to prescribe us for medicine and you know there is a good deal of humbug for wine being necessary in sickness." They resolved: (1) to view with pain and indignation any encroachment to do as they please; (2) to protest impeachment of their respectability by being lumped with rum, gin and brandy and other low or gutter beverages; (3) to consider a pledge of total abstinence an insult for those who can take care of themselves and thus need no such restriction; and (4) deep sorrow for the disregard of teachings of St. Paul. "Drink ye no longer water, but take a little wine for the stomach's sake."[21]

Alcohol abuse was no respecter of army rank, position in society, financial status, race, color or religion.

> The Parson said, "Where is the drunkard?" The honest Deacon rose with face red from frequent draughts of his favorite drink. He steadied himself as well as possible on the pew rail saying "Here I am!" "And now where is the hypocrite?" Deacon leaned over his pew to the Squire whom he tapped on the shoulder while addressing him, "Come Squire, why don't you stand up? I did when he called on me."[22]

From the pulpit of the Reverend Henry Ward Beecher came charges that the use of tobacco was hazardous to your health. Indiscriminate use led to thirst and drinking.

> The cup and the cigar are well acquainted with each other. The use of tobacco wastes the nerve-force and the brain-force. It squanders life by leakage right from the center. You do not know whether you

are the one in five that will be poisoned and prematurely destroyed. It is repugnant of every feeling and its pleasure illusive at best. It is a poison leading many a youth to the cup. Is it worth your while to spend your moneys for a habit that incommodes others, annoys those about you, has a bad influence on your health, and will probably injure your morals? Abstain from it.[23]

Another bane of the Christian right was the "hard swearer" or profanity. It was all too common in streets and public places. "We wish all addicted to the habit could understand how vulgar it is and how it is accepted as proof of a bad cause and a week will." Politicians seemed especially addicted: "the fierceness of their profanity is in inverse ratio to the affluence of their ideas and a chronic weakness of intellect. The utterance of noise may present a sound in an otherwise vacuum but is no indicator of sense."

Two Reverends and the Bishop of Boston filled the thousand-seat chapel of the Christian Commission. They encouraged soldier prayers, gave speeches on religious revivals and conversions to God, and sang patriotic songs with the spirit and enthusiasm of the camp band.

Concerts were given with string and wind instruments with players from the Sanitary Commission and hospital. Music was provided by McKelvey's Coronet Band, Orchestra and Glee Club, and admission was $.25. The tunes in one concert were *Grand March, Wedding March, Tenting on the old camp ground, Sounds from Home, Prize Banner Quickstep, Read me a letter from home, Voluntary, the Long, Long, weary day, Do they think of me at home?, Break it gently to my mother,* and *Sweet Home*. "They played on a cool rainy evening amidst slush and snow for a mostly male audience though quite a number of ladies were present. Performers were all amateur and quite excellent. The repeat performance the next Wednesday for Christmas was better than the previous one."[24]

Sermons

For those steeped in the Old Testament, the world was bound by God's will: the nation's war was also His. The army chaplain had the dual role of assisting individual soldiers and binding the fighting men to a higher authority, thus consecrating a holy war that ultimately served God. The nation need be reminded of its spiritual destiny and moved towards greater national devotion. This was an obligatory rather than voluntary war for survival, and no one was excused from serving.

Weekly sermons covered a multitude of human endeavors and frailties summarized in the hospital paper. Clothing was given to those in need, not those just in want. Those too lazy to wash socks did not get another dozen. Charity and generosity were Americans traits.

> We have asylums for the deaf, blind, inebriate and incurable. Our public schools are carried on at immense expense. We are taxed with extravagance but charity keeps pace so the needy are not overlooked. The country is in greater danger from worldliness and vices of its citizens than from the power and malice of its foes. Divine judgments have not led to repentance. The pressure of woe has not brought soberness of feeling. The peril of national bankruptcy and ruin does not incite economy. Great religious revivals are needed to arrest and subdue these fearful evils.[25]

It was the poor or financially challenged soldier and young maidens who had virtue and achieved ultimate success in happiness, love and life's other enriching experiences. The following was about *being rich*.

I am a ruined man. "We must leave the large house; the children can no longer go to school. Yesterday I was a rich man and today there is nothing I can call my own. This war has compelled us to call our creditors together as our ships have been seized and we are utterly ruined!" "Dear husband," said his wife, "we are still rich in each other and in our children." He is a father of eight, how could he be poor? They left the large house, sold its contents and discharged the servants. His wife's economy astonished him. She embroidered, performed needle work, raised flowers, and made prints for booksellers. All family members were at their post busy, cheerful and healthy. Economy and industry was emphasized and nothing wasted. They thrived and then declined to return to the great house. The youngest said, "Father, all we children hope you are not going to be rich again for as little ones we were shut up in the nursery and did not see much of you and mother. Now we all live together and learn to be useful. We were none of us happy when we were rich and did not work. So father, please do not be rich anymore."[26]

How Much Owes thou to the federal government and army? Who defended rights and property of libraries, colleges, churches, financial and art institutions, newspapers and charities? There was an incalculable debt and gratitude owed for this service. "It doesn't take a Christian to hate slavery; a decently tamed wild beast could do that! It doesn't take a generous man to praise our Army arranged in our defense and our homes, against the greatest Rebellion in Time! The man with a paving stone for heart need ask how much owes thou."[27]

The chaplain's audience, the valiant volunteers, were praised, encouraged, and prepared for the exigencies of life. There was "less immorality in the army than anywhere and nothing tries a man's religious stamina as military service." The Reverend Henry Clay Trumbull of the 10th Connecticut Volunteers declared,

> The moral standard is far higher in the army than out of it. Each soldier is lifted above his corresponding fellow outside, the lowest going highest by the very nature of the service. When the army disbands and throws back to society its soldier missionaries, it will be a fine day. I dread for the men the temptations of home and social life when they go north on furloughs and long for their return to the pure atmosphere of camp and field. If I had a son or brother for whose soul I was anxious I would sooner put him in the army than elsewhere in hope of his improvement and conversion.[28]

The triumphs at Gettysburg and Vicksburg during the first week of July 1863 were discussed the following Sunday by Chaplain Potter of New Bedford, Massachusetts.

> It is easy to glorify the national flag and the soldier's skill, devotion and valor. Evil dies hard, but our cause is just. Have hope, faith, unflinching courage and manly fidelity. Battle and disease has claimed thousands of brave hearted victims. The nation stands glorified because it has been crucified. It has borne the pangs of mortal agony that it may wear the crown of immortal life. It has given its hands, and its feet to the cruel nails, the country is purified and redeemed by tears, blood and sweat.[29]

He then quoted Dr. Henry Bowditch, a pulmonary expert from Harvard Medical School, who spent weeks in large hospitals and ambulances near Antietam and whose son Nathaniel died from unattended abdominal wounds. "I was amazed at the quiet, uncomplaining fortitude displayed by our suffering soldiers. It was a most interesting psychological phenomenon, and it was all but universal. It raised my estimate of human nature and raised my own individual nature to a higher grade of existence. The memory of those suffering so nobly born will ever be a stimulus for me to bear serenely the greatest ills of civil life."[30]

The realities of war were faced by those on the front line.

> Many delight in war for its valor, apparent magnanimity, the self-command of the hero, the fortitude which despises suffering, the resolution that courts danger, superiority of mind to body. Soldiers seldom delight in war. The picture should be that of extreme wretchedness of the wounded, the

mangled, and the slain. Avoided are the heaps of slaughtered. The peaceful sovereign is received with faint applause. Men assemble in crowds to hail the conqueror perhaps a monster in human form whose private life is blackened with lust and crime and whose greatness is built on perfidy and usurpation. It is the surest and speediest road to renown. War will never cease while the field of battle is the field of glory and the most luxuriant laurels grow from a root nourished with blood.[31]

What of death, heaven and the beyond? In *Eternity have no gray hairs,* "flowers fade, heart withers, man grows old and dies, but time writes no wrinkles on eternity. The ever present unborn, un-decaying and undying is the endless golden thread entwining destinies of the universe. Earth has its beauties but time shrouds them from the grave. In the dwelling of the Almighty, there can be no footsteps of decay."[32]

Death is inevitable, part of life's trajectory. It is ruthless, the king of terrors, strange, incomprehensible, and respecter of neither wealth nor rank. "The poisoned arrows of swift destruction break the brittle thread of life and give entrance past the iron gate of death." For the Christian with faith, this is a welcome messenger. "The sweetest music is not the peal of marriage bells, or tender singing in moon-lit woods, nor trumpet notes of victory. It is the soul's entrance into heaven."[33]

Indians, Mormons, Irish, Jews

The quilt of American society was strengthened by ethnic and religious groups foreign to these shores. Society's evaluation of their virtue was influenced by folklore, fake science and prejudice.

Humorist Artemis Ward was lecturing in New York on *Life among the Mormons.* He sent complimentary tickets to editors inviting them to come to his show but bring only one wife.

There was an Indian chief in Newport, this past summer who seeing a banker riding with four horses asked if he had eaten so much dinner they required four horses to carry him.

Annals about the occupation of this continent by the Anglo-Saxon race, present us with some of the most daring instances of individual valor that can be found in the records of mankind. The white man often fall victim to his stealthy adversary who were always a mortal enemy. It was victory or annihilation on either side, both aimed at the destruction of the other. The shadow of the *Tawny Savage* could darken his pathway at any instant. These were men of expedience and courage: the situation demanded instant and artful action to outwit the cunning of the dusky adversary. A white man inspecting his property goes to the forests to collect money and is attacked and shot by Indians. One Indian was of Herculean size bearing a like sized tomahawk. A smaller Indian is first shot and killed. The unarmed white man faces the large Indian and in the struggle, the Indian is stabbed with his own blade and dies.[34]

There are no people in the world with which eloquence is as universal as the Irish. When Leigh Ritchie was traveling in Ireland, he passed a man who was a spectacle of pallor, squalor, and raggedness. The sight made his heart ache, and he turned to address him.

"If you are in want, why don't you beg?"

"Sure, it's begging I am your honor."

"You didn't say a word."

"Of course not your honor; but see how this skin is spakin through the holes ov me knee trousers! And the bones cryin' out through me skin! Look at me sunken cheeks, and the famine that's starin' in me eyes! Man alive! Isn't it beggin', am I not a thousand tongues?"

Nations cannot escape the penalties of wrong doing any more than individuals. The Jews incessant mutterings of discontent caused them to wander forty years. Their rebellion led to righteous judgment of the guilty; they demanded a king and got tyranny and civil strife; they forsook altars and yielded to idolatry. The result was God's vengeance just as in this war.

Two New York soldiers were sentenced for some trivial offense and taken for police duty cleaning up the camp. Moshe and Sykesy were immigrants with dialect to match. They had worked well and were seated on a log awaiting the sergeant of the guard to relieve them.

MOSHE: Saay, Sykesy, what you goin to do when yer three years is up? Goin to be a vet, say?

SYKESY: Not if I know myself, I aint no! I'm going to be a citizen I am. I'm goin back to New York and lay off and take comfort, bum around the engine-house and run wid der machine.

MOSHE: I'm goin home to New York, and as soon as I got my discharge take a good bath and get this Virginia sacred soil off me. Then I'm goin to have my head shampooed, my hair cut and combed forward and oiled, and then to some up-town clothing store and buy me a pair of togs. I'm goin to get a gallows suit too-black britches, red shirt, black silk choker, stovepipe hat, with black bombazine [silk] around it and a pair of shiny leather buttes. Then I'm goin up to Delmonico's place and order jest the best dinner he can get up and all he has on his dinner ticket. I'll be a citizen then and won't have to break my teeth off gnawing hard tack. After I've had my dinner I will perch my feet up on the table, drink my wine, smoke my cegar, read the New York papers, and wonder why the Army of the Potomac don't move.[35]

On Blacks and Slavery

Hymn for liberty described a world darkened by slavery which must be overthrown by all good Christians. Join a crusade where the slave no longer dreads the lash and can now burst his chains! Maryland freed its slaves and her soldiers were now on the side of freedom. The sin of slavery was a declaration of war against freedom.

A sermon proclaimed that opposing the monstrous evil of slavery was the duty of every man. Those who owned no whips or slaves were not free from the crime of oppressor. In a republic, every man was responsible for corruption and abuses. All men shared rights and the pursuit of happiness. You are your brother's keeper and are responsible for his injustice and oppression. Self-interest closed the eyes of the North and South against the crime of slavery, and they were all being bitterly punished for it. For the puritanical North, arresting the criminals was required for men to be righteous and enter the gates of heaven.

"All the lawlessness which has infested our country should be put in the account of slavery and its tendency towards illegal measures."[36] The very nature of slavery was to foster lawlessness. Men trained in the stern, unyielding discipline of the camp would not hastily violate the law of the land. Men could not at the same time repudiate the authority of the laws and next claim their protection.

The uneducated often made more sense than the privileged and cultivated. A Negro's head was examined by a phrenologist who deduced smaller brain, little intelligence and an inability to survive without a master. A volume of arguments could scarcely have conveyed more than the fellow's homely speech: "It's hard, massa, to tell what meat is in de smoke house, by putting de hand on de roof."[37]

The distinguished orator Wendell Phillips was questioned by a man of such rotundity that he seemed to carry everything before him. He asked Mr. Phillips what was the object of his life.
"To benefit the Negro."
"Well then, why don't you go down south to do it?"
"That is what we are thinking of. I see a white cravat around your neck, what is the object of your life?"
"To save souls from hell."
"May I ask you if you propose to go there to do it?"[38]

Parson Brownlow originally a Southerner was asked what being a d—d old Lincoln-man thought about arming Negroes to fight white men. "Yes sir, I would. And if I had the power I would arm and uniform every wolf and panther, cougar and bear in the mountains of America; every crocodile in the swamps of Florida and South Carolina, every Negro in the Confederacy and every devil in hell's Pandemonium."

A farmer from Kentucky was fearful that his slaves might leave and enlist in the army. He asked his senior and wisest slave Ben as to what he would do. Ben asked what the result of the war would be. The master replied colored men would be free. Said Ben, "We wanna be clear for we think if de war is goin to make us free, we oughta fight; but if it's foe the Union and the Constitution as id was, we think massa, you oughta fight."[39]

A private in one of the negro regiments guarding rebel prisoners at Point Lookout Maryland received a letter from the daughter of his former owner suggesting that as he is now earning money for himself, it would be a fine thing for him to send five dollars for which they were in great want, and as for herself she would be much obliged to him if he would give her enough money to buy a new gown.

"Our army is strengthened with 60,000 colored troops. One third is ready for any offensive operations. They are good enough for garrisoning towns and fortifications, guarding depots and protecting line of communications. They fill the places of an equal number of white troops required for the same service."

The *Nashville Times* reported, "General Chalmers alleges in excuse of the Fort Pillow massacre, that the rage and indignation of his soldiers at the sight of black troops could not be restrained." There is one way to restrain it—knock their infernal brains out.

President Lincoln has said it was our duty to protect colored soldiers the same as white soldiers in reference to the slaughter at Fort Pillow. The president reiterated that the government would not fail to visit retribution when the acts were clearly proven.

On July 4, 1864, the colored people of Baltimore gave the President a copy of the Holy Bible, an Imperial quarto of the American Bible Society bound in purple velvet with heavy gold mountings engraved in walnut case lined with white silk at a cost of $580. It is engraved "To Abraham Lincoln, President of the United States, Friend of Universal Freedom, from the loyal colored people of Baltimore as a token of respect and gratitude."

Charles Brown a Negro was in a fight with German George Fink both prisoners in deserters division. The Negro ran passed [sic] the picket line and was shot in his back and right side inflicting a dangerous wound that proved fatal.

In Texas one of our colored soldiers with money for the first time could not tell the difference between one, two or five dollar greenbacks and yet paid ten dollars for a watch. His lieutenant seeing the purchase asked the time of day.

"Lord, cap'n replied the darkey [they call every officer cap'n.] "I dunno, how d'ye suppose I can tell?"
"Then why did you waste your money for a watch?" asked the lieutenant.
"Why Cap'n I bout it so dey couldn't keep dis chile on guard duty ober two hours."[40]

Romance and Marriage

A guide for the search and seizure of a lady's heart found an eager audience.

A young beauty witnessed a two horse vehicle running out of control. She was horrified recognizing the two gentlemen of her acquaintance. She screamed "Boys jump out quick, jump out—especially Tom." Her sentiments as to Tom were no longer secret.

When thou art buying a horse or choosing a wife, shut thine eyes and commend yourself to God.

There are many cases of "popping the question" under singular circumstances, the eccentric, the abrupt, the businesslike, and the silly. Of the eccentric is a well-known merchant dining at a friend's house sitting next to a lady with rare charms of conversation.

"Do you like toast, Miss B___?"
"Yes," responded the lady

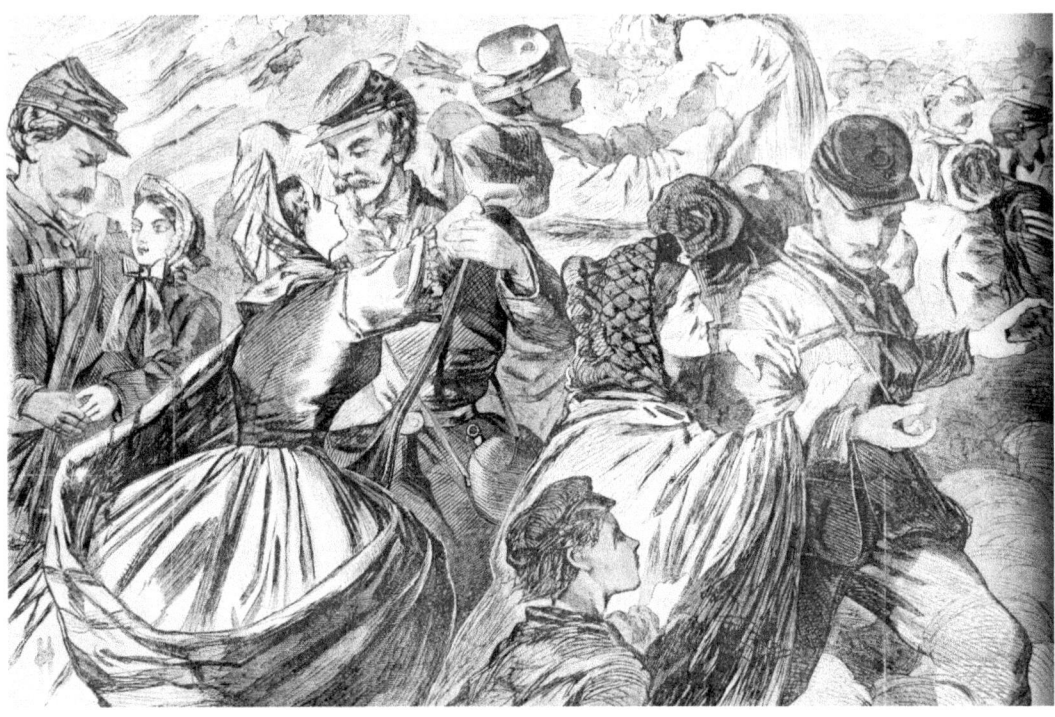

Winslow Homer, "Home from the War." *Harper's Weekly*, **June 13, 1863.**

"Buttered toast?"

"Yes."

"Buttered on both sides?"

"Yes,"

"That is strange; so do I. Let's get married."

They were married a month later.[41]

Of the abrupt sort is a retired gentleman of age 40 with a beautiful house dining with a friend who said "you have everything here that the heart and desire but a wife."

"That's true. I must think of it." He left and went to a neighbor's house and asked for the housekeeper.

"Sarah I've known you for years and have just been told that I want a wife. You are the only woman I know that I should be willing to entrust my happiness with and if you agree we will be instantly married. What is your answer?"

Sarah knew him and that his offer was serious and well lay [sic] out and answered him in the same spirit.

"I agree. So?"

"Will you be ready in an hour?"

"I will."

"I shall return at that time."

His dining partner accompanied them to the clergyman for a marriage for a successful marriage of many years.[42]

A young businessman, ill cultivated, realized he needed a wife to take care of the women's department and a few thousand dollars to stock it which would aid his goal of happiness and prosperity. He goes on a horseback journey meeting an elderly gentleman and confides the situation with him. The latter has three daughters "all good girls as ever lived," and invites him for dinner. He returns for dinner the next day and is charmed by Kate the youngest also rosy cheeked and blue-eyed, joyous and pretty. He confides his choice but is rejected. The father must first marry off his eldest daughter but the young suitor declines that choice and her $5000 dowry. He leaves disconsolate and is met down the road by young Kate. Her dowry was $3000. He and Kate married two months later.[43]

An example of the absurd was Zachariah Peebles an industrious, stout and sober farm hand who spoke little and was smitten by the charms of a bright eyed only child of Widow Brown who also exhibited the same traits of silence. He helped her with whatever chores were required and was a constant visitor at her home though scarcely ever speaking. Two years passed and there was still no marriage. On New Year's Eve he was allowed a stout jug of cider. A few moments later he rose up to his full height of 6'2" putting his head up the chimney so that little was seen above the waist and delivered an oration, at least for him. "If somebody loved somebody as well as somebody loved somebody, somebody would marry somebody." Zachariah remained in the chimney silent as death until with earnest solicitation of the widow Brown he removed himself showing a reddened face. Zach and Sally were married a few weeks later.[44]

A lady and gentleman acquainted but one week was walking in Philadelphia being shown by the lady the streets of the city as he was a stranger. They noted a wedding party entering the church and sat in as witnesses. The gentleman then took the lady by hand to the altar and presented her to the astonished minister requesting they be made one. In ten minutes the knot was tied.

Artemus Ward viewed matrimony as survival by subservience.

I have attempted to reorganizin my wife once. I shall never attempt it again. I'd bin to a public dinner and had allowed myself to be betrayed into drinking to several people's health; and wishing to make 'em as robust as possible, I continued drinking their health until my own became affected. The consokens was I presented myself at Betsey's bedside, late at night with considerable liker concealed about my person. I had somehow got persesluun of a hoss-whip on my way home and rememberin' some cranky observashuns of Mrs. Ward's in the mornin', I snapt the whip putty lively, and in a loud voice said, "Betsey, you need reorganizin! I have come, Betsey," I continued—crakin' the whip over the bed—"I have come to reorganize you!" That night I dreamed that somebody had laid a hoss-whip over me sev'ril times; and when I woke up I found she had. I haint drunk much of anything since, and if I ever have any reorganizin job on hand, I will met it out.[45]

The newly widowed and childless parents suffered the most painful sacrifice. At the Sanitarian Fair in Washington, President Lincoln spoke of the role of women.

Nothing great or glorious was ever achieved in which women did not act, advise or consent to. The chief agents in these Fairs are the women of America. I am not accustomed to using the language of eulogy and have never studied the art of paying compliments to women, but if all that has been said by orators and poets since creation in praise of women were applied to the women of America it would not do them justice for their conduct during this war. God bless the women of America![46]

Soldier weddings became commonplace especially in New England.

In one village in Connecticut where a wedding is a rare event, no less than twenty-seven occurred since last thanksgiving. The high bounties of veterans and recruits make them sound investments in the matrimonial market. The brave carry off the fair, Mars and Venus unite amongst goodly piles of greenbacks where even the clergy profit. A bounty and pension cuts away difficulties from many a love match. Weddings appear on short notice. The villages and towns in the interior of this state are almost depleted of marriageable girls, some converted into war widows by the sons of Mars. The best way to conciliate these Dixie damsels may be to furnish them with good Union husbands.[47]

There were two suitors for one beautiful gal: one a prince in clothing and manners, the other dumbfounded by the ladies' presence. George, the "stupid fellow looked instantly as red as a beet and as expressionless as a pumpkin." "Prince" Henry got up to leave and was asked if he was going to war, "Not I, indeed. I believe this goodly town did me the honor of drawing my poor name from its autocratic wheel but I have already cancelled the obligation. I shall remain here attending to my own affairs." George claimed he had a horror of being drafted. Nettie exclaimed, "Oh but if I were a man, why I'd act like a

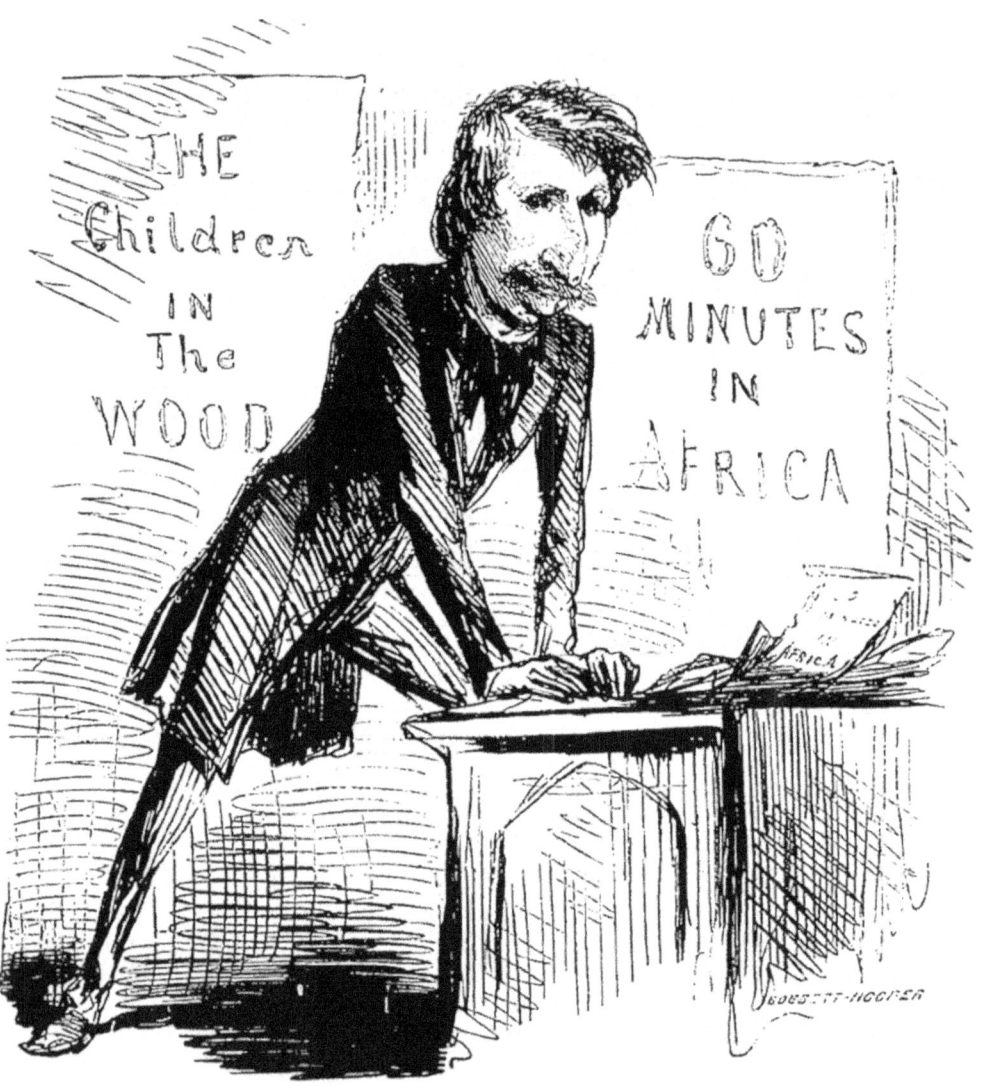

Artemis Ward (Charles Farrar Browne). Political and social satirist (1834–1867). *Vanity Fair*, May 4, 1862 (courtesy Connecticut State Library).

man." George sent a letter expressing his love for Nettie but said that his country called and he had already entered the army. He said his name would never be on the draft list because he had previously enlisted. Nettie and Captain George would be married when he came home on his first furlough.[48]

> Hattie Hayden sat near Dan Hartley sewing socks for soldiers. He had eyes only for the delightful young lady in *Soldier gets the girl*.
> "I wish I was a soldier," said Mr. Hartley.
> "Why aint you then?" asked Hattie.
> "I am not able to endure the marches. I have been weak of body for the year past. Your mother knows. She recommended a tonic for me last spring, cherry brandy. I found it very beneficial."
> She finished her sewing exclaiming, "the last of last order, mother. I wonder what poor fellow will wear them."

"When they wear out, what will he do for another pair?" asked Mr. Hartley.
She put a note with the socks, "Dear Soldier, When you need another pair write me and you shall have another. May your feet carry you straight to victory and may they pause only upon the platform of unconditional surrender."
Dan confessed "you are the best company I ever knew."
"I know better and that is Company A, 1st Massachusetts Regiment."
Her sister intervened; "You should marry a soldier."
"I intend to," said Hallie.
Her card reached the 1st Massachusetts Volunteer Carl Wunenburg. As his socks wore out, he requested another. Hattie lost her family becoming homeless at age twenty. Driven by necessity she became a governess in Boston for a haughty wealthy family with four children. Despite all provocations she remains reserved. The brother of the difficult mistress was Captain Wunenburg, a kind and sensible man with inner strength and fine character. He was engaged to a beautiful debutant. With her hopes of happiness slim Hattie asked if the captain knew a private with same name since she was the knitter of his stockings. They became one.[49]

In *A Woman Alone,* a mother traveled by steamboat down the Potomac in search of her sons. Armed guards reviewed her papers. "I hope she finds her two boys but it is doubtful; twenty are dying a day." She passed through the door of the hospital. If her sons had been spared in the Battle of Fredericksburg, would disease be a worse enemy than the sword and shells?

"Is Robert H--- better?"
It was the nurse's hard duty to tell her the sad tidings.
"He died last night."
"And Edward," gasped the stricken mother.
"He died this morning."
They pointed her to a mound outside beneath which Robert lies, then visited her last son Edward's grave. The soldiers lead her back to the boat, knowing her true comfort awaits in heaven.[50]

The following were notations found on articles submitted by women for unknown soldiers:

This blanket was carried by Milly Aldrich (93 years old) down-hill and up-hill one and a half miles to be given to some soldier.
My son is in the army. Whoever is made warm by this quilt which I have worked on for six days and most all nights let him remember his own mother's love.
This blanket was sewed by a soldier in the war of 1812. It may keep some soldier warm in this war against traitors.
This pillow belongs to my little boy who died resting on it. It is a precious treasure to me but I give it to the soldiers.
These stockings were knit by a little five years old and she is going to knit some more for mother says it will help some poor soldier.
This box of lint was made in sick room where sunlight has not entered for nine years but where God has entered and where two sons have given their mother good-bye as they have gone out to the war.
This bundle of bandages is a poor gift but is all I have. I have given my husband and my boy and only wish I had more to give but I haven't.
These eyeshades were made by one who is blind Oh how I long to see the dear old flag that you are all fighting under.[51]

Prisoners of War

After Lee's retreat from Gettysburg, Union prisoners from West Virginia were paroled and sent walking from Richmond to Union lines, a distance of 100 miles. They struggled, hungry and faint, through Martinsburg, where loyal women tried passing food to them through rebel ranks but were repulsed by rebel guards. "They armed themselves with loaves and pies and with these amiable weapons, shelled the prisoners, over the heads of the guard in spite of their most vigilant efforts to prevent it."[52] Some were barely able to walk absent shoes, and some were almost naked. "They are now at home, wrecked physically but unbroken in spirit having braved the perils of the traitor's sword, the loathsome and galling bitterness of the tyrant's dungeon and the taunts, jeers, and inhuman barbarity of the dupes of treason and secession."[53]

Makeshift facilities functioned as a hospital. As soon as Union prisoners arrived, everything of value was taken. They were immediately stripped of canteen, haversack and blanket. Such behavior was commonly reported by others in the same predicament.

A surgeon left in charge of a hospital at the Battle of the Wilderness reported the capture of 800 wounded and their transportation to rebel lines from which he escaped. He described soldiers lacking everything, including surgeons to dress their wounds. The rebels were destitute of medical stores and were surviving by stealing hard tack from their dead and wounded.

By the summer of 1864, the number of union prisoners confined in Libby prison in Richmond from the beginning was estimated at "97,000." A great number contracted diseases from which many died. Yankee ingenuity resulted in an escape in which 109 prisoners tunneled out, 26 reaching Washington. They dug with forks, spoons and plates and used spittoons, Havelocks and shirts to remove the dirt. The tunnel was 60 feet long and opened into an old tobacco shed beyond the line of guards.

In the spring of 1864, the War Department determined that there would be no further exchange of prisoners, except man for man, irrespective of color. The South refused to parole black soldiers, and Grant declined any exchange. General Wadsworth went to Fortress Monroe to suspend a recent arrangement under which 75 Union soldiers were exchanged for 100 grey. General Benjamin Butler, called by some "beastly, brutal and inhumane," resumed an informal system of exchange in May 1864. He was credited with "natural business qualifications and a vast fund of valuable experience" ending with resumption of some exchanges and a "triumph of what most worthy officer may well be proud." Butler understood money as a lubricant for the machinery of politics, business and bribery.

Attempts were made to soften the blow on the prisoner's family. Written authorization from the prisoner was required to draw pay for his wife, the guardian of his children, or widowed mother. The application must be sent to the senior paymaster of the district by his regiment, along with a certificate from a federal court judge. The Sanitary Commission offered this service without charge and published their investigative narratives of *privatizations and suffering of United States officers and soldiers while prisoners of war in the hands of the rebel authorities*. An eyewitness account appeared during the Presidential election of 1864 concerning Private Terry of the 82nd New York Volunteers.

> All blankets, haversacks, canteens, money, valuables of all kind, extra clothing and in some case the last shirt and drawers were taken. Rations were beyond light and facilities crowded. The projection of a foot or finger beyond a "Deadline," brought deadly bullets of the sentinel. Escape attempts were in vain in the face of prison walls, vicious guards, protecting woods and bloodhounds. Water dark and foul-smelling was filtered through remnants of haversacks, shirts and blouses. Wells were dug but produced diarrhea or were so limited in quantity to be of no use, and camp police was limited. "Is this hell?" Rebel authorities never removed any filth and seldom were visits made by officers in

charge. It was common belief that General Winder issued orders that any guard who shot a Yankee outside the deadline would have a month furlough. Some who were shot were in a melancholic and despondent condition and suicidal. Hundreds lay about motionless or walked vacantly to and fro, with poor food, no clothing and no shelter. Letters seldom reached us and few had means of writing. Letters arrived in large batches and soldiers were charged ten cents each that most could not pay. At Andersonville, a gang of desperate men preyed on their fellows with robbery and murders. A criminal court was established by General Winder upon their complaints resulting in eighty-six arrests and six hangings. Private Terry was a hospital clerk under Dr. White who with very limited means did all in his power with twenty-five assistants. There were thirty to forty deaths daily, reaching a high of 146. Leading causes were starvation, diarrhea, dysentery, pneumonia and scurvy.[54]

These facts were legitimate fodder for the election. How can you negotiate with such monsters? A visit to Libby Prison produced another ugly report. It was three stories high, 80 feet wide and 110 feet long. In charge was a Colonel of an old Virginia family known as a "Negro whip and Negro trader." The floors were rough planked, the windows narrow, dingy and dirty, the rooms overrun with vermin and damp mold, and the atmosphere cold and tainted. Rations were small, the guards foul-mouthed and brutal. A 12' by 12" room held 15 to 20 inmates. Minnie balls were found in the window sill. "The boys practice once in a while on the Yankees; rules forbade coming within three feet of the Windows. Sometimes they do, and then the boys take a pop at them."

Charges of cruel and inhuman behavior were given credence through various news items. At the battle of Bean Station in Tennessee, rebels stripped bodies and shot all personnel coming near the battlefield to show attention to the dead. The body of a little drummer boy was left naked and exposed. Two little girls but 16 resolved to give the body a decent burial. At night they took hammer and nails and boards and from their own scanty wardrobe clothed the body, made a rude coffin for the dead and dug the grave. The noise of the hammer brought some of the rebels to the spot, but the sight was too much for them. Not a word was spoken, and no one interfered. The little drummer boy then slept undisturbed in his grave on the battle field.

Deserters

The Confederacy had a mandatory three-year conscription law that yielded murmurs of mutiny and deserters who began infiltrating Union lines.

The Canadians were disgusted by the presence of so many miserable Union bounty-jumpers. The *Toronto Globe* said: "It is a great pity that men engaged in such swindling operation cannot reach the punishment they richly deserve. They are closely watched by the police and promptly arrested on the slightest infraction of the laws. Some are escaped prisoners; half of these were never prisoners but imposters who managed to slip through our fingers."[55]

Canada became a receptacle of criminals, traitors and malcontents. The stream of émigrés included runaways from the South too cowardly to fight, refugees from the North dreading to fight, and the timid from both who feared loss of property. The Southern fire-eater in faraway Canada could "whip five detestable Yankees at a time, pound tables and make oaths of violent retribution." His clean linen and honest face created a false image of respectability, cooking up schemes and plots more desperate than harmful.

Among the barking and snarling Canadian visitors were disappointed office holders, place seekers and copperheads. They declared "the south will never return to the Union on any terms" and did not consider themselves defeated. They were content to remain in Canada, insisting return to the South was impossible.

Exchanging identity with a corpse was one way out of the carnage. George Benjamin of Bennington, Vermont, a member of the second Vermont Regiment, put his letters and papers in the pockets of a man just breathing his last, then "skedaddled" to Canada. His estate had been administered, and friends had mourned his death.[56]

A large area was built several miles from Augur Hospital to house under lock and key deserters of all stripes. Guards in the Deserters' Camp were offered "fees" as high as $100 for passage through the lines. Watches, jewelry and large sums of money were involved. Arrangements were made for a pass to Washington on a fixed day, and the client was allowed to "run the guard" and then switch to civilian clothes. The bribes were reported to and then confiscated by officers, discouraging further attempts. On one occasion three deserters paid the sentinel $30 for permission to run the guard. They were allowed through and then arrested and placed in the guard house.

Some deserters were shot attempting to escape and others imprisoned. Most escapes failed. An extraordinary bounty jumper was Jack Sheppard, who collected 16 different bounties before being placed under strict surveillance. Two hundred guards covering three shifts a day were needed to deal with deserters from the Camp and Augur Hospital. Passes were required and small sentry boxes erected to protect the guards (invalid soldiers) from inclement weather. A notorious bounty jumper attempted to escape from the guardhouse in Camp by running into a barracks and hiding under a bed. He initially went undiscovered but when he thought the coast was clear he ran out the door, only to be apprehended. Another deserter was part of a detail assigned to rack wood for the quartermaster. Three were missing at roll call. They had racked themselves with the logs but were dislodged and arrested.

A bunch of deserters full of "bold villainy and being audacious scoundrels" robbed fellow passengers who were recruits and convalescents on transport from New York to Alexandria. They took money, pistols, and watches, having their own banker and receiving officer to handle the money. The ring was arrested and stolen items returned to the rightful owners. In a separate but similar event, hundreds of convalescents arrived from New York and on route several gangs tried to rob them but were overcome.

Adam Hill was a deserter working on a road party near a Veteran Reserve camp and was shot while attempting to escape, a not uncommon event. The guard challenged his attempt and warned him not to pass. Hill replied with threats, then received a gunshot wound to the thigh, initially thought serious but not dangerous, and was "doing well" in the hospital until he died.

Two privates from New York held in the Deserters Camp were found climbing out the window and were challenged by a guard who was "met with abusive language." A shot was fired, hitting a man asleep through the chest and wounding one escapee. Both were sent to the hospital. Another deserter from New York was shot in both legs while attempting to escape. The decision to amputate was made but because of his condition delayed till the next day. He died the next morning before surgery was attempted.

A volunteer from the 15th Connecticut Volunteers wrote that the reason for executions was "we are not dying fast enough so they decided to start shooting us." Private John Thompson of the 1st Ohio cavalry was found guilty of deserting to Mosby's notorious gang and assisting them with attacks on the persons and property of Union men. He was publicly executed on camp grounds, an event "well attended with the usual martial ceremonies and witnessed by a large concourse of citizens."

A novel experiment was tried in Deserters Camp to exterminate the vermin infesting other inmates. "The subjects were ducked in a pool of spring water in the rear of camp. The experiment provided salutary results and afforded infinite jest to the innocents who have kept their garments free from pollution."[57]

Not all were guilty. In May 1864, 250 alleged deserters against whom there was no substantial proof of intentional law-breaking were released and charges cancelled if they were "willing to proceed to the field and vindicate their character as soldier with valorous patriotism on equal footing with their comrades who sinned not." The rate of desertions dropped to five a month. By June 1864, there were 138 deserters left in camp. They still required constant and heavy guarding due to the viciousness of some and attempts at escape. Many were sent out as charges against them were weak (and bodies were required for Grant's offensive).

Health Care

Each issue listed the general hospitals in the department: 17 in Washington, five in Alexandria and two just outside. It was emphasized that the federal government provided state of the art health care for veterans. "There is a widespread impression that the general government neglects the wounded and sick soldiers with inadequate general hospital accommodations, insufficient medical and hospital supplies as well as food and clothing. Nothing could be further from the truth. By May 1864 the Union had 192 general hospitals with 80,213 beds."[58]

Surgeons were held in high esteem, and some were presented with sword, sash and belt, and in one case a silver set of bowls, spoons and goblets. Men detailed to Augur Hospital gave Dr. G. Sutton "two beautiful saddles and their accompaniments for him and his wife." The cost was $188. The next day the doctor treated his detail men to an elegant fruit supper. Captain Mahoney, commanding the Veteran Reserve Corps, was recipient of a gold watch worth $150.

Gratitude extended to nursing as well. The splendid present of a photo album costing $75 was presented to Mrs. Eliza Shearer from the Veteran Reserves for "kindness to their unit." She was regularly at the bedside of the sick and wounded, offering cheerful assistance.

In September 1864, a number of hospital chiefs of staff were removed from command and placed under arrest or furlough in the search for corruption, though none was found. Dr. Pliny Adams Jewett in New Haven and Dr. Valentine Mott in New York were examples. The presidential election was in two months, and charges of corruption in the medical department and Sanitary Commission were leveled in many newspapers as a reason for changing administration. At Augur Hospital, Dr. Sutton was relieved of command while a board of examiners investigated. After a 15-day furlough, he resumed his duties as no financial corruption or malfeasance was found.

How many men seek the almighty dollar was a sermon addressing the difficulties of medical practice.

> Some toil with no remuneration coming in dollars but gain in other forms. The physician works hard and long for the relief of suffering humanity, going about doing good, finding work the first thing and

work the last thing, toiling on from day to day, exposing himself for the benefit of others and barely realizing more than a comfortable living. He is not confounded by the apparent success of the quack or the money grubber. His pay is competency of living, the society of educated men, blessings for the poor, recompense with gratitude from the rich, boundless fields for intellectual exercise, access to the rich stores of knowledge and the glory of the Creator.[59]

Two medical treatments were promoted. Sun stroke responded to pouring cold water over the head and wearing a damp cloth inside the hat as a preventive measure. The addition of quinine to whiskey was considered health-restoring, especially in the warm months.

Amputations by "saw-bones" were commonplace. To obtain a government sponsored artificial limb required an application stating that the limb was lost in line of duty, signed by the commanding officer and the surgeon in charge, with discharge papers and details of place and manner of losing limb. Any of five manufacturers could be chosen, in New York City, Rochester, Washington D.C., Chicago, and Philadelphia. Commissioned officers were not entitled to benefits. The federal government allowed soldiers to take the $75 instead of the artificial limb.

An interesting couple was a soldier with both legs amputated at Gettysburg and another with both arms lost from an artillery blast in Charleston. The leg amputee could not attend church regularly. They wished to purchase a velocipede to go out together and attend church but had no money and no home or relatives to help. They kept in good spirits; the armless carried the legless upon his back whenever they went out.

Handbills were posted around camp, offering to insure the lives and limbs of soldiers killed or injured in battle so they could "eat, drink and be merry." Life and limb insurance placed a value on elbow or thumb flexors or a phalange. The loss of an arm was $500 a year, a finger $100. "The subject needs infinite questioning, more tiresome than entertaining and might puzzle the ingenuity of even our Wall Street lovers of the soldier. The company president name is Blunt. Uncle Sam is a better insurer; not concerned over price but the care of the whole soldier."[60]

A young boy had ulcerations on each heel with exposed bone and tendon and a wound in the fleshy part of the left thigh, missing half a pound of flesh and muscle. Both wounds were full of maggots. Turpentine was used by the surgeon to get rid of the maggots, yet the brave little fellow bore the intense pain like a martyr and said: "I suffer very much, but am willing to be torn piecemeal, joint by joint, while living for my country and for liberty." [Maggots have been used for centuries to clean up infected wounds as they eat only dead tissue and are painless.]

Members of the medical community were sometimes among the deceased and warranted an obituary. Nineteen-year-old Private George Lamsom from Stowe, Vermont, was hospital steward, having served for one year. In March 1864, he died from typhoid fever contracted in Augur Hospital.

There was a monthly Chaplain's report on hospital medical activities, including deaths, chapel services and burial in the Soldiers cemetery located in the back of the hospital, usually the day after their demise. For the week proceeding March 14, 1864, there was an admission for a badly fractured leg, one typhoid fever and two fevers of unknown cause, all of whom died. The hospital census was 324 patients, 93 admissions, 47 return to duty, 23 desertions and four deaths. For the week ending May 4, 1864, the following deaths were noted: pneumonia (two), scarlet fever (one), measles (four), and gunshot wound (one).

After the devastating Battle of the Wilderness, 500 men were dispatched by the federal government with entrenchment tools and coffins to decently bury the remains of the many exposed soldiers. The surgeon notified the regiment of each soldier who died in the hospital, who in turn notified the paymaster. Providing financial support for next of kin while avoiding attorney and agent fees was enabled by government auditors.

Getting the remains of soldiers home required a death certificate and a request for provision of interment signed by the hospital surgeon and sent to the adjutant quarter master, embalmer, express office, railroad depot, steamboat landing or other point of departure. The coffin need be enclosed in a separate box brought to the hospital before removal from the premises. The government furnished boxes for officers but not privates, for $5 each. Pennsylvania provided a transportation ticket for the box and one other person. New York furnished part of the transportation fee. Friends of soldiers of other states had to pay all other costs. Railroads required "good embalming" (absent signs of decomposition) or they would not transport. "They have been compelled to put the coffin off and bury them by roadside when not embalmed well."[61]

Ulysses S. Grant

The Governor of Illinois was interviewing candidates for military positions, most muscular and over six feet fall. One slight fellow appeared in homespun and was asked his resume. "I was educated at West Point at the country's expense and served in Mexico. I was sent to Oregon, though I returned to the country an equivalent for my education and resigned. The country is now in trouble and I wish to serve." Later the need for an officer knowing minutiae of regimental organizations arose, and Ulysses S. Grant was hired. He eventually became a subscriber to this newspaper.

General Grant's visit to Washington was met everywhere with enormous enthusiasm. His reception at the White House was the "most furious, coat-tearing and button-bursting jam that was ever witnessed in the East Room." The following day was spent with Secretary of War Stanton and General Halleck. The day after, he visited the Army of the Potomac and headed west. A grateful and expectant Congress gave Grant a gold medal for his victories. His profile was outlined with a laurel wreath. The name and year of each victory was surrounded by a galaxy of stars. On the reverse was a figure of Fame and the American eagle with outspread wings ready for flight. In the right hand was a symbolic sword and in the left a scroll with the names of battles. A caption read "Proclaim liberty throughout the land."

Senator E. B. Washburn spoke of his Spartan simplicity and energy at Vicksburg. He traveled light and took little with him. "His entire baggage for the six day I was with him was a tooth brush. He fared like the commonest soldier partaking of rations and sleeping upon ground with no covering except canopy of heaven. How could such a soldier fail to inspire confidence in an army and lead it to victory and to glory?"

He was described as fair, firm, resolute, and definite. He was glorious not for his appearance but for his deeds. He was the best executive and administrative officer in the army and the best fighting general in the world. His strategy and military judgment were extraordinary, showing more caution than any other military officer. His record was 31 battles, of which 14 were in the Mexican War and 17 in the Civil War. As of May 1864, he had captured 90,000 prisoners and 472 cannon. His command showed no jealousies, bickering, or quarrels among his officers and no Court Martials and no man shot for desertion, unlike the Army of the Potomac. His devotion for duty was exemplary, his character flawless. He sent no foolish proclamations or edicts against the press, accepted no flattery, and graced victories with humility and humanity.

He ate with his staff, expenses divided among the ten in equal proportions. They used plain crockery, hard cots without mattresses, few wash basins at the table, and no show or parade. There was no liquor or wine permitted. His baggage was cigar, telescope and tooth brush. He was plainly clad with threadbare clothes and an untidy look. Flannel shirts were practical and kept clean, fancy clothes were not needed. He went everywhere and saw everything himself. He never swore, rarely laughed and had a sort of grim humor. He rode his horse in the rain with one aid, no carriage and often got soaking wet. Other generals rode in a carriage with 12 dragoons as escort, while he rode with one or alone.

For Grant there was no retreat. "Our regiment has been under fire twenty-three days in succession, fighting more or less every day. We have been whittled down pretty much and have eighty men left." Another volunteer remarked, "Grant makes the bandbox soldier fight. White collars and patent leather boots are played out. He fights his men for what they are worth. He has their full confidence; all orders, charges, marches are cheerfully obeyed." [At the Battle of the Wilderness, there was no cheering, not with 28,699 casualties and 3,723 deaths.] Another reported: "We are enjoying ourselves in the usual way. We have fight for breakfast, dinner and supper; twice between meals and three times during the night. In short it has become a second nature. It is said a man who will leave his meals to fight loves it. In that case the Yankees must love to fight for it is an everyday occurrence to jump up from coffee and hard tack and give the Johnny's a round two."[62]

In May 1864, there was heavy fighting up and down the Rapidan River. Newspaper headlines shouted:

Highly Important News
VICTORY!! VICTORY !!
GRANT OUTGENERALS LEE,
ARMY OF THE POTOMAC TRIUMPHANT,
Unparalleled Slaughter on Both Sides, Heavy capture of Artillery and Prisoners.[63]

The spring offensive brought many casualties:

The graves of our men, buried by the enemy in immense trenches are visible near every road. In many places scores of skulls grin horribly at the mournful observer. A forest of trees were cut down by solid shot and shells, pierced and scarred by bullets. Generals Grant and Meade were in the saddle constantly personally directing movements. Rebel prisoners assert that Lee ordered all his wounded men able to hold a musket to take their places in the ranks again for today's battle.[64]

Grant wrote his own press release. "We have now ended the sixth day of very heavy fighting. The result to this time is much in our favor. Our losses have been heavy as well as those of the enemy. I think the loss of the enemy must be greater. We have taken over 5,000 prisoners while he has taken from us but a few except stragglers. I propose to fight it out on this line, if it takes all summer." Secretary Stanton declared, "the government is sparing no pains to support him."[65]

On Lincoln

Harriet Beecher Stowe, the little lady who started the Civil War according to Lincoln, was firmly in his corner, along with the abolitionist movement.

Little did the convention know of the honest, fatherly patriotic man standing in his simplicity on the platform at Springfield while asking for the prayers of his town's men. God's hand protected him first from the danger of assassination in Baltimore, bringing him safely to the nation's capital. Lincoln is a strong man, not aggressive so much as passive, not a stone buttress but a wire cable whose strength sways to every influence yielding on this side and that for popular needs yet tenaciously and inflexibly bound to carry it to great end. He is surrounded by traitors, and half-hearted men of Border States, Free State men, radical abolitionists and conservatives. He weighs the words of all but remains inflexible to honest purpose. He is the most abused man of our nation. Like Moses leading Israel through the wilderness, he had seen the day when every man seemed ready to stone him and yet with steady perseverance holds on looking for God's help.[66]

Lincoln's positions were like granite in resolve. He addressed the House of Representatives, receiving a great deal of applause: "we will not re-enslave such persons as are made free by the Emancipation Proclamation or by any act of Congress. The war will cease on the part of the government whenever it shall have ceased on the part of those who began it."[67]

After the Emancipation Proclamation, some political observers became hugely supportive. Edouard Laboulaye, a liberal French political writer, opined: "Americans don't appreciate Mr. Lincoln at his proper value. No monarchy in Europe could carry on such a colossal war in front while harassed by so many factions and fault finders in back. You don't give him his due."[68] He saw the American conflict decisively shaping the struggle of free men and popular democracy worldwide against the privileged few holding for themselves all rights and justice.

A White House visitor was troubled by the policies of the administration and got this reply.

> Gentlemen suppose all the property you were worth was in gold and you had it in the hands of Blondin to cross Niagara River on a rope. Would you shake the cable or keep shouting out to him "Blondin stand up a little straighter, Blondin stoop a little more, go a little faster, lean a little more to the north or to the south?" No, you would hold your breath as well as your tongue and keep your hands off until he was safely over. The government is carrying an immense weight. Untold treasure is in their hands. They are doing the very best they can. Don't badger, keep silent, and we'll get you safely across."[69] [Blondin was a French acrobat and high wire act, the first to cross Niagara Falls in 1859.]

In March 1864, Lincoln called a draft for 300,000 more troops. Foreigners

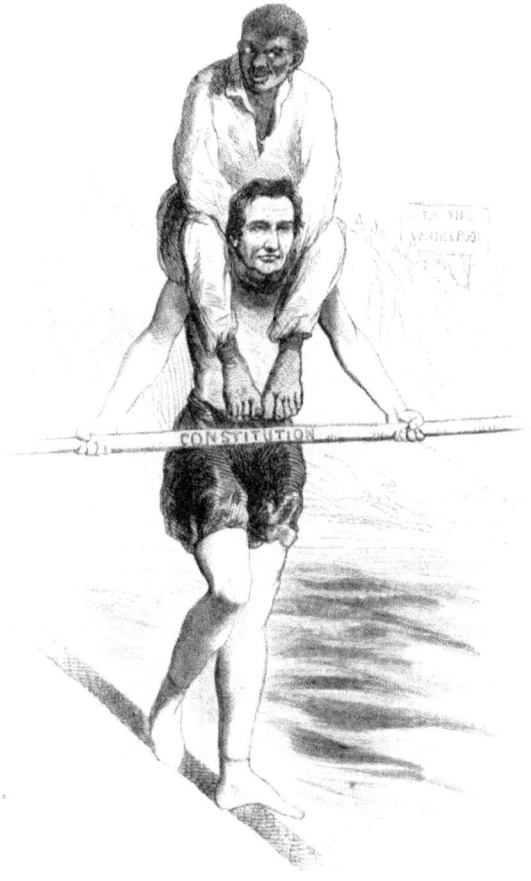

"The Coming Man's Presidential Career, à la Blondin." Crossing Niagara Falls. *Harper's Weekly*, August 26, 1860.

and those who had already served were exempt but could act as substitutes. Some signed up just to get the bounty, then departed before the sun set. If caught, the charge was desertion and the penalty death. Lincoln directed that deserters condemned to death by court-martial and whose sentences were not otherwise acted upon should be sent to the Dry Tortugas in Florida, imprisoned until the close of the war. This was one of the few places still endemic with yellow fever, carrying a mortality rate of 50 percent, half that of a firing squad. Executive clemency from civil law and acquittal was pitted against martial law and execution. "The decision to suspend executions for desertion and send violators to Florida was noble in being just and divine in being merciful. The edict added the luster of humanitarian and philanthropy to his just and patriotic administration."[70]

Lincoln had regular meetings with individual public citizens. A widow whose only son was drafted asked for his release. He advised that an only son relied upon for subsistence exempted him from service and referred her to the Provost Marshall. An Irish woman had a son in the penitentiary for stealing and wanted him released for her support. "Can't help that, ought not to steal." The next in line exclaimed: "We have no particular business but merely wish the pleasure of shaking hands with you." He rose to his feet quite cordially and conversed freely. "We were favorably impressed. He is not slow drawling or dragging kind of man. He is quick in movements; articulation is distinct, sharp and rapid. He appears to be care-worn and painfully anxious but when he speaks and interacts with people seems brilliant and pleasant. There is an indomitable energy, honesty and truthfulness. These are the secrets of his success in life."[71]

As a well-paid attorney for the railroad, his expertise on right of way on land or water determined landmark court decisions. Many of his speeches were steeped in religious lore, though his church had no walls or ceiling and his bible was a well-worn King James edition. During a deputation, an over-regarded clergyman was styled "a pillar of the church." Lincoln's clear-eyed reply was, "they would've done much better to call him a steeple."

> I once knew a good sound churchman named Brown who was on a committee to erect a bridge over a dangerous and rapid river. Architect after architect failed and finally he found a friend named Jones who built several bridges and might build this one. "Yes, I could build a bridge to the infernal region if necessary," declared Jones. The sober committee was horrified and to reassure them Brown replied, "I know Jones well, he is very honest and a good architect and if he says he can build a bridge to Hades-I believe it! But I have my doubts about the abutment on the infernal side." Lincoln went on, "So when politicians said they could harmonize the Northern and Southern wings of the democracy, why I believed them. But I had my doubts about the abutment on the Southern side.[72]

He addressed the Sanitary Fair in Philadelphia in June 1864.

> "It is a pertinent question when is this war to end. I don't wish to name a date, lest the ends should not come at the given time. We accepted this war that we did not begin. We accepted it for an object and when that object is accomplished the war will end; and I hope to God it never will end till that object is accomplished. We are going through with our tasks if it takes three years longer. I shall discover that Grant may be greatly facilitated in the capture of Richmond by rapidly pouring to him a large number of armed men at the briefest notice. Will you go? Will you march with him? Then I shall call upon you when it is necessary!" The crowd roared its approval after each question.[73]

In August 1864, a peace conference with the rebels was reported a possibility in Niagara. Lincoln would meet with "any proposition which embrace the restoration of peace, the integrity of the whole Union and the abandonment of slavery and which comes by and with an authority that can control the armies now at war against the U.S." After the election, the unyielding goal was reunification. There would be no negotiations for Southern independence, and Congress would abolish slavery by constitutional amendment. He proposed taxation to meet the debt of $1,000,750,000 and a limited amount of tax exempt securities to be issued not liable to seizure for debt.[74]

Later that summer, a gentleman remarked to President Lincoln that nothing could defeat him but Grant's capture of Richmond, which would then be rewarded with nomination and acceptance at the Chicago Democratic Party Convention. "Well, I feel very much like the man who said he didn't want to die particularly, but if he had to die that was precisely the disease he would like to die of!"[75]

November 24, 1864, was proclaimed by Lincoln as the first national day of Thanksgiving for "many a signal victory over the enemy who is of our house hold." He gave thanks for the health of the armies, increased population, and new resources of wealth opening up for our people. "Almighty God has filled the hearts and minds of our people with courage and resolution in the great hour of trial to the Republic. Thanks to the ruler of all the earth for his goodness and mercy on this day of our national peril."[76]

Politics

As advertised in its opening statement, politics would not be pursued in this paper but could not be ignored.

> When politicians get elected they often become oblivious of their antecedents, but seldom forget relatives.
> An army chaplain preaching to his soldiers exclaimed: "If God is with us, who can be against us?" "Jeff Davis and the devil!" promptly exclaimed one of the boys.
>
> To negotiate with the enemy, look in their eyes, the windows of the soul. They speak a language of their own. Beware a cold glazed look, or an evil eye, the lighthouse for an evil heart.

No presidential election was more consequential than November 1864. An officer with two crutches and one leg gave his appraisal. "Armistice, certainly I go for an armistice: but only after Richmond and Petersburg and Charleston have fallen, after Mobile and Wilmington collapse, after the last rebel has keeled up in the last rebel ditch. Oh, I love armistice, but I want them to come from the rebel side and not from ours."[77]

Some patterns of behavior seem unaffected by time. A correspondent spent an hour watching Congress and filed this report.

> All is apparent confusion and excitement in a perfect Babel. A dozen members clap their hands calling pages, one talking most earnestly and shaking his fists above his head as if ready to pound his ideas into their craniums if they didn't see it as he did. Others read papers with feet on top of desks while a Senate messenger reads from a paper that nobody pays attention to. On one side a member is delivering a harangue. They seem to know when a vote is to be taken and ready with yea or nay. One gets the conviction that for decorum, dignity and dispatch of business there are many village debating societies equal if not superior to the lower house of Congress. In the Senate it is quite different: dignity, courtesy, and deliberation characterize its proceedings.[78]

A gadfly in the House of Representatives was Congressman Fernando Wood: "We of New York sent fourteen regiments into Pennsylvania when she was invaded." A witty Republican from Pennsylvania replied, "Yes you did Fernando: the muskets that you sent to Georgia when the war broke out came back to Pennsylvania at Gettysburg. Fourteen regiments of your friends and more brought them."[79] He was Tammany Hall's Mayor of New York City at the outbreak of war, proposing that the city leave the Union to preserve its trade and profits with the South and "disrupt all bonds binding her to a venal corrupt master and consider an open alliance with the confederacy." He lost a bid for re-election in November 1864.

Divisions between parties were so deep that compromise became impossible. There is a modern ring to the policy that whatever you are for, we are against.

There is a class of politicians in this country whose highest ambition seems to be the defeat of any measure, however commendable, proposed by their opponents. They are willing to incur any risk in order that their end may be accomplished. The commutation system needs to end so you can no longer buy your way out of serving. A system is needed that brings men instead of money in support of government. Some politicians deem the success of party more important than the pacification of the country and are determined to defeat the measure and deplete our armies, bringing ruin and bankruptcy upon the nation. Copperheads who once opposed $300 commutation because it offered protection to the rich and oppressed the poor now oppose its repeal and substitution of men on the same ground. In their unpatriotic attempts to embarrass the government, they have forsaken every principle of political virtue and become the supple tools of their parent serpents; the devil and secession.[80]

What of the descendants of this conflict, the sons of the brave volunteers? "America's Agincourt will mark their father's nobility. The glorious coat of arms might show one sleeve hanging empty. My father fell at Gettysburg. My father went down in the Cumberland. My father was rocked into the long sleep below the waves in the iron cradle of the Monitor." Those who would have no part in glorifying our fathers were rebels. Other sons would steal away muttering with bitterness of soul, "God help me! *My* father was a *copperhead!*"[81]

The Democratic Convention in Chicago showed that many Union people were tired of the expense and suffering of war and supported concessions, compromise, and armistice—anything to end the conflict. Others viewed them as delusional, crying out for peace when there was none to be had without disunion. "In opposition to them I expected to be smeared from head to foot with copperhead's lines, to be called a seeker of notoriety, abortive negotiator and a meddlesome volunteer diplomatist. Smash their peace party into one million fragments so that our mission to Richmond is not a failure." A toast at a revered battle site by a Hoosier Dutchman gave his colorful perspective. "As for domestic traitors; may day hang by de edge of de moon wid dare fingers greased!"[82]

Some declined to make sacrifices. A Union man's neighbor was a "growler" about taxes. He opposed the war, considering it the work of politicians; brother against brother was a terrible mistake. His 1862 income tax bill in Philadelphia was $43.21.

"That's all right," I said.
"That's all right? I have been robbed of $43.21."
"You have been protected in property and person and granted the privilege of citizenship. Your income is a form of rent of property. To defend property from General Lee could cost what? Your store on South Wharves—what if it burned to the ground?
"I am more than ashamed of myself. My neighbor in Carlisle had rebels take six horses, six cows and oxen, two hundred bushels of grain, burned down his barn and lost thousands of dollars."
The government provides security at home and abroad, defense against enemy, and stops desolation of home. Some gave an arm and leg to the cause without word of complaint. Thousands have given sons and wives given husbands. Be righteous![83]

State agents were sent to gather in the soldier's vote. Department passes were required and civilian inspectors were sent to insure the election was fair and that no political speeches or harangues would be permitted in the large tents erected for voting.

Some states sanctioned absentee ballots and others did not. The state constitution needed to approve explicitly or take the impractical route of amendment, which required a prolonged legislative process. The Governors of Pennsylvania and New York petitioned Secretary of War Stanton to furlough home their soldiers from hospitals who were fit for travel. Augur General Hospital received orders to furlough convalescents from Maine, Massachusetts, New Hampshire, Pennsylvania, Ohio and Illinois.

"An enthusiastic political meeting was held in the chapel of Augur Hospital on Monday night last with addresses by Dr. Sutton [chief of medical staff] and others sustaining the Union candidates. The object of the meeting was to have a social political chat with the men about to go home on furlough." Sutton's goal was to have all necessary papers ready, giving each recipient 20 days' leave, but cautioned: "Much depends on the energy and loyalty of the governors and state agents and when any of these fail in kindness or duty to their soldiers they should receive censorship for their neglect."[84]

Polls opened in camp for Pennsylvania and Ohio troops who under their state laws were allowed to vote in the field. Hospital patients and members of the Veteran Reserve Corps voted at the same polls within a circuit of one mile. The results for Pennsylvania were: Union 365, Democrat 61. The results for Ohio were Union 96, Democrat 6.

The first issue of this paper declared in its prospectus who was the sworn enemy. Calamity was predicted for the South. A yellow fever epidemic broke out in New Berne, North Carolina, with 1,200 citizens dead. Rebel soldiers were eating tallow candles and others were digging up roots and plucking buds from trees for food. Rumors held that rebels made a chemical mixture called "sneezing compound," which they injected into hiding places on board blockade runners, in order to discover any individual who might be surreptitiously endeavoring to leave the South. Confederate prices became unaffordable with wheat $30 a bushel, corn $24 a bushel, flour $150 a barrel, and lard $5 per pound.

A voice of the Democrats, the *Chicago Tribune*, took issue with the oft repeated statement "the rebellion is on its last legs." How many legs have the rebellion? "There is a leg in Ohio called Vallandigham, one in Chicago called the *Times*, two in New York, the *Journal of Commerce* and *The World*, and one in Cincinnati, the *Enquirer*, besides two very lame legs at Richmond and Atlanta. The Northern legs are the most serviceable."[85] Elections have consequences and need to reckon with facts on the ground. Clement Vallandigham, or "Valiant Val," was an outspoken copperhead, ex-congressman and one-time newspaperman who opposed the "despotism" of "King Lincoln." He planned a race for Ohio governor in the fall of 1863 but was rejected and advised to seek employment in the Confederacy or Canada.

> The majority ruled. The country has passed through the most exciting and animated political contest known to its history. Four years of death and desolation drained the entire able-bodied male population while women and children in many cases widows and orphans were left to pass a cold and half-starved existence in homes formally luxuriant in every comfort. Slave bearing properties have been lost. Their lesson has been a bitter one and the bitterest part is to come. Their cup of iniquity is full. The election chose that the union should be maintained at any and every hazard and that slavery its criminal assailant shall die the death its treason merits.[86]

What was due their leaders? Jeff Davis, "his supreme highness," lauded by his own press as the most "cool and dignified statesman of his age," became an imbecile President and receiver of stolen goods. He tried to "rekindle the fires in southern hearts" and then lost Vicksburg and Gettysburg. The Southern armies were decimated by desertion, disease and wounds. "Despite his protests the people have their own deep-seated convictions wrought by four years of hunger, deprivation, and desolation of unsuccessful warfare in a bad cause. Our Armies are outnumbered, out fought and out officered leading them to huddle in their misery."

With the war's end, hard questions needed to be addressed. The dead would not be dishonored. Arlington National Cemetery already had 5,000 union and rebel soldiers interred. On each marker of the Confederate soldier was the painted word "rebel." This would be changed to "Confederate" or "C.S.A." "We cease fighting or condemning a man after his death." The time for reconciliation would soon be hand. This did not apply to the abolitionist John Brown, considered by some a martyred hero and by others a vicious terrorist.

> John Brown made war upon what he believed to be a wrong and not in support of a crime. He was not educated at the expense of Virginia. He had never sworn to support the Constitution and its laws. He never enjoyed high honors and emoluments at the hands of the Commonwealth upon which he made war. Where John Brown was innocent, Robert E. Lee is guilty. He was educated at the cost of the United States, enjoyed rank and other benefits its bestowal, bound by oath and his honor to stand by his government and failed both. Robert E. Lee shed rivers of blood. John Brown was merciful and kind toward prisoners who fell into his hands. Robert E. Lee allowed Belle Isle, Libby prison and Andersonville. Robert E. Lee lent his name to statements he must have known were false whereas John Brown refused to tell a lie to save his life.[87]

> What shall we do to them? Some say try and execute at once. Others say let them go into exile. They must answer at the bar for their crimes and if found guilty by a jury of their peers they must be sentenced to death. The President could pardon or commute any sentence.

> The question of restoration of the union requires time, patience and care. To do this it would be well to imitate the wise surgeon in his treatment of a fractured limb. Let the parts be *cleansed of all morbid surroundings;* let the general system be soothed and allayed and freed from febrile symptoms; but the diet be of peace and fraternity; place the broken portions in connection; direct all our skill in nursing and nature will soon accomplish the good work.[88]

Sacrifice

Whose son, whose father, whose brother did the fighting and the dying? The hero did not give up, because "our war for democracy is for inalienable rights, liberty and equality for all, and immutable universal justice."[89] For the Reverend Barton of Boston, the martyr surrendered all while paying a heavy mortgage covering all he was worth, including body and soul, as the price for freedom and justice. He waited not for conscription but volunteered and "with certainty and satisfaction achieves the purpose of his maker and attains the love of his community and mankind."[90]

The virtues of soldiers are eternal. In Cromwell's time, society feared they could not absorb all the veterans when the war ended but did so because men were better because of the experience. "The war has made the stripling ennobled, more worthy, and put a little manhood into them. The once idle now blasted their trumpet while covered with wounds and glory. Heroic manhood now stood erect absent frivolities. The war developed what was in us: humanity, generosity and courage."[91]

The volunteer was self-reliant, knowing precisely what to do and then doing it. They groomed the tent with evergreen boughs, policed the area, made their own dinner, and were ready to march at once. The first enlisters showed thrift and enterprise deserving the $100 bounty that late-comers to war received, but was denied the original volunteers. Despite being tired of war, old troops renewed and re-enlisted wholesale. After two years of field service, the army became home and trade.

> Veterans like sitting around camp fire discussing old battles and look forward to the shock of battle with haversack full of pork and crackers, canteen of good water, chewing tobacco, rifle and ammunition. Large bounties of federal state and municipal government are important no doubt. But they would not barter away their liberty and sell their lives for a few paltry dollars. Old soldiers can't be bought and sold like sheep. They are unwilling that others should step in and carry off the laurels won by their valor and endurance.[92]

The volunteer seldom got the honor or reward. The iron-hearted soldiers won victories and deserved private affection and public gratitude. He fought for his country and offered his blood and life as sacrifice for maintenance of the Union and the Constitution.

Battle

The blast-iron furnace of battle tests the mettle of its participants. No soldier is "eager for the fray" or "burning to be led against the foe" or "spoiling for a fight."[93] Entrance to a Pennsylvania sharpshooter regiment required hitting an object from half a mile. If you could see it, you should hit it. Opposing armies often chattered to each other and exchanged goods. The following dialogue was overheard during picket duty:

> "I say, can you fellows shoot," asked a Vermonter.
> "Well I reckon we can. Down in Mississippi we can knock a bumble-bee off a thistle blow at three hundred yards."
> "Oh, that aint nothing to the way we shoot up in old Vermont. I belonged to a military company with a hundred men and we practiced every week. The cap'n draws us up in single file, and sets a cider barrel rolling down the hill and each man takes his shot at the bung-hole as it turns up. It is afterwards examined and if there is a shot that didn't go into the bung-hole, the member who missed it is expelled. I belonged to the company ten years and there ain't been anybody expelled yet."[94]

Some described battle as a detached, predictable event where the good guys always won. The uninitiated attempted to imbed with and experience the dangers of being a soldier, but artillery shelling was serious business.

> There is a remarkable coolness and indifference displayed by soldiers under fire. We asked an officer if the loss of life had been great from rebel shells.
> "No we take them as a joke; there will be one along directly and you can see. What time is it? Just fifteen minutes since the last time. Here she comes, hello old fellow!"
> Splash! And the shell buried itself, exploding in the ground throwing dirt over the tent and some of the pieces falling within reach of us, a hole twenty feet from the door. They laughed heartily but why we could not tell; it was anything but amusing to us. We were about to bid them good day then when they kindly invited us to stay and see another.
> "It will not be long gentlemen. There will be another in fifteen minutes."
> We did not see it in that light and sped on our adventurous way. Had the ground been hard or rocky the shell would in all probability exploded on the surface then there would have been two enlighteners shot.[95]

The Battle of Chickamauga cost 16,170 lives for the Union and 18,454 for the Confederacy. The fighting took place over 16 hours and 30 minutes. That came to 2,200 casualties per hour.

Poems about battle told of drums beating and bayonets gleaming amidst a deafening roar and rattle. Who would survive the charge with a lion's courage, amidst slaughter rife? Who would become torn and mangled? The battlefield for both defeated and victorious was a "wail of orphanage and widowhood, a chill of woe and death broadcast across the land. See the charred earth, pools of clotted blood, and festering heaps of slain. Nature has never made such horrors! And when those fattening bones shall have long moldered into dust, she will spread out luxuriant harvest to hide them forever from sight."[96]

And what of the ocean of patriotism witnessed in the beginning after the bombing at Fort Sumter? Was there now enough to drown a mouse? There was little waving of handkerchiefs and flags, and few outbursts of welcome as veterans passing by was an everyday occurrence no longer awakening the enthusiasm of the early war years.

"Our veterans should know they are appreciated but can't fail to note despairingly the contradiction of the silent and barren reception they now receive with how they were formerly honored. Let us cheer the soldiers."[97]

Is patriotism merely a name? There is a reason for love of country. It belongs to humanity and cannot be severed. Its virtue warms the blood, strengthens our best purposes, and adds to our sense of personal dignity. Our country is our larger home in which fellow citizens are kinfolk. The oak is the constitution and the Union is the fountain of prosperity wetting our lips in hot weather and sustaining us. Beware of short sighted and mean selfishness that governs some of the more active political spirits.[98]

A mother teaches her child to love their enemies not destroy them as all wars are wrong. Be ever on the side of peace and good will to men and not the side of hatred and destruction. Her twenty-four year son old wishes to join the army imploring; "Shall we tamely submit to see this nation destroyed and its flag shot at, rent and trampled. Love of country is next to love of God. Our neighbors have gone off to war." She replies; "Do your duty. Be brave and God bless and keep you." She gives consent much to her amazement. "I give him to his country and pray that God will make him equal to his duty. To lose him would be fearful but to find him a weak coward in the day of battle would be far worse." Her son's regiment goes into battle and heroically saves the life of his Captain at mortal risk. With courage, endurance and self-sacrifice brave hearts will prevail.[99]

Four legged creatures, like the volunteer, had the character traits of being loyal, brave and faithful, hoping for the reward of gratitude from the two-legged master. Man's best friend was just that.

A Washington woman sold a slightly worn dog named "Sailor" to a family for twenty-five cents. The new owner carried supplies for sick soldiers and brought the dog as company. The dog liked military life and remained with the Rhode Island battery. At second battle of Bull Run, wounded and dead were removed under flag of truce. The field of battle was five miles long and three miles wide covered thick with living and dead. Six of the wounded lay under a tree for shade but the ambulance could take just four. One left behind had an open head wound and another soldier, John Barry a broken leg. He sent the loyal dog to Georgetown forty miles away with a note of desperation in its ears tied behind the neck: "I am wounded and on the battle field," and signed his name. Sailor ran to his old family, howling and acting strange to alert them of his note. After a day of dog pleading and anxiety the strings were cut and the note found. A return note indicating help was on its way was relayed by the dog. By this time John Barry had been taken from the field and his leg amputated. But Sailor found him anyway and delivered the letter. If all those standing on two feet, who have been engaged in putting down this rebellion were as brave and faithful as Sailor the rebellion would have ended long ago![100]

An ugly looking specimen of the genus canine was a great pet of both our own and rebel pickets. The dog had been trained to carry messages between pickets. A rebel paper would be placed in his mouth and he would scamper off to the union lines to deliver and return with a northern paper.

He was entrusted with packages of coffee and tobacco and always delivered them properly and safely.[101]

The black shadow of mortality gave shivers to the denizens of battlefields. The remedy for paralyzing fears was denial, desertion or confrontation. There were numerous literary attempts to explore this common and inescapable event. Truth and fancy, patriotic lore and propaganda were mixed to be sorted out by an experienced and anxious reader.

> His brother went off to war, thought too good, too true and too brave to die. At Bull Run he was on the list of missing. Months passed and a letter from his captain arrived: "I alone saw him fall and heard him say, 'God protect my sister and our country.'" His only brother slept on a distant battle field without a stone to mark his grave. His last breath was a prayer for his living brother. "Do not forget those who poured out their life blood upon this soil. We must mourn our dead, whose voices are hushed and will never come again."[102]

> One woman made three offerings for sacrifice. Her husband was a born leader. His insignia of authority had been God given and everywhere his fellow men recognized his right to command. "His glory was mine. I followed newspapers for casualty listings with names of killed, wounded and missing. My husband's name was on the first list. I was blinded, fainting and died with him. The General was laid to rest at the state capital with tall guards motionless like carved statues at his head and feet with the pageantry of a military funeral. Victor my only son fell assaulting Richmond."[103]

> A fifteen year old drummer boy of the 17th New Hampshire died at Fort Sumner Army Hospital. He was the first of his family to enlist. His father died with the 10th Maine at Lynchburg. A second son fought at Gettysburg with the same regiment and was missing. A third son was also wounded at Gettysburg with a severe head injury and discharged for disability. Because his mother was in financial need the drummer boy re-enlisted. "The country needed them and it was only right they should go," said the mother. His drum sits silently at home.[104]

> Lieutenant Dietrich of the 59th Massachusetts was a witness of true heroism at the battle at the Wilderness. A man was struck by solid shot cutting one of his legs nearly off and was bleeding to death. Private Broad volunteered to fetch him off the field despite being exposed to almost certain death. "I have neither wife nor child to suffer if I am killed." He put him on his shoulder and brought them to safety. He laid down his burden saying "I may have saved your life, but I have lost my own." He was shot through the brow and died soon after. He was as brave a man as ever lived.[105]

Disabled Veterans

There were 25,000 troops in the Invalid or Reserve Corps. Finding them employment was an important issue. "It should be the present and future policy of the government to employ its disabled veterans in or out of service to the exclusion of those who sacrificed nothing."[106] The Discharged Soldiers and Sailors Association was started in New York City, with offices in Boston, to procure work for discharged soldiers and sailors by bringing together employer and job seeker. Of 252 applicants mutilated in service by loss of leg or arm, only one-fifth found employment.

What to do for the newly discharged soldier besides a pension? Making fans and knick-knacks had its limits. Opportunity and training in other areas were needed. Government policy had been to grant land as bounty to discharged soldiers.

> Confiscating Confederate property appears not doable, but there are millions of acres of public lands in the great west. Emigration should be encouraged to settle the country and our treasury needs the revenue which the settlement of new wastelands would yield in taxes and productivity. Many youth who became volunteers had neither time nor opportunity to acquire trades or even gain an education. They have served three years and more. They gave up great opportunities to serve the country and deserve more than tedious apprenticeships.[107]

And what of the South, what should their role be? In 1865, a Pollyanna view of the future was shattered by the cruel reality of assassination. The defeated did not throw rose petals before the conquerors, engage in harmonious cooperation or accept the notion of freedom and justice for all.

> Southern people will think like free men after the war is over. Their new dignity and aspirations will demand schoolhouses. New prospects will make them forget the past. The downfall of slavery will open the road to prosperity for the poor laboring man. The great landed estates will go to pieces and fall into the hands of the poor laboring man. We shall soon see neat white cottages rather than mansions. Thousands of northern men will again invade not with musket and bayonet but with spade, plow, machinery, capital and knowledge. These invaders will be peaceful neighbors and all will be one people. The immense resources of the soil will spring to light under the magic touch of free labor. They will say "Blessed be you brethren of the North! We were sick and wretched and you have made as well! There will be peace and reconciliation, obedience to the great moral laws of the universe and progressive spirit of our age, harmonious cooperation, mutual benefit, and goodwill to all men."[108]

In June 1865, the capital of the United States held a grand parade across Pennsylvania Avenue from the Treasury building a mile east to the Capital. The procession was 30 miles long, 150,000 strong and took 12 hours. The uniforms were faded and weather-stained, and banners tattered. "The only national debt we can never pay is the debt we owe to our victorious Union soldiers. It was a vast host of moving heroes united into one undulating mass in marching cadence decorated with bayonet, gun barrels and sabers, a river of life and manhood." Windows were ablaze with banners. Garlands of flowers and especially roses adorned soldiers, horses, guns and cannon barrels. Silk banners glistened, some shriveled and shredded from the fighting. "The rank-and-file marched twenty deep with buoyant rhythmic tread and stride. These were veterans of desperate combats whose trials and work were done with victory fairly earned. And where were their comrades, missing ranks with empty boots?"[109]

The last issue recorded the closing of the hospital. Two hundred sixty-six men were transferred to Philadelphia. For the week, 120 had been admitted, 20 returned to duty, one deserted and three died. There would be no more occupants for the remaining 911 beds after June 11, 1865.

Four

The Cripple

The Department of Washington included five hospitals in or outside Alexandria, Virginia, overseen by chief of staff Surgeon E. Bentley. Claremont General Hospital was reserved for eruptive fevers such as smallpox that required quarantine and was located three miles southwest of Alexandria. L'Ouverture Hospital was located in Alexandria on the corner of Prince and Payne Streets and was reserved for black soldiers and American Indians, its name derived from the celebrated Haitian leader Toussaint L'Ouverture.[1]

The 3rd Division U.S. General Hospital was the largest of the three and the only one to create a newspaper, *The Cripple*. [See Appendix II.] The hospital had five branches spread out over five contiguous streets in Alexandria. As was standard elsewhere, the names of admitted, returned to duty, transferred, furloughed, discharged, deserted and deceased were dutifully listed in each paper's issue, and by February 1865, their state of origin and Congressional District.

Across Cameron Street was the bustling Third Division Hospital. Enclosed spaces were filled with rows of tents near a sutler's shop and a "large quaint looking collection of buildings all combining to form a hospital." A 38-year-old brewery converted to a seminary was now devoted for hospital use. Long rows of beds ran down each side with little stands between them.

Headquarters was a rectangular structure made of imitation brown stone with a hollowed-out square in its center built 100 years before. It was used as a storage facility, converted to a hotel with dumb waiter and finally a 500-bed hospital. All the wards had connecting walkways with cover per federal regulations. A large, multi-storied brick building had five rooms on the first floor. The second floor was used for office space. A long, one-story building ran north to south with a courtyard, and an archway connected a two-story, old-fashioned brick structure with lyceum and astronomy observatory in the rear from which a ten-piece band played nightly.[2] One-story barracks in open, "healthy" locations were converted to hospital wards because they were easy to keep clean and lighted and cheap in construction.

Circular number 7 declared that medical records were an important facet of treatment and that the Bed Card would be the foundation for every patient. They were filled out by the attending surgeon or for greater legibility by a clerk from the medical officer's dictation and were signed and forwarded to headquarters, providing documentation for furloughs listing date, diagnosis, treatment, duty status, and pertinent clinical information. Medical officers and guards would ensure that all soldiers wore hospital clothing and especially dressing gowns when on the wards. When outside the hospital, all inmates wore army uniforms. Officers required the usual salute from all men.

Inspection day at the hospital was for some worse than field duty. The "dust of ages" and cobwebs were decimated with direct frontal assaults, showing dirt and vermin no mercy. Weapons of choice were the scrub brush, mop and pail. Like Sherman's bummers—a commonly used phrase describing soldiers General Sherman sent out to obtain food and supplies from the southern landscape—they fought, scoured, polished and swore to make floors white, tins bright, faces clean, toilet heads empty, and any signs of vermin obliterated. Ward masters determined the intensity and duration of these hygienic assaults.

During winter months, fighting was minimal and as a consequence the mortality rate was low. Private Dory Longwood of the 7th Indiana Infantry wrote his parents in December 1864, about convalescing in Alexandria. "I am in the same place and getting along fine. My health is still improving and I have a better appetite than I have had for a long time and can get all I want to eat. It does not appear like there is more than three sick in this building and they are wounded men. There are five or six hospitals within sight of here. There is not a great many sick in any of them at present."[3]

The Cripple was published every Saturday at headquarters from October 8, 1864, through April 29, 1865. Subscriptions for one year, payable in advance, were $1. In its salutatory address, the appropriateness of the paper's name was discussed. The institution was designed for sick and wounded soldiers, many of whom were "disabled, deficient or otherwise flawed. We will try our utmost to conduct it so as to deserve a better name." The paper was to be politically impartial and "nothing of a political character inserted." Contents would be about friendship, information and literary matters in the form of poetry, sketches, brief communications and commentary. The paper would provide "a new source of energy to pull the hospital forward and fight error to the death, throttle prejudice, and inspire confidence in us. It is your papers as much as ours."[4]

The Cripple's small office was stocked with skilled printers, editors, and necessary materials for publication. It was sold throughout New England, including Cattaraugus County, New York. Although expounding Christian beliefs and tradition, the editor was Leopold Cohen, who in January 1865 married the daughter of Samuel Misch of New York City, officiated by Rabbi A. Adler.

A unique feature was the column *To Correspondents*. Critiques of submissions to the paper were published. Being rejected was painful enough, but in public was even more so even if anonymously.

"Dr. P. we are happy to welcome you among our correspondents."
"Dr. N., our thanks and please continue to contribute to our paper."
"Miss Sarah, your poetry received with thanks, will be published next number."
"Nom de plume is OK."
"Very pleased to hear from you: but do so in short pieces in small doses."
"We are happy to add the name of such an able writer to the list of our correspondents."
"K.K. you have hit the nail on the head and will succeed by writing often."
"Sketch received. We are very glad to hear from you at last, much obliged."
"Very beautiful will be in our next number."
"K.K. your submission *To some of the ladies of Alexandria* is declined though very good. It is too personal for our paper. Don't be discouraged."
"*The dying soldier* would be good for a nine year old girl. Practice makes perfect, try again."
"You have dropped off entirely from the original subject and converted it into a personal matter. Please send us your real name as evidence of good faith."
"Need to keep within the limits of decency and respect and it is too long."

The Cripple. Division III U.S. Army General Hospital. Alexandria, Virginia (courtesy Connecticut State Library).

"Respectfully decline-not interesting enough but don't be downhearted."

"C.K.H., your letter is too long for our paper."

"Had to make considerable alterations to render your poem suitable for our paper, next time favor us with prose."

"*The Rose* is rejected. Poetry is not your forte so try prose."

"We cannot accept your poetry as it is not original. We know your real name and have read the same under another author some time ago."

A primer on submissions was succinctly labeled *Hints to Correspondents,* although *Twelve Commandments* would be more accurate.

Write with good ink on paper with ruled lines, leave one page of each sheet blank, use ample margins, number pages in order, write in plain bold hand with less respect for beauty, use no observations that can't be printed, punctuate properly, underscore for italics, be sure of spelling of names, use no unintelligible words, place directions to printer at head of sheet, and never write a private letter to the editor on the printers copy but always on separate sheet.[5]

The printer's devil was the apprentice in the printing office, often the target of teasing in prose, not to be confused with the real Satan. "At a festival of lawyers and editors a lawyer gave a toast: 'The Editor always obeys the call of the devil.' The editor replied: 'Of the Editor and the Lawyer-the devil is satisfied with a copy of the former, but requires the original of the latter.'"[6]

Subscriptions were purchased by officers, hospital stewards, soldiers and citizens alike. "Our goal is to relieve the monotony of sick and wounded in hospitals and not to hurt anyone's feelings." The editor, who worked only part-time on this endeavor, thanked the surgeon in charge for his generosity and assistance. The first issue was commemorated with poems using first letters of sentences to plug the hospital's title.

> *Poetry for* The Cripple
> Acrostic, No. 1
> Tired, leans he gladly
>   On his crutch and cane;
> How he thinks and murmurs sadly
>   They will never come again;
> E'en the days I gamboled
>   By my mother's knee;
> Cheerily through the woods I rambled;
>   Gathered pebbles by the sea.
> Rushing to the battle,
>   When of strife I read,
> In the midst of smoke and rattle,
>   And the clash of blade to blade;
> Pierced by minie flying,
>   Prostrate faint was I;
> Pain o'er came me; I was dying,
>   But He willed I should not die,
> Life indeed, what's living
>   For support to beg;
> E'er to seek a pittance driven,
>   For they have cut off my leg!

Another unique feature was *Life in Alexandria*, which explored features of the confederate town founded in 1747: attractions and distractions, places to see and others to avoid. It was no longer a sleepy Southern town but a metropolis with trains, ships and an occupying army.

> The well-known though inglorious Alexandria still exists, its site unchanged by the onslaught of its enemies. This is a busy bustling place of ten thousand; full of migratory birds, hawks and vultures. There are scores of cheap clothing shops with gentlemen's furnishing, stores lining the thoroughfare with "right smart" prices. Tobacconists, stationers, newspaper venders, photographers, soda water and ice cream saloons, restaurants, theaters, sutlers and peddlers of all sorts of wares springing up like mushrooms. A black boy offers to shine shoes for a dime. There were hawkers for opera and theater, even a Shakespeare saloon. There were so many deserters from rebel army this city could be called a "deserter's home." Citizens in slave holding states seem to despise labor because "white fingers dislike soil. The ladies would not putt their heads in from the windows if it was raining. They would need to call a servant to do it.[7]

A throng of carriages seeking trade shouted, "Carry your trunk?" Newsboys announced great battles real or imagined to encourage sales. "Rebels are defeated!" The wide Potomac River was lined with endless wharves for shipping, abundant warehouses, and government buildings filling in the gaps. The streets abounded with confederate "damsels with brothers absent," fathers in the old capital and mothers playing "carry and fetch" with confederate agents "all loathe to swear or affirm allegiance to the United States and by hook and crook avoid the loyalty oath."

The nearby fish markets advertised with their distinctive smell. Unchanged were the post office, bank and fire department, blacksmith shop, and grain elevator. Railroad depots were crowded with carpenter shops, crisscrossing tracts, piles of ties, rails, pile drivers, and cars including sleepers sat everywhere. Old hulks were sticking out of the mud. There was a cavalry camp nearby in tents on barren treeless ground, "cheerless and uninviting." A shanty town was built around it, filled with "rows of contraband dwellings." Crime was rampant; an intoxicated soldier was murdered one evening for $25, and no charges were ever brought. The caution to outsiders was to stay out.

Pickets guarded the periphery and passes were required. The Loudon and Hampshire Railway ran northwesterly, and from its junction the newly erected dome of the Capital building in Washington was visible. A stone's throw away was Georgetown, with many more shanties, sheds, broken brick kilns, gas works with ruddy smoke stacks, and an entire block for the Quartermaster department.

The lighthouse at Jones Point was the most beautiful spot in the city. It was surrounded by an artillery battery with six brass pieces, a 25-ton gun throwing 400-pound shots. There were bucolic scenes of rolling brooks, trees, and farm houses, and a Catholic cemetery where "rest in peace" signs abounded for the many that came from Ireland. Just opposite and set apart was the cemetery for colored soldiers, simply an enclosed piece of ground with not a tree to shade it.

The City of the Dead was the cemetery for Protestants and soldiers. The Quartermaster department organized the beautified soldiers' cemetery, shaped as a parallelogram with longitudinal paths, chapel, bell tower and a view. "A very neat little corner is set aside for those of the Jewish persuasion and the Hebrew characters add a peculiar interest to the place. There are 40,000 Jews in the Federal army. Is it assumed they eat their pork rations?"[8]

Only the Armory Square Hospital in Washington offered discount embalming. For the edification of its readers, the delicate subject of care for the dead was outlined in a compact army regulation posted in April 1865.

> *Circular number 11.* When an officer or soldier dies in the hospital, quartermaster shall furnish hearse, coffin, and place of internment upon requisition of the surgeon in charge. Permanent records will be kept in books. An escort will be furnished by Garrison or Veterans Reserve Corps. Bed card will be attached to each coffin giving name of hospital, deceased name, rank, company, regiment and date of death. On the death of an officer inventory of his effects will be forwarded to the adjutant general. The nearest relative will be at once notified by date and cause. After two months, articles not called for by authorized persons can be sold at auction and proceeds sent to the adjutant general. Swords, watches and trinkets should be labeled.[9]

All the streets were unpaved (much like Washington) and in rainy seasons, seas of mud abounded. The garbage dump, "Smellifluous Hill" or "Odoriferous Hollow," was fed from the offal produce and sinking pool of the city "replete with putrefaction." Dead animals, sewage and detritus of all varieties ended there. Nearby was "another nuisance, the block long irregular sheds of the negro shanty which detracted from the beauty of city. People must live be they black or white."[10] With Sherman's sweep through the South, thousands of slaves became refugees, the north creating shanties to house them.

Blacks

The creation of a hospital just for Negroes and Indians invited comparisons of the two races: "peculiar crispy hair, jet features, broad projecting mouths, thick lips and shambling gait of the Africans," versus "the long straight locks, broad copper colored countenance and generally stooping posture" of the Indians. "Negroes from long continued habits idle away most of their time and particularly are steady eaters, always punctual at meal time. The Indians are busy continually making curious baskets and picture frames. This hospital would be excellent school for ethnologists."[11]

The notorious slave auction house or "Slave Pen" was nearby with a center portion and two wings. The office below was used as a prison for women and others. It became "synonymous with degradation and punishment." Prisoners were placed in an enclosure with the sky as the roof and bricks for the floor, and thus exposed to snow and rain. They were bound with ball and chain, absent fresh air. The number of deserters was large and accommodations small. Some were in confinement six months and more. "If not hardened before they arrive, they became so."

The relationships with slaves, contrabands and free black men were revealed in fictional stories, jokes, puns and actual accounts. Frederick Douglass gave a lecture on "Unity of the races," but only a small number of whites considered non-whites their equal.

The Freedmen of Vicksburg went to the Jeff Davis plantation on July 4 and had a grand jubilee celebration. An aged and reverent darky offered a prayer: "Massa Jesus, save Massa Jeff 'fore it too late. Oh Lord, Take him by de nap of de neck and shake him over the fiery furnace until he squeals like a pig in de fire. But don't let im drop, but fetch him to repentance, and save him soul in de eberlasting kingdom, 'fore dem Yankees make him dry bones in a box."[12]

A contraband from North Carolina marches up to officer of the day.
"What's your name?"
"My name's Sam."
"Sam, what?"
"No sir, not Sam Watt, I'se jist Sam."
"What's your other name?"
"I has got no other name suh, I'se Sam dats all."
"What's your master's name?"
"I'se got no master now. Massa dun runned away. I's free now."
"Well, what is your father and mother name?"
"I'se got none, nebber had none. I'se just Sam nobody else.
"Have you no brother or sister?"
"No, never had none. No brudder, no sister, no fadder, no mudder, no massa—nothing but Sam. When you sees Sam, you see all dere is of us."[13]

Tom, a man of pure African descent and not very hefty on work, was found crying in the kitchen by the lady of the house.
"Why Tom what is the matter?"
"Dey sez my brodder had been gone and mar'd a wite woman!"
"I should think you would be glad."
"Wy missus I feel jes as bad bout my brodder marr'in a wite gal as you'd feel ef you brodder 'don marr'd a *culled lady*."[14]

A sermon in the Church of the Slawtered Innocents it was said: Mankind is the most perverse and unreasonable ov the human family. Wile they may assent 2 a principle, they never will put into practix if it bares hard onto em as indivijules. Tu wit: leckturs on divinity of slavery are based in inferiority of wun 2 anuther, strong over weak. What if apply the same rule to white northern fok. Those who cud lift 600 pound owned the rest as slaves being superior to the inferior. You can tak my furniture, sell my children, make me your concubine. Is like being slammed with a chair. Northerners take unkindly to being inferior ones[15] [by Petroleum V. Nasby].

German

A number of immigrant groups were both volunteers and draftees in the Union army, and upon their shoulders much of the war's success would depend. Their speech patterns, cultural features and stereotypes were fodder for amusement. Large populations of Germans contributed from Pennsylvania, New York and western states. In *Mince Pies versus religious tracts*, a Union soldier taken prisoner outfoxed the slave owner over dinner.

> A rebel lady visits a Nashville hospital accompanied by her Negro servant carrying a basket with white linen cloth. She approached a German volunteer asking, "Are you a good Union man?" "I ish dat," was the laconic reply with hopeful glance at the basket. The lady replied, "That is all I wanted to know" and passed to the opposite side of the room where a rebel soldier was asked the same. He replied "Not by d—d sight." She uncovered the basket and laid out a bottle of wine, mince pie, pound cake and other delicacies devoured in the presence of the non-participating union soldiers.
>
> The next day another lady with covered basket asked our German friend if he was a Union man. "I ish by got; I no care what you got: I bese Union." She gave him her tray full of religious tracts but no edibles. "I no read English and beside dat rebel on dish oder side of dis house need tem more den me." Later on a third rich lady asked the same question. "By Got you no got me dis times; vot you got in basket." She demanded an unequivocal reply. "If you got tracts, I bese Union: but if you got mince pie mit pound cake unt vine, I be sech like de ribel."[16]

Irish

Large numbers of Irish immigrants also served as volunteers or draftees. Prejudices against them and Catholics in general were endemic. Stereotypical traits included slovenliness, loyalty to Rome and intemperance.

> There's a man in New York so opposed to Catholicism that he won't travel on crossroads. There is a man in our city that won't eat beef for fear that it might be a portion of the Pope's last Bull.
>
> *Sound of sunset.* A warship arrived firing their guns at sunset. An Irishman inquired of the sailors, "What was that noise." "Why that's sunset," was the contemptuous reply. "Sunset, holy Moses!" exclaimed Paddy, with distended eyes. "And does the sun always go down in this country with such a clap as that?"
>
> A friend said to an Irishman: "It's pretty slippery this morning." Be jabbers, it is; for I slid down three times this morning without getting up once!"
>
> *Liquor and bigamy.* How common is it for the poor wife to excuse the sins of her husband on the grounds that if it were not for drink, he would be the best husband ever? Such devotion aught make a man ashamed of his beastly habits and conduct. An Irishman was brought before the court charged with bigamy and was asked how many wives he had. A little woman by his side replied, "shure, and that's not the question yer honor should be askin him. He knows that he has only one and that's me, but when he gets a draft too much, he thinks he sees me in all the women. He's as true a man has ever lived, and he luves me better than all the world besides. It's his licker that gets the other wives for him."[17]

Temperance

"Rum and ruin the social evil is here, an ulcer upon the community spreading disease and death." In tracts and sermons, intemperance was the vice which "betrayed the hidden faults of a man, and showed them in odious colors and faults to which he is not naturally subject. Wine throws a man out of himself and infuses qualities into the mind making him a stranger in his sober moments."[18]

A short story outlined the downfall of fools and drunks who claimed, "*I couldn't help it.* I am a wretched man! I am a victim and martyr." As an infant his nurse kept dropping him in a spittoon or coal bin. A brick thrown at rats knocked out his front teeth. His fiancé lost her engagement ring, forcing him to buy another. He took out a loan for a gold ring but got brass. The bride, while cutting the wedding cake, cut *his* finger. A bawling infant soon arrived, catching her finger in a door jamb after rolling out of her cradle. His wife, startled by shrieks, accidentally poured boiling water on his legs. "I am sure I did not mean to bother you about my troubles, *I couldn't help it*."[19]

A gentleman asked a poor drunkard to give up the intoxicating cup, "where was it you took your *first steps* in this intemperate course?" "At *my father's table*," replied the unhappy young man. "Before I left home to become a clerk, I had learned to love the drink that has ruined me. The first drop I ever tasted was handed me by my now brokenhearted mother."[20]

A landlord discovered one of his customers drunk and sloshing about in the mire, tried to set him upon his feet, and asked if he was sick or what was the matter? "No, I ain't sick. No, I ain't drunk. But I'm mighty discouraged."[21]

Even celebrating the end of war was no excuse for drunkenness. "Exception must be taken for those using intoxicating liquors. There is nothing manly in a drunken man. He disrespects his country. It is a crime to get drunk and it is a disgrace to the man, his friends, family and a stain on his country's escutcheon."

Intemperance was linked to profanity. Circular number 5, issued by the Surgeon in Charge, declared that profanity opposed the spirit of army regulations and ordered it discontinued. Objection was raised about tobacco, either smoking or chewing, considering it an exceedingly disgusting habit. Carpets had become a large spittoon. Even in churches, one saw "pools of liquid filthiness. It injures the body, weakens intellect, adversely affects the nervous system and blunts moral perceptions." In New York City, more money was spent on tobacco than on bread. Sermons on tobacco were unequivocal. "It is a powerful, bitter, acrid and unpleasant smelling substance. It is poisonous and positively injurious to those who use it, more especially those who use it to excess. It impairs digestion, brings on nervous disorders and enfeebles the whole system resembling delirium tremens. In some cases it has brought on insanity."[22]

Sermons

The surgeon in charge oversaw the paper's operations. His wife had traits of the common soldier and was considered a religious person with "grace, fortitude, and an ability to withstand suffering with resignation." Her death was announced with black bunting framing the printed page.

Divine services were held every Sunday at each of the five hospitals, directed by five different chaplains. Audience rooms were well ventilated, a feature designed to promote health and wakefulness during presentations.

Sermons about profanity, philanthropy, the importance of home and the hereafter were intended to show the righteous and holy way. Goodness sanitized mind and body. The cheerful lived longest and were most likely to enter heaven. In the same newspaper issue, one column over, was a cautionary note: "it is a bad habit to carry your pins or your religion in your mouth." Humorist Josh Billings was forthright: "Sekts and creeds uv religions, ar like pocket cumpesses, gud enuff to pint out the direckshun, but the nearer the pole you git, the wuss tha work."[23] His real name was Henry Wheeler Shaw, a popular writer and lecturer born in Lanesboro, Massachusetts, in 1818. His father, grandfather and uncle were all Congressmen. He was allegedly expelled from Hamilton College for removing the clapper of the campus bell, and by 1858 was a journalist in Poughkeepsie, New York. He wrote in the slang of the period with wit and common sense, using phonetic spellings. Social and political satire was delivered in lectures, newspaper columns and books.

The search for happiness and salvation was a common topic for Sunday service.

> An eccentric wealthy gentleman put a sign upon his estate with the notice "I will give this field to any man who is contented."
> An applicant appeared. "Are you a contented Man?"
> "Yes sir, very."
> "Then what do you want with my field?"
> The applicant did not stop to reply.[24]

A church officer both penurious and stingy was married to a "crazy woman" who one Sunday morning exclaimed to a crowded church: "Do you see that man? You could blow his soul through a humming bird's quill into a mosquito's eye and the mosquito would not wink! They won't have to open the door of heaven but a precious little crack; if they let him in!" While she may have had the potential for the madhouse, her derangement did not dull the keenness of mind.[25]

Adam and Eve in the Garden of Eden illustrated how *man is the cause of his own misery and woe*, his sufferings, injustice and falls. Eating the fruit from the forbidden tree of knowledge put thorns on roses, gall with nectar, sorrow with joy, and despair with hope. Getting wisdom and becoming God-like was tricky business best left to professionals or would risk "wallowing in the mire and clay of wretchedness" with the serpent.

The Thanksgiving Day sermon offered prayer for the terrible results of slavery, praise for gains by armed forces in the field, and firmer establishment of free institutions and schools. Jefferson Davis should have a monument of "skulls heaped high and at the apex be his." Thanks were offered for the beneficence of the Boston public, who supplied all the hospitals in Alexandria with poultry and other edibles for Thanksgiving dinner.

The chaplain supported the war but was opposed to the death penalty. Doctors claimed long-term solitary confinement was a terrible punishment but could give no hard evidence. It cost $760 to execute a bounty jumper for desertion. If he had a God, it was Mammon; the true God he worshipped not. He shed no blood yet military

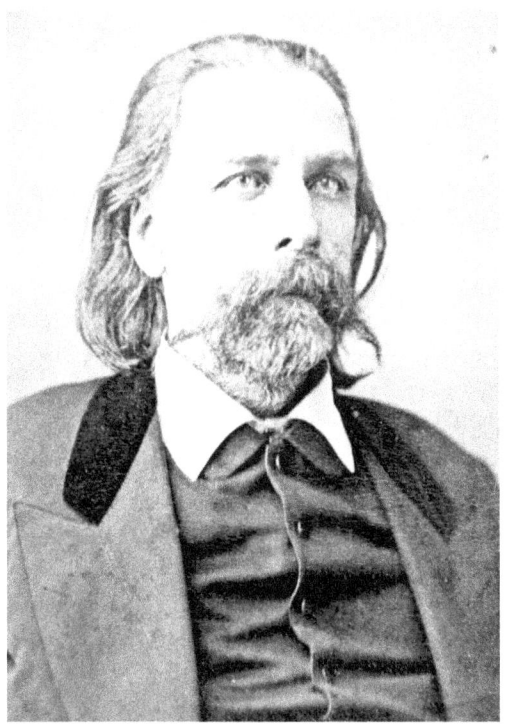

Josh Billings (Henry Wheeler Shaw). Political and social satirist (1818–1885) (personal collection).

law said he must die. What was gained by this death: a terrible punishment and deterrence? But did it deter? Military justice destroyed. "Execution of criminals only adds to them and creates a thirst for notoriety. If instead criminals labored, all would gain. In the end we should save and preserve. With love the sinner may be won from his sin. In wrath, remember mercy."[26]

A written reply to the "reformatory philosophers" quoted scripture that demanded the death penalty for various offences by stoning, impaling, consuming fire or sword, claiming deterrence by example. Society's goal was to uphold civil law and not the goals of the criminal.

> *"Why men do war* in the face of the Christian doctrines: peace on earth good will's towards men; thou shalt not kill, and love one another. War is man's hobby and ambition. He spends years of toil perfecting machinery that makes slaughter easy, no longer an outbreak of angry passion, but an exact science. If within the past thousand years we spent as much wealth and wisdom on fixing the social condition of our fellow man, instead of their physical destruction, we should now be in the enjoyment of the millennium. What of the alarming paradox that wholesale murder is not murder at all. A man cannot kill just one, but a nation can kill many. A man leaves his happy fireside, throws aside his wealth, load him-self with back-pack, toils daily on dreary marches, sleeps under the stars eating ill cooked food to gain opportunity to kill one another. War is often necessary, and some are even just and in the right. What God doth is right, though we may not be able at once to discern his purpose."[27]

Politics

A rebel deserter described their version of conscription. "They take every man who has not been dead more than two days." Charleston Harbor was bottled up, causing "great distress" with blockade runners making up its only viable business along with war matters. Bodies were being exhumed and stripped for their rags. The paper's general news section declared Lee's army worn out and saw signs of exhaustion everywhere. For the upcoming election, the *London Times* predicted a Lincoln majority of 500,000. Hotel board in Richmond was $50 a day and bacon $10 a pound.

By the fall of 1864, there was good news from the war front. "Our troops are in good condition, no sick or wounded are now sent north. Iron clads are on the move, reinforcements arriving for Grant, and Sheridan has the valley checked. Our resources are still great, our population is still large and growing and our patriotism is still in the ascendant."[28] General Sherman advanced and the rebels retreated. He seemed inscrutable and invincible.

> General Sherman at a battle at Kennesaw Mountain thought he saw a signal light and asked his artillery officer to make a hole through it. The captain turned to the corporal and said: "Corporal do you see that light?"
> "Yes sir."
> "Put a hole through it."
> "But captain, that's the moon."
> "Don't care; put a hole through it anyhow."[29]

On November 8, 1864, some states assembled large tents between Cameron and Queens Streets so its soldiers could vote. Ohio soldiers voted in each hospital in a booth made by the military agent of that state. The New York men sent their votes home.

A Pennsylvania volunteer described a one-hour train ride from Washington to

Philadelphia requiring tickets and furlough papers. There were no empty seats as newsboys hawked papers, crying out headlines. Passengers were all homebound voters—government clerks, Washington employees or political appointees. A crash involving a cattle car caused a derailment and hours of delay. A surgeon treated a fractured leg, a chaplain gave last rites, and drunken soldiers shouted much of the night, some drying greenbacks by a fire. They arrived in Philadelphia 23 hours after departure, "but we voted that day."[30]

Newspaper accounts of death or injury from railroad accidents was common. Company reports blamed drunks walking on tracks or falling off trains as the commonest cause. Derailments from defective rails or connectors, bad roadwork and plain human error were also at play. Collisions and running off the track were "unavoidable perils of the road. What can't be cured must be endured." One wag proposed that passengers carry certificates signed by doctors and other prominent people; "P.S. perfectly safe, D.T. dangerous in tunnel, and S.R. safe and respectable."

Large numbers of soldiers sent home to vote were slow in returning. An order from the War Department terminated furloughs of all men fit for duty, and on November 14 rendered liable to arrest all who overstayed that date. The reasons given for the order was "to secure the efficiency of the army."

The editor was surprised by the election results and disappointed that his man McClellan lost. For this editor, there were only two possible explanations for the results. The army's faith in their former commander had diminished, or the election vote was fraudulent. It was alleged that a woman in Carthage, Illinois, committed suicide because her husband voted Republican. "What a copperhead! We suppose she must have bit herself and died."

David Ross Locke was from Broome County, New York, a printer's apprentice from age twelve to 19. During the war he was a journalist in Toledo, Ohio, and he died in 1888. He was a Republican who used the pen name Petroleum V. Nasby, a cartoon-like Copperhead with a semi-literate vocabulary using the phonetic spelling popular at the time. Nasty Nasby portrayed a loud, opinionated pro–Confederate who deserted the cause while making no personal sacrifices. He was in turn lazy and intemperate, an embezzler, a bigoted opportunist who mostly wanted a political appointment to a lucrative postmaster position and little else. Lincoln was a fan of Nasby and boasted, "if he will communicate his talent to me, I will swap places!"

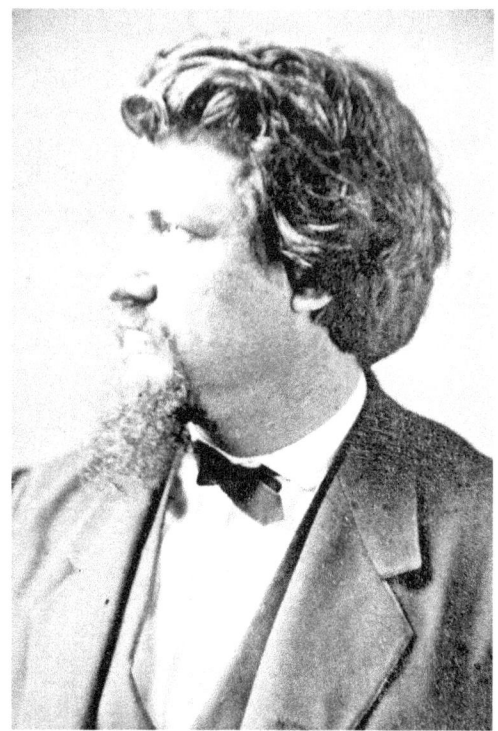

Petroleum V. Nasby (David Ross Locke). Political and social satirist (1833–1888) (personal collection).

The Last of Copperheads compared Sherman's taking of Atlanta with Moses who "lit up with pillars uv fire and smoke, only the fire an smoke wuz behind him. And the people uv the 'South lift up their voices and becoz ther niggers are gone is bitter in the mouth as a Dimokrat is Qwinine, but more bitterer is Fedral victrys. Plaid out is Davis and Dimocrisy has follered soot. For though John Brown's body lies all mouldy in the grave, his sole is amarchin on. I ain't the rose uv Sharon, nor the lily uv the valley but the last uv the Kopperheds! I bilt my polittikle howse on sand-it hez fell and I'm under the rooins. Uv pollytix I wash mi hands, I shake its dust orf mi remainin garmence.[31]

As Pastor of the Church of the New Dispensation, Nasby switched from copperhead to anti-slavery with blinding speed. "The harder the wurk yoo dew fer the devil the moar death yoo git fer wgis. We laboard fathefully in the servis of slavery. We dismist our conshenses, went back on our record, swoar black wuz white and vicy versy, even goin so fur ez 2 go 2 tew wars 2 perpetooate it. What iz the result? Linkin hez abolish it bi proclamation. The Konferisy wich was institootid 2 presarv it, is perosin to throw it overgoard ez the prise uv recognishen and without stopping 2 enguire wat iz tew bekum uv us northern dimokrats who have tied ourselves 2 it. So Jonah was hoisted in 2 the billin waves 2 save a set uv marinors who wuz not profits. Wood that I bi gobbled up bi sum friendly whale and in doo time vomit me out on dry land. Ez for me I'm anti-slavery man from this time out. Mi conshense won't allow me 2 support it no longer and besides it don't pay."[32]

A volunteer penned the name *Knott R. T. Miss Ward* as an imitator of Artemus Ward, making several contributions to *The Cripple* under *Sense and nonsense-Mi deer Crippull*. The real Ward was Charles Farrar Brown, who died in 1867 at age 33 of tuberculosis. He was born in Waterford, Maine, starting out as compositor and later contributor to newspapers. The "Artemus Ward" series began in *The Plain Dealer* in Cleveland, Ohio, and spread across America and England with lecture series and book collections of his wit and drollery of folksy spellings. Another Lincoln favorite, his *High-Handed Outrage at Utica*, was read to the Cabinet before he presented the Emancipation Proclamation. Work of his imitator follows.

The Congress fellers ar makin laus az fast az tha kin. It'll take a Fillydeify lawyer ter keep track en em caus tha go from 1 thing 2 anuther without enny distinction to party, but I guess twill cum out awl rite. Abe knose his biz. Generul Grant had a coppy ov the Alexandry Crippull in his poket which was red loud 2 the meetin with congress. Generul Hancocks goin 2 raze a knew army corpse entitled the Vetterin Army Corpse, composed ov awl the olde solgers who hev laust bleed and dyed for there Kountry.[33] [The writer was promoted to corporal and transferred to Grant's headquarters.]

Hope for an end to the nightmare war was the keynote in many sermons. "Four years after Lincoln's first election, thousands have fallen resting below the sod. Thousands are crippled crutching their way through life and widowed thousands bedew their cheeks with tears, while orphaned thousands bewail those who return not. Oh God how long, how long! Let us take hope as morning always breaks."[34]

New York's Broadway unashamedly flashed signs of wealth and prosperity with virtually no evidence of war. Merchants, boot blacks, walkers-by, opera houses and theaters were "rife with gaiety." Few soldiers were on furlough, and only an occasional amputee was seen, but being so common would hardly be noticed. Soldiers bearing crutches or slings do not bring cheering crowds with hugs or kisses. In Washington, salaries were up (except for soldiers), and army contractors were prospering. Alexandria was still under martial law, requiring passes for entrance or exit. Large numbers of new immigrants lessened the effects of war on the native populace as they had little to no family to mourn their passing.

Romance and Marriage

As a medication for boredom, pain and suffering, love and romance have few rivals.

"What is your consolation in life and in death?" asked a clergy catechizing a young woman. She had no answer. The clergyman insisted. "Since I must tell, it's a young printer named Peter, on Spruce Street."

> If you in lager find no bliss,
> And loathe cigars, no child to kiss,
> No wife to love, no gal to hug,
> Don't seek oblivion in the jug.
> And if you haven't any sister,
> Just ask some chap to lend you his,
> After spark for a little while—then "splice,"
> And all the rest will come to nice.
>
> The greatest fun, my paper friends,
> Cannot be found in beer.
> Cigars, nor babies of each sex,
> Nor wives, who prove so dear.
> But ah, the best, the *nonpareil*,
> The creamiest sort of sport,
> Are semi-weekly meetings with
> The girl you love to court!

Once the chase is initiated, how best to catch the golden ring: frontal assault, flank, siege or bombardment with flowers and candy? "The ladies greatly surpass the best artillery; they carry balls a great deal too far." Josh Billings added his colloquial patter on courting and marriage.

> Courtin' is a luxury. I'm in favor of long courtin'; it gives the parties a chance to go find out each uther's trump kards. It iz real good exercise and iz just as innersent as two merino lambs. Fist yu want to git yure system awl rite. Nest find out how old she iz. Begin moderate, increasing the dose as the patient seems to require it. Court the girl's mother a leetle. Don't swap photographs oftener than once in 10 days less yu forget how the gal looks. Look sorry and draw in occasionally so the girl will see what ails yu. Evening meetings are a good thing tew tend. Don't brag on uther gals. Don't court for muny, nor buty, nor relashuns. These things are just about as kerosene is to refining bizziness. Court a gal for fun, for the luv you have her, for vartue and kizziness there iz in her, court her for a wife and for a mother, for strength, court her in the kichen and parlur and over the wash tub. Let me know how it works out. Write me.[35]

> Az a ginral thing, wen a **woman** wares the britches, she has a gud rite to them. Woman's inflooence iz powerful-espeshlly when she wants anything.

> Woman will sumtimes confess her sins, but I never knu one 2 confess her faults.

> Yu ask me which is the most best, the married or the single condishun? Most every boddy, at sum time in their life, haz tried the single state. I hav tried both states and am reddy tew sware that if a man can git a woman who kan fri pankakes on both sides without burning them, and dont hanker tew be a wimmin's kommity, the married state iz a heaven and arth awl at onst. But after awl, the married state is a good deal like falling out ov a cherry tree, if a person don't happen tew git hurt it is a good reazon for not trying it agin.[36]

Other stories on romance poked fun, instructed, advised and entertained the sick, the wounded, and the soon to be discharged.

> "Git out, you natty puppy-let me alone or I'll tell your ma!" cried out Sally to her lover Jake.
> "I aint techin you, Sal," said Jake.
> "Well perhaps yer don't mean to nuther, do yer?"
> "No I don't."
> "'Cause you're too darn scary, you slab-sided, lantern jawed, pigeon toed, goggled kneed owl you aint got a bit of sense."
> "Now Sal I love you and you can't help it and if you don't let me stay and court you, my daddy will sue yours for that cow he sold him t'other day."

"Jake if you want to court me you'd better do it as a white man does, not set over their as if you thought ai was pizen."

"How on airth is that, Sal?"

"Why side right up here and hug and kiss me as if you really had some bone and sinyou of man. Do you spose that a woman's only made to look at you fool? They are made for practical results to hug and kiss and sich like."

"If I must, I must, for I do love Sal," laying his arm on her shoulders.

Sal said: "That's the way, that's acting like a white man orter."

"Oh Jerusalem pancakes!" said Jake. "If this aint better than any applesass ever marm made. Crackee! Buckwheat cakes, slapjacks and 'lasses aint nowhere long side of you Sal. Oh how I love you." Their lips came together and the report that followed was like pulling a horse's hoof out of the mire.[37]

A young gentleman was wooing his beloved and heard a loud shout. The entire plug of a barrel had escaped, and beer came pouring out. She plugged it with her fingers and screamed for help. "Why don't you put in the bung and stop your squalling?" Though relieved it was solved, the gentleman was so mortified of the ladies [sic] knowledge box being so bare he cancelled their engagement. He then met a good-natured shoemaker who had two holes in his door, one larger than the other. One was for a cat and the other a kitten. Our friend suggested just one hole would suffice, and the cobbler resolved "to cut the little hole out." He then came across a farmer trying to get his cow to eat off the moss.

The idea of gathering it and bringing it to the cow had not occurred to him. A sailor with a too long bit of rope proclaimed, "If it was too short I would splice it here but I don't know what to do." After contemplating all these short thinkers, he decided to restart the marital engagement, but another had won her hand. In despair he added suicide to the gains of evil, a Miss-fortune; a Sue-I-sighed resulted. Lesson: short-sighted people should wear spectacles as it "helps to see."[38]

The foibles and joys of marriage were prominent in hospital literature, providing an instruction manual for the inexperienced and hopeful.

"A horse team or other couples are well matched if one of them is willing to do all the work and the other is willing he should."

Why is it that beautiful ladies often take up indifferent husbands after many fine offers? A friend asked her to walk through a field with reed and flowers and pick the most handsome. She did pick one and was asked if that was the handsomest one she had seen? "Oh no, I saw many finer as I went along, but I kept on in hopes of finding much better until I had gotten nearly through and then was obliged to select the best that was left."[39]

An old maid, who was over-nice in regards to cleanliness, once scrubbed her sitting room floor until she fell through to the cellar.

Health Care Providers

Hospital stewards were mostly on-the-job trainees, some previously chemists though "some did not know quinine from chalk." *The Caduceus* was a small, semimonthly paper devoted to the interests of Hospital Stewards and hospital attendants, published by an executive central committee in Washington D.C. Its motto was "we propose to fight it out on this line." They submitted a petition asking stewards, surgeons and assistant surgeons to support their pay raise, claiming the Surgeon General supported the measure. A brevet second lieutenant of artillery received $112.83 a month and no exam was required. The veterinary surgeon and brigade band leader received $75 monthly, twice their current salary. The steward could not even make sergeant pay.

Members were directed to contact their respective congressmen and solicit support by sending $2.50 to help usher the bill through Congress. This was considered lobbying, which is legal, rather than bribery, which is customary. The editorial board of *The Cripple* was enthusiastic about the *Caduceus* but would not support the bill even though some of its members were stewards. "It is the finest and neatest appearance of any paper we have seen in a long time and deserves our hearty support. But sacrifices need be made and the paper does not recommend the raise, just the right to ask for it."[40] Awarding them lieutenant status would make them equal to assistant surgeons; they had asked for too much.

The standard for the medical profession in ethics and conduct was summarized by Dr. E. Neal for the benefit of *The Cripple's* readers. First was the *responsibility* of being a guarding angel of the tree of life, alleviating the pains of the dying and diminishing the sufferings. Guard both the entrance and exit of life as the great and last friend of frail humanity, while conducting government and private business with beneficence and integrity. Second *practice as science and art:* the public was not qualified to judge medical ability. The ignorant and susceptible public could make false assumption of knowledge which does not exist. Remain a student from cradle to grave to absorb new science. Lastly, *Duty and moral obligation* meant to work in scenes of great suffering, watch terrible and incurable disease, treat both mental and physical disorders, remove suspicion, be confidant, prudent, kind and circumspect, stifle emotions, and offer consolations on religious nature on occasion.[41]

Understanding the human condition and how to improve it sometimes came with experience. The study of patient outcomes was elusive and humbling.

A physician walking down the street said to his partner. "Let us avoid that pretty little woman you see there on the left. She recognizes me and casts upon me the look of indignation. I attended her husband."

"I understand you had the misfortune to dispatch him."

"On the contrary," replied the doctor. "I saved him so that she did not get a chance to get another."

Bolus, the doctor who was very angry when any joke was passed on his profession, once said, "I defy any person whom I ever attended to accuse me of ignorance or neglect." "That you may do safely, doctor," replied a wag. "Dead men tell no tales."[42]

"How many deaths?" asked the hospital physician going on rounds.

"Nine."

"Why, I ordered medicine for ten."

"Yes, but one wouldn't take it."

A Union soldier prisoner was asked what he had done.

"I took something."

"What do you mean?"

"One morning I did not feel well and went to see the surgeon. He was busy writing and said, 'you look bad, better take something.' He then went on with his writing and left me standing behind him. I looked around and saw nothing I could take except his watch, so I took that. That's what I am in here for."

A peasant sold the village Aesculapius a sack of wheat and called for payment.

"I have no money," replied the man of Physic.

"Well then give me back my sack of wheat."

"Impossible it is eaten up."

"Then give me a chair, table or something."

"I have none, I'm flat broke."

"Then put some leeches on me anyhow."
The doctor did as was requested and the peasant departed satisfied.

Dear Doktor Hirsute, Hair Purswader in Salvashun Bitters.
Yur hair greese placed on an old brush grew hair in fifteen minutes, tis really wonderful. I rubbed a drop or two on the head of the cane which has been bald for five years and now I have to shave the cane daily. I put some on the cat's tail, and now she looks like a fox. Some men are born great, and some become great and some have greatness bestowed upon them. Dr. UR all three of these men in one. Your vegetable trinity of sassafras, poke root and elderberry is a great vegetable tonic. Although whiskey ain't one of the vegetables, it is of the tonics. People love their tonics. The more vegetables you get the greater amount of whiskey. The Christian world loves vegetable bitters. Let the cod liver, the patent trust men, the pill men and the plaster men rave and rant. You have what the world wants. That is an herb bitter with a whiskey basis.[43]

A distinguished New York surgeon whose love of the art was such that he would at any time sooner amputate a leg than eat his diner, performed such operation and was expatiating with great delight on the subject to some friends at Bellevue.
"Then the patient is recovering?" said one of them.
"Bless the man!" replied the doctor. "Why no patient can survive an operation like that. No, he is dead, but the operation itself was a beautiful success!"[44]

Empty sleeves and pant legs created an industry to deal with its consequences. "The limbless soldiers of this hospital sent a petition requesting the $75 government grant be given directly to them for direct purchase near their homes enabling quicker and easier adjustments if necessary." The paper agreed with this proposal only if the money was not spent for other things. Most of the upper extremity prostheses and some of the lower were never used because of discomfort, especially in hot summers, and absence of functionality. Humor, often self-deprecating, could be as effective as peer pressure.

If some men had their limbs broken they would be cripples for life; their bones would be too lazy to knit.

A little girl, busy making a pair of worsted slippers for her father said to a young companion near her. "You are very lucky; your papa has got only one leg."

"No pain will be spared," said the quack when sawing off a poor fellow's leg to cure him of the rheumatism.

A reaction to the heroic treatments of the nineteenth century and its bleeding and purging, and running the bowel were less intrusive therapeutic modalities such as hydropathy, magnetism, and naturopathy. Homeopathy used minuscule doses of chemicals to treat all conditions. Symptoms were the disease, and its cause of no relevance. According to *The Cripple*, homeopathic theory was "If a patient has a broken head, hit him again with a brick bat." Quacks abounded as the public seemed enamored with cure-all pills, potions and electro-magnetic machines.[45]

Dr. A says he daily cures numbers who have been to all the so called doctors in the city and receive no benefit, and his terms are more moderate than theirs. Ye lame, ye halt, ye blind why tarry ye? Here is the all healing physician. But Dr. B offer to cure you at once, even if declared incurable by other physicians. He's the only one in the city offering speedy relief. He does not use Mercury or any other dangerous medicine. If you are at a distance, he will treat you by mail.

If one doctor fails the other is sure. They were made for each other. They cannot however be everywhere. Then nobody would die, except those taken suddenly ill. All the rest would recover by seeing the doctor or by mail. What is the use of all our hospitals when such blessings are within calling distance and cures in one to three days? Let's not forget one modest practitioner who says that his success "has been considerable." I believe that man.

Woe unto your tonic bitters, Indian vegetable pills, cough syrup, bronchial troches and your kin; for

Drs. A and B are omnipotent. They cure without you. Patent medications are no longer the benefactress of mankind. Your medicines take too long to cure. Dr. B cures you in 48 hours.

Advertisements

A standard practice to move merchandise was to shade the truth. "Fool me once and tell a lie disgustingly leaves more in the bill than in the play. Who benefits is apparent to all." Let the buyer beware, advised a critic!

> Advertisers are seldom modest praising their wares. Booksellers can sell everything and at the lowest prices anywhere; get any book for the lowest price. Dry goods are the same. Get perfect satisfaction at the lowest rates. A clothier offers endless variety of the finest goods and at the lowest prices. Others have the largest stock offering a more than fair deal. Sewing machines have magic skills, even self-adjust with prices hard to believe. Visit the finest billiard saloon in the country, the best restaurant in the city, drink the best liquors. The same establishments making the same claims means at least one is lying.[46]

Disabled

Members of the Veterans Reserve Corps staffed hospitals as guards, attendants, nurses, cooks or clerks and could not be relieved or transferred except by order of the Secretary of War.

In New York City, a bureau of employment for disabled and discharged soldiers and sailors was organized. The goal was "to lessen pauperism and crime, save productive labor for country, aid those who served honorably, and prevent need for costly charitable institutions as exist in Europe."[47] Many employers thought the disabled totally incapable of work. Some who qualified for the Reserve Corps chose employment in the civilian sector because salaries were much higher. Knot R. T. Miss Ward explained the advantages further: "I've jined the Vetterin Preserve Corpse. I took precowshun to jine this, cause u kno that wee air preserved 'during this orfull crewell war.' The Yuneunn and the Constitushunn hev both got to be preserved, and is why I peal 2 u gentle reeder. Why shoodn't thay preserve us, their noble offenders—*that' what I want 2 kno*."[48]

Volunteers and Sacrifice

For the average fighting soldier, it was a tough slog with no relief in sight. Advance then retreat, hurry up then wait. "Hurry up boys, quick march for the fun ahead. Tired, hungry and sick men were gallantly lead against an enemy who fired a parting salute and quickly skedaddled," according to correspondent Captain Gregg. The war was hard tack for soldiers and hard taxes for citizens.

Sad reflections described "heavy and sorrowful hearts; faces grown pale in death's cold embrace, parents at premature graves, the victims of an unholy and fratricidal war, a bloody sword of treason and brother against brother." In January 1865, transferred troops described their camp as "not a desirable place for leaky boots as the grounds were soaked from heavy rains and melted snow."[49] It was cold inside and out, so they huddled around a fire drinking hot coffee. On picket duty the cold pinched their toes despite thick-soled boots. They washed in a cold stream, soap and towel in hand. Breakfast was hot coffee, hard tack and cold pork which was barely palatable. Periodic formations were interrupted by a solitary sniper shot. Guns were slung across shoulders, knapsacks over the back, and tired feet trod to the last places of the day.

The editorial board was certain. "Each and all should strive to bring this accursed rebellion to a speedy termination because the cause is noble, sacred and just. The man who loves not his country is worthless and unchristian. An able man who will not fight and defend it is a coward."[50] *Our soldiers* left home, surrounded by loved ones, hearts filled with sorrow, children clinging to him as "his bosom heaves with emotion, scalding tears come unbidden and with a choked utterance he says good-bye," then receives a father's blessing, a mother's prayer, and a God bless you from his wife. Dreams and memories can be shattered by stern reality.

Satiric anti-war sentiment opposed flag waving and sermonizing. Be sensible, claim exemption and dodge the draft.

> I am willing to serve but am compelled to forego the pleasure and honor of wearing the "blue." I have no father, brother or sister. I am the only son of my aunt. I am her defense against stale bread, cold ham, or extra pies. I am her right hand man and only support at the breakfast table. If I left she would have no one to love, none to caress and no one to be her banker. I have been too tenderly raised to make a soldier. The fear and ire of a soldier would not agree with me. I snore. When I see any fighting I always recollect it. I fear that in the excitement of battle I would go rearwards and demoralize my comrades. How would my aunt replace me? It is necessary to have some of our best men at home to gallant the ladies while their husbands and brothers are far away. Some influential swear men must remain at home to plan campaigns and battles and tell those in the field how to gain glory, win victories and conquer the rebels. If you hear of any officers needed where there will be no danger, plenty of glory and big pay, telegraph me at once.[51]

The relationship of an officer to his men and their duties was subject to serious discussion. One measure of the character of each regiment was the degree of interest and involvement of the officers in the well-being of their men. "The ordinary soldier may search for amusement leading him to ruin but officers must do their duty. They must study their characters, interest him in their pursuits, enhance confidence in their counsel, praise every good effort, sympathize with them, offer consolation in affliction, and be their friend on earth never deserting them."[52]

There were three key attributes of the true soldier. *True courage* required seasoning with wholesome fear: recognize danger and overcome it. The first duty of a soldier was *willing obedience* without hesitation or grumbling. Having the *patience to endure* tested the soldier's response to hardship. He received wounds, marched long distances, and had no idea where he was going, the distance to be traveled, or the objective to be conquered. He knew nothing of what he was going to do and nearly always was ignorant of what he had done. "All men are soldiers after a sort, fighting the great battle of Life."[53]

Camp Stories were vignettes of the soldiers' life. They "slept under the soothing crack of a picket's rifle and the harmonious hum of a thousand blood thirsty mosquitoes."[54] Soldiers sat round a camp fire, discussing chaotic battles and the endurance and requisite skills demanded for survival.

> We marched through swamps in Virginia with many falling asleep and were kept from falling by our comrades on each side. Some marched until their strength failed, then fell dying by the road side. Wounded men begged others to help them on but no help could be given.
>
> Rain, wet clothes and shoes full of holes made our feet resemble moving shovels full of mud. With empty haversacks, hungry and tired, we marched along-watching for sutler's wagon or commissary

team. We spotted supply trains and got coffee and hard tack and then built breast works and did some skirmishing. Rebels advanced raining down shell, grape, canister and shot. Our gunboats opened and sent two hundred pound "mess pots" chasing them back. They rallied but were slaughtered like sheep. Wagons were ordered to keep in the road with artillery and infantry on one side, cavalry on flanks, front and rear. Instead artillery and wagons cut roads for themselves or crossed lines. Infantry marched everywhere as ranks, arms and colors were in a motley mass and chaos was never better represented. Generals ignorant of their commands, colonels without regiments, captains without companies, men carrying muskets upside down and down side up, sick and well, wounded and whole all traveled along in one grand mixed up mass, all bearing towards one common destination. Some asserted it had no end, others were sure it was the wrong road, and some were tired and pitched tents. The majority kept on, emerging out of the woods into an open field where officers cried out their units name to reorganize. It was like a railroad depot with station attendants shouting the next stops."[55]

At Harrisons landing, a barn was taken apart for its boards to act as beds and grass as mattress. Following rain, the mud was ankle deep, making even the horses useless. Several short limbed fellows got both feet stuck and were unable to pull out, falling hopelessly on their faces needing rescue by their longer limbed comrades. During and after pay day a number of soldiers with more money in their pockets than brains in their heads used rubberized blankets to establish a gambling den. The Provost with fifty swords broke it up, giving them two days of work in the trenches with pick and shovel. Sutlers arrived after pay day with cans labeled "spiced oysters" that contained no oysters but villainous whiskey at $2.50 per can.[56]

At Yorktown, the rebels buried torpedoes in every direction. We had to step carefully around it as if traversing a swamp. Roads were filled with water through which we plunged ankle-deep. There were no fences, barns or branches, nothing but water soaked ground. I found two old barrel staves, serving as a bed for the night. If anyone thinks it is pleasant to sleep all night in wet clothes on two barrel shingles in a wet field by the side of a cold river, it is anything but. The sun came up the next day so we dried ourselves and clothes out. We found oysters in the river and soon had a bagful sitting without a stitch of clothes on. We made a fire, cooked and ate them as our clothes dried.

One poor fellow with his arm torn to shreds by a shell begged for water so hard that I gave him a drink and in a shorter time than I can tell you my canteen was empty. Here I saw a sight I never wish to witness again. Coming furiously up from the rear was one of our batteries running over the wounded and dead killing some and mangling others and commenced firing. Some of the wounded lay under the very mouths of the guns and it was agonizing to see the poor fellow's helpless and dying hold up their hands for help when none could be given them. The Captain of the battery sat on his horse coolly smoking a cigar and ordered firing at a little white church in the distance. A Dutch man observed the rebels had been firing horse shoes, bits of iron and other such things. Suddenly came rushing through the air a sledge hammer which killed a man and then struck the ground beyond. It was dug out and the Dutchy observed, "Mein Gott, der black schmit shop come next."[57]

Those who survived life-threatening experiences often reported a kaleidoscope of memories flooding their consciousness, ranging from events of childhood to parenthood. Life on the battlefield was unforgiving, unpredictable and relentless.

Three Soldiers
Three soldiers sat in their tent one eve,
    Sat in their tent as the sun went down;
Each thought of who loved him best,
    And the many kind woman friends in his own native town;
For men must fight, and women must weep;
    Though the bullets are thickly flying.
Three wives sat in the cottage door,
    And prayed to God as the sun went down;
Prayed that the loved one gone to war,
    Might again return to their native town,

For men must fight and women must weep
    There's a country to save, a union to keep;
Though the bullets are thickly flying.

Three corpses lay on the battle field,
    On the battle field as the sun went down,
And frantic those women are wringing their hands,
    For those who will never return to the town
For men must fight and women must weep.

Wounded

Am I awake! Or is it but a dream?
Why am I here upon the hard damp ground?
Why do I so weak and nerveless seem?
Why is all so dark and still around?

Ah! I remember now—the rebel traitors came,
And with stout heart we fought them long and well.
But in the midst of battle, smoke and flame
A whizzing bullet struck me and I fell.

Would you were with me mother, sister, now
That I might see your dark, loved forms again,
That your soft hand might cool my fevered brow;
And your kind voices sooth away my pain.

The very weak! This pain o'er tasks my strength
I'm fainting!—oh we fought them long and well,
And victory shall be ours at length—at length—
I'm going—mother—comrades—all, farewell!

The Dying Soldier
By L. H. S., Hartford, Connecticut

Upon a southern field
A dying soldier lay.
The breeze around him played,
In the pleasant month of May
He lay sadly thinking there,
Of his dear young wife at home
And his little children fair.

Of his mother, when she blessed him,
When he left her at the gate,
Oh! How sadly she would miss him,
And how vainly watch and wait.
He raised his eyes to Heaven,
The sunshine brightly smiled
And gilded all around him,
Like some sportive little child.

And the God who dwells in Heaven,
Upon his great white throne,
Saw the soldier as he lay there,
Dying all alone,
And he sent his angels down
From their starry home on high,
And they came and stood beside him,
Come to see the soldier die.

Nostalgia

One treatment for nostalgia or homesickness was a letter from home. Soldiers were warned about money from home being stolen. "A large number of packages arrived at the Washington Post office with the wrappers destroyed; or the address so mutilated that they cannot be forwarded. It is officially suggested that persons sending packages write on a card the full address, and fasten it securely to the contents of the package inside the wrapper and this will secure prompt delivery."[58] A soldier from New Hampshire who lost an arm and leg sent letters and funds to his aged mother, living in the poor house, who never received them. A villain absconded with both letters and funds, discovered after the fact by the superintendent of the poor house, who hoped the thief would soon be brought to justice.

Some hospitals had photographers on campus. Sending pictures to loved ones back home boosted morale as in this letter to the editor. A head holder was routinely used to prevent motion but produced sharp images of stiff, unsmiling subjects.

> *Blues versus pictures.* Did you ever have the blues, Mr. Editor? I found the best cure is picture gazing, better than lovemaking or even filly hunting and a great deal surer. Not paintings or sketches. People dress up in style and sit before the camera. They put on their good clothes, brush their hair and put their hands in the most awkward and unnatural possible position. He is bolt upright as if an iron rod ran through his head to keep itself poised. The result is a stiff unnatural picture as unlike the original, as the old woman's children who all look alike but are not. The carte de visit should be labeled cart physic.[59]

Pet stories concerning faithful and courageous canines were especially popular. The 11th Ohio Volunteer Infantry received a spaniel dog from a young woman. He was wounded on three occasions and went missing for weeks, returning emaciated, but recovered with all fours. He was shot in the right shoulder but survived with a noticeable limp. "He is still suffering from his last wound yet wears a cheerful look. Around his neck is a clasped steel collar placed three years ago: I am company A's dog; whose dog are you!"[60]

Prisoners of War

In October 1864, there were 2,000 military prisoners in Alexandria, and in Andersonville 11,000 had died. There was no protection from rain, sun or cold, and the little food was bad or poorly prepared. The odyssey and sufferings of individual volunteers provoked national clamor for recourse.

> I was home at last after three years at Andersonville and Libby prison. It was time for exchange. John was taken with the rest, barely able to move but returning home to his daughters who were wild with joy. "He's coming, father's coming!" The wagon arrived, but the father does not kiss or hug or recognize them. He sits upright, unmoving, unsmiling, skin ashen, eyes fixed ahead not seeing. He doesn't speak except to mutter "Bread! Bread! Oh, give me some bread." He is but a crazed skeleton.[61]

Sacrifice

The consequences of war on the average soldier were discussed by special correspondent "Knot R. T. Miss Ward."

Az for noose I am holy destitoote, havin only the passin events of the fewtcher. If the Pungkintown fowkes had ownly let mee gone on 2 Washington in '61 this ere war wood knot hev cum; butt they C thar folly now and begin 2 repaint. Over 10,000 of our fellers CTcents have bean kild since then, yew no we awl have fort, bled an dyed for hour Kountree! It is beeond the power of yre imar-generation how bad it is 2 C sum of hour poor fellers kummin out, sum without Annie Lakes, Arms or heads.[62]

The national consensus on the war's outcome was divided. The "croakers" predicted collapse of financial markets followed by general bankruptcy. Others believed that if a storm occurred, it would be short-lived and a unified nation would move forward.

Prayers were answered: Richmond fell and the war was over. "Religious people believe in redemption and being magnanimous. The people of the south, our poor unfortunate brothers, have been deluded. Extend the hand of charity and forgive their sinning that was forced upon them. Their leaders are alone to blame and justice will be served in its most terrible form."[63]

Alexandria was full of life with the Union men doing the most rejoicing. Peace bells rang across an exhausted, blood-soaked landscape amidst song, cheers, embraces and tears. The blue sky was background for the red, white and blue flag as cannon boomed with glee for a spontaneous mass meeting. A procession with cavalry, infantry, light artillery, the Veterans Reserve Corps, the medical staffs and workmen in general marched to the patriotic strains of several bands. Fire companies followed, bearing flaming torches and fireworks. A mob of marchers with the usual lot of drunken men cheered along the whole route. It was a merry and noisy procession including ambulances and wagons. Many but not all windows were decorated with lights and wreaths; the disloyal families realized this was the beginning of the end. The celebration lasted 48 hours.

Lincoln

None rejoiced more than the gaunt leader, aged far beyond his years. "Why is Abraham Lincoln like a bad Christian? He takes his Todd to church."[64]

An elderly gentleman who knew Lincoln in Illinois visited Washington to get a job but failed, despite having credentials. He called upon the President, who gave him this prescription. "Take three pounds of petticoats, four smiles, two tear drops, with gammon at discretion; stir briskly, apply while warm to the blind side of a secretary, and you have a never failing prescription for getting office."[65] Who dared say that Mr. Lincoln was not shrewd?

Black formless clouds moved in, a nation stricken with impenetrable gloom. The blessing of peace and the end of hostilities ended with a cursed assassination. Blackened borders were the new uniform of hospital newspapers. The deep emotions of anger and despair flew off *The Cripple's* pages. "It is with mingled feelings of horror, sorrow and indignation that we record the assassination and death of our much loved president. It is as if the firstborn in all the land were slain. Our mourning is like that of David for Absalom: "Would to God I had died instead of thee." The loss was irreparable and inconsolable. "Traitors, men of treason struck him down and so doing have slain their best friend. Who can tell what an enraged and incensed nation now will do?" Cries for mercy were replaced with shouts for justice and vengeance. "Banish every man and woman who refuses to swear allegiance. Punish all who commit treasonable acts. Death to traitors! Let suffering never cease for those who destroy our noble men and seek to destroy our noble country."[66]

Brave men wept manly tears for their friend who was no more. Lincoln sprang from the common people, the laboring class. A self-made man, plain, honest, sincere and kind, he sought the greatest good for the greatest number. His sole purpose was the good of the nation, to do right, ready to consider the cause of poor and humble as well as rich and exalted. "He firmly pursued the course his clear and accurate judgment had pointed out best, regardless of the frowns or applause of enemies or friends. We can now see the wisdom of his councils, the justice of his measures, the clearness of his judgment, the expediency of his policy, and the firmness of his purpose in pursuing the right. He felt the need to ask for divine aid and guidance asking his friends in Springfield to 'Pray for me.'"[67]

Valedictory Closing

In February 1865, the Department of War consolidated the hospital network in Alexandria to cut expenses and send troops home. The soldiers' rest facilities became the Rendezvous of Distribution. Barracks were altered to accommodate fewer patients. There would be better accommodations, more easily administrated and without paying rent for the sick and wounded soldiers. One by one, each of the five hospitals closed.

A steady stream of soldiers wearing blue arrived at rest stops heading north, and those wearing grey heading south. Business and profits in the city would decline absent the free-spending soldiers. "But that's scarcely a consideration of ours. There will be fewer scarred faces and armless sleeves and the like seen in the streets. The familiar

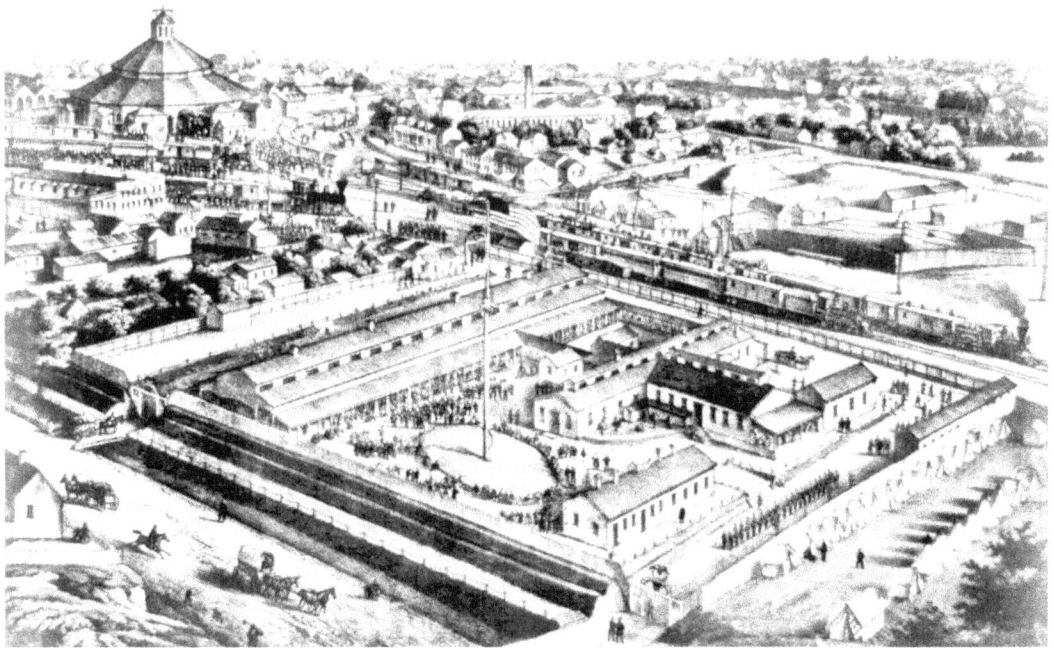

Soldier's Rest, Alexandria, Virginia. Crowded Union camp near railroad station with Sanitary Commission Lodge for Invalid Soldiers. Used as hospital from May 28 to October 4, 1864 (Library of Congress).

clunking of crutches up and down the thoroughfares will almost cease and Alexandria will be nearly freed from its great hospitality."[68]

A hospital circular was issued in the spring of 1865 that "no burials will hereafter take place on the Sabbath." There was no more need. The shooting had stopped and the volunteers went home.

Five

The Crutch

The Middle Department contained 11 hospitals with a bed capacity of 6,189. The largest was Division No. 1 U.S.A. General Hospital of Annapolis with 1,562 beds. Surgeon B. A. Vanderkieft was chief medical officer, also commanding the officers' hospital in that city whose bed capacity was 409. The third hospital in Annapolis was nearby Division No. 2 with 600 beds. (See Table IV.)

At the start of the war, the Naval Academy in Annapolis was 16 years old. Because of Maryland's Southern sympathies, midshipman, officers and instructors were transferred by ship to Newport Rhode Island. They were replaced by the Union Army and three hospitals. Rows of pavilion-like buildings received sick and wounded along with recently paroled and exchanged Union soldiers from Confederate prisons. It was located on the Chesapeake Bay, in the rear of St. John's College, 20 miles east of Washington, accessed by the Annapolis and Elkridge Railroad.

The main hospital had six sections divided into 38 wards. There were 11 acting assistant surgeons, two full surgeons and one medical cadet. Some brick buildings were divided into patient wards. Walls were clean and white, the floors neatly polished. Checkered walkways were shaded by trees and adorned with manicured shrubbery, while broad commons sloped towards the sea, cooled by its breezes and illuminated with stunning sunsets reflecting off the bay.

The officers' hospital was established on March 29, 1864, in the precincts of the Naval Academy. The portion known as Section III was selected for sick and wounded officers, thoroughly renovated and prepared for their reception. General Order 127 authorized the surgeon in charge to requisition the medical purveyor for medicines, hospital stores, and furniture, and to hire nurses, cooks and laundresses. He would have custody of hospital funds and collect, disburse and account for same. The Surgeon General office charged officers $1 for each day as a hospital patient. A special attendant cost 30 cents a day more. [Privately owned hospitals in New York City charged the government $4 a week for enlisted men and $7 for officers.] Officers were considered "on detached service without troops," and costs were deducted from their regular pay. If short of funds, an officer could obtain a certificate of indebtedness. Upon hospital death, the amount was deducted from his pay as formulated by the hospital treasurer, who was a medical officer.

Some considered that making officers pay for rations at $1 a day was excessive. "The government ought to furnish a caterer to every officer in the Army and especially officers in the hospital and if this is not done before Congress adjourns all of our best officers will resign as sure as fate. Perhaps we should pay their board as well."[1] Wounded and convalescing officers represented 250 different Union regiments.

On a long low strip of land just to the south of Horn Point was Section Six, the hospital for contagious diseases (smallpox), exposed to a fresh medicinal breeze from Chesapeake Bay and sufficiently distant to offer quarantine. It was a horn of plenty with vegetable patches, peach and pear orchards, and fresh vegetables delivered daily to kitchens, including strawberries when in season. Given to the state in 1745, it had livestock, including pigs, ducks and geese. Free issue of necessary clothing was made to soldiers returning to duty from this hospital, including one pair of trousers, one blouse, one shirt, one pair of drawers, and one pair of socks. Clothing worn on arrival was burned.

Sister Tyler was the directress of ladies acting as nurses. There were two chaplains, the Reverend Henries serving just the hospital and the Reverend Sloan representing the Christian Commission. The chapel had as altarpiece the bible, wine cup and cross. Stained glass windows were surrounded with displays of circling stars that glittered in reflected light. A bald eagle gracefully festooned the national flag with the motto "God and Country." There were arches of evergreens with scrolls on which were listed the most important battles. The windows were adorned with shields, flags and wreaths. Religious services were held every Sabbath at 2 and 7 p.m., prayer meetings Wednesday at 7 p.m. and bible class Thursday at 7 p.m.

Hospital visiting hours were 12 noon to 6 p.m. daily. Mail arrived daily at 10:00 a.m. and 8 p.m. and departed at 2:30 p.m. and 9 p.m. Letters awaiting pick up at the Post Office were listed in the newspaper. The library was open daily from 8 a.m. to noon and 2 p.m. to 8 p.m. All the books from the Naval Academy library had been shipped north. Replacements came from religious organizations, the Sanitary Commission and the lay public. A pass was necessary for all but officers. All articles brought in for use of patients had to be deposited in the hospital store room unless special permission was granted by the officer of the day. From 11 a.m. to 2 p.m. was the Board of Examination for Invalids, composed of one doctor and three regular army officers who determined disability and discharge status.

The Crutch was first published on the grounds of U.S. Army General Hospital Division Number 1 on January 9, 1864, and continued through May 6, 1865, a total of 71 issues. Subscriptions were $2 a year or five cents for each issue. The motto was E. PLURIBUS UNUM (out of many, one), the logo a bald eagle. This was a weekly news and literary paper devoted to the interest of the soldier. Distributed every Saturday, it would "relieve tedium of hospital life with good reading" on subjects thoughtful or action packed.[2] This was to be a "readable paper," letting the patient's friends and family at home know their goings-on. All articles in *The Crutch* would be original to *The Crutch*.

A detailed medical directory for both visitors and residents of all hospitals and especially medical departments in and around Annapolis included each ward and its surgeon, rules for visitors, and the names of other hospitals in Annapolis: St. John's College Hospital (Officers only), Division Number 2 Hospital, Camp Parole Hospital and U.S. General Hospital at Annapolis Junction. All men admitted, discharged, furloughed, transferred, deserted or deceased were listed, along with editorials, literary pieces, summary of news, original contributions, selections from the best authors and extracts from other public journals. Various general orders new and old were posted: furloughs for paroled POWs, re-enlistments for a $300 bounty, board examinations for invalid soldiers, and addresses of hospital medical directors allowing disabled soldiers on furlough to report for authorization and continuation of leave.

The soldier needed *Mr. Crutch* for cheer, comfort and support. It would get "new

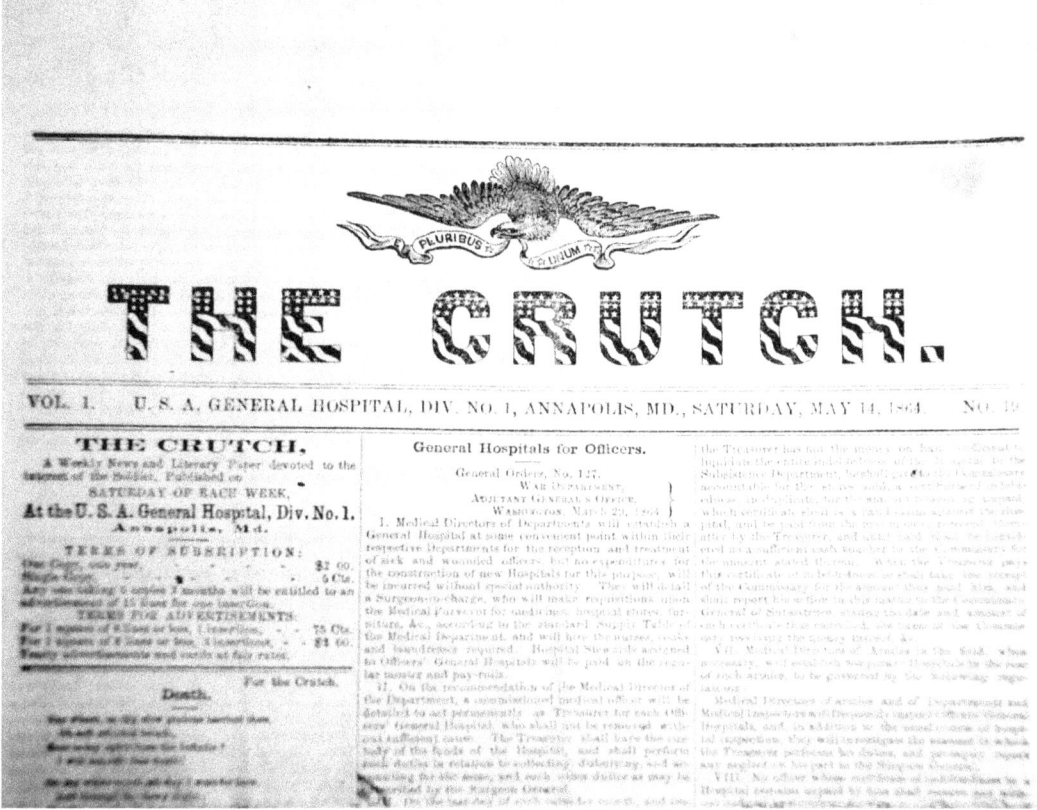

The Crutch. Division I U.S. Army General Hospital. Annapolis, Maryland (Maryland State Archives).

ideas in and false ones out" and be entirely devoted to the interest of the soldiers in the hospitals and not simply a record of hospital news. Its name was both positive and accurate, though some did not think it appropriate. Other titles were suggested but none seemed as expressive of the intended design. "*The Crutch* implies lameness, disability and lack of beauty that attracts attention. It also suggests usefulness and not being just ornamental. It is a helper and supporter of the weak and disabled. We trust it will meet with favor among the soldiers."[3] For those who disliked the name and requested a change, an answer was forthcoming. "What a vandal, you are! Change the name? There is not a more popular word in the English language than the crutch; it has weight in meaning and enters into the practical and useful economy of the times. Philosophers, poets, artisans, and everybody but the lazy and timid look upon it reverently. What do you suggest; The Harp?"[4]

Others defended *The Crutch as* an angel of pity, binding the wounds of battle and strengthening the fallen ones, a heavenly enterprise on a holy mission. "When I first saw you I thought what a queer name for a paper. Why do you think I am a cripple that you must come to offer me your help? Have I a spinal affliction or rickets? You do not offer support to the strong but always lend a hand to the weak in the guise of the angel of pity. You give relief to the victims and are beautiful. If you are a crutch, I honor thee and thy scars, thy beautiful maiming, and glorious infirmities!"[5]

Another paper, *The Knapsack*, was published quarterly by the lady nurses and was composed of lectures and debates given at the Lyceum, which included a miniseries on intemperance. They supported the name of *Crutch* and were contributors. As to crutches, they admired "sterling qualities of kindness and self-sacrifice, always ready to be used in the service of the suffering and weak." They encouraged soldiers to persevere and choose liberty or death. "Never give up! It is wiser and better to hope than despair."[6]

For some exchanged papers, there are few to no surviving copies to review, which included *Finley Hospital Weekly, The Haversack,* and *The Convalescent*. The last was published at the Camden Street Hospital in Baltimore, issued semimonthly "with a large amount of original and selected reading" mostly submitted by its patients. The General Hospital in Jefferson Barracks, Missouri, submitted a paper also called *The Convalescent*. The *Hospital Register* of Satterlee Hospital in Philadelphia was recognized as an "original, solid, reliable and staunch pioneer in the new and adventurous field of hospital literature."[7]

The Crutch was not to be a political paper. "This is simply a hospital register by sufferance of military authority. We cannot make it a channel for discussion of questions relating to the government or candidates for presidency. Letters about the upcoming election will not be published." As in other hospital newspapers, this policy was ignored.[8] This remained a military hospital and due diligence was maintained as to who was in command, issued orders and made policy.

In its 16 months of existence there were three publishers and editors: Charles N. Burnham, Alonzo Colby and Charles Boswell. A loyalty developed for civilian volunteers, especially in nursing. Two such figures were featured in reminisces on the deaths of Mr. Young and Miss Billings. The latter was from St. Lawrence, New York, and died just two weeks after becoming ill. Her will stated, "If I die in this hospital, may I be buried here among my boys," and she was.[9]

At its peak there were over 600 subscribers from every state. To save money, papers were left at the post office for pick-up Saturday morning. Lithographic views on "good quality paper" of U.S. General Hospital Division Number 1 and 2 were put on sale. Ads were encouraged if promptly paid.

As in other facilities, the U.S. Sanitary Commission offered free help for war claims and pensions, bounties, arrears of pay, and prize money. Tents filled with supplies for the relief of recently arrived regiments were the work of state agents for all camps and hospitals in Annapolis. The Sanitarians offered places to stay and religious services on the Sabbath at their House of Delegates. For Christmas of 1864, they presented a cooking wagon with "many compartments and multiple boilers" to make tea or coffee.

On the last page were advertisements for products likely to appeal to its readers. The Holland House restaurant for food and drink was "reasonably priced," as were American House Hotel and Restaurant, a dry goods store, a watchmaker and clocks, jewelry and spectacles, billiards and bagatelle, a bowling saloon, cigars and tobacco, stationery, dry goods, general stores for soldiers, hats and gloves, boots and shoes, guns and pistols, military vests, leggings, pants, overcoats, caps, Havelock, undershirts, shoulder straps and J. Bernstein's military clothing emporium. A help ad from a hospital surgeon read, "Wanted! Colored man or boy to take care of two horses and attend to some other like business."[10]

The printers and compositors brought skills learned before the war and as a group were proud, insular and partial to dark humor. One issue was dedicated to "married" and the next to "died" or "killed." Rules were established concerning those daring to enter their inner sanctum, the Printing Office. Enter softly, don't inquire for the news, subscribe to the paper and pay in advance, read the news yourself, engage in no controversy, keep six feet from the table, do not touch the type, do not talk to compositors, and do not touch the manuscript or proof sheets. Observe and fear not the "devil."[11] [The printer's devil was traditionally the apprentice who fetched type, mixed ink and as a consequence had darkened or black skin. He was the source of blame for mischief in type, misspelling and absent lines. Mark Twain, Benjamin Franklin, Artemus Ward and Petroleum V. Nasby started in that job.]

Other proverbial truths were issued for those failing insight from the first set of rules. Never ask the editor for news; it is his duty at the appointed time to give it without asking. Never write lengthy articles or ask him what he thinks of your piece as the truth may offend you. Never ask the identity of an article's author on subjects of public concern. Never look at copy in the hands of the compositor or on file or he may knock you down with his stick. Never examine proof sheets for it is not ready for thine eye and thou may not understand it.[12]

Blacks

The relationship of the black race within American society was multifaceted, serving as source material for political and social commentary often addressed with humor.

A Negro preacher observed to his hearers at the close of his sermon: "My obstinate congregants, I find it no more useful to preach to you than it is for a grasshopper to wear knee pads."

Chaplain and contraband.
ARMY CHAPLAIN: "My young colored friend can you read?"
CONTRABAND: "Yes sah!"
ARMY CHAPLAIN: "Glad to hear. Shall I give you a paper?"
CONTRABAND: "Sartin, massa, if you please."
ARMY CHAPLAIN: "Very good. What paper would you choose now?"
CONTRABAND: "Well massa, if you chews I'll take a paper ob terbacker."

The chaplain sighed and passed on.[13]

A frightened Negro tells of an advancing heavy artillery skirmish after which Negro Jim was not seen for a whole day. He came out at night and when asked where he had gone rolled his large eyes and said: "Oh! Massa, I heard something coming through the air, saying, 'Whar's dat nigger? Whar's dat nigger?' And pretty soon that ting busted, and little debils went skirmishing all around arter dis niger, and I run away!" Those persons who have heard shells, whizzing through the air will readily see that Jim's description of them is perfect.[14]

NEGRO FAITH: *Dialogue between an "aristocratic female" and a colored woman:*
ARISTOCRATIC FEMALE: "The niggers will never be free. They are too ignorant and indolent to be of any account." Colored woman: "Do you think all the prayers and cries to the good Lord won't have effect? Haven't they been offered in faith, and don't you know de good Lord can do everything."
ARISTOCRAT: "But the Lord will never free the niggers nor restore the union." Colored woman: "Why bress you honey, don't you see the good Lord has two great keys in his hand what holds de union together."
ARISTOCRAT: "No. I never saw the Lord's keys."
COLORED WOMAN: "Well you see honey, de Lord has two great keys in his hand. One is Dar-key, with that he has unlocked the union, so all de niggers, as you call them, will come out free. De other is de Yan-key, and with that the good Lord will lock the union up again."[15]

"How do I look, Pompeii," said a young dandy to his servant, as he had finished dressing himself.
"Elegant, massa; you look as bold as a lion."
"Bold as a lion, Pompey! How do you know? You never saw a lion."
"O, yes massa, I seed one down at massa Jenks in de stable."
"Down at Jenks, Pompey? Why you abominable fool, Jenks hasn't got a lion; that's a jackass."
"Can't help it, massa, you look just like him."[16]

"Niggerism." Massachusetts is known as the "nigger" state. Why such a small state should receive such an odious epithet is surprising. Are not all minds created equal? Is liberty for all and the union inseparable the face of our history? There are designing ambitious party politicians who are raising a standard throughout the free and loyal states whose rallying cry is "up with the traitor—down with the Nigger, why should we falter now?" Are we so infatuated and so cowardly and intoxicated by the delusive, treacherous, poisonous melody of that siren song of "peace on any terms," so as to sheath our swords and stack our arms whether our country shall be free or not.[17]

A philosophic elderly darky served at Fort Donaldson and was interviewed by a reporter for the Cincinnati Gazette.
"Did you stand your ground?"
"No suh, I ran."
"That wasn't very creditable for your courage."
"That ain't my line. Cooking's my perfeshun."
"Then you have no regard for your reputation."
"Reputation nuffin to me by the sins of life."
"Do you consider your life of more value than other people's?"
"It's worth more to me, sah. I value it very highly, more than 1 million dollars for what be wuth with the bref out of me. Self-preserbashum am de fust law wid me. Different men set different values upon dar lives—mine isn't in the market."
"If you lost it you would have the satisfaction of knowing that you died for your country?"
"What satisfaction that be to me when de power of feelin' was gone?"
"Then patriotism and honor are nothing to you." "Nuffin, whatever sah—I regard dem as among de vanities."
"If our soldiers were like you, traitors might have broken up the government without resistance."
"Yes sah, dar would had been no help from me. I wouldn't put my life on de scale gainst no gobernment dat eber existed for no gobernment could replace de loss of me."
"Do you think any of your company would have missed you if you had been killed?"
"May be not, sah—a dead white man ain't much to dese sogers, let alone a dead niggar—but I'd miss myself and dat was de pint wid me." It is safe to say that the dusky corpse of that African will never darken the field of carnage.[18]

Irish

The following two stories play on the stereotype linking Irish and the grape.

An Irish drummer now and then indulged in a noggin of right good spirits was asked by an impudent young ensign.
"What makes your nose so red?"
"Plaze, sir, I always blush when I spake to me officer."[19]
Mr. Dodge the celebrated electricity physician was lecturing on health and particularly the evil of tea and coffee had morning breakfast with a son of Erin.
"Perhaps you think I would be unable to convince you of the deleterious effects of tea and coffee?"
"I don't know, but I'd like to be there when you do it."
"If I convince you that they are injurious to your health, will you abstain from their use?"
"Sure, and I will swear."
"How often do you use coffee and tea," asked the doctor.
"Morning and night, sir."

"Did you ever experience a slight dizziness on the brain on going to bed?"
"Indeed I do."
"And a sharp pain around the temples about the eyes in the morning?"
"Truth I do, sir,"
"Well," said the doctor with assurance and confidence in his matter. "That is the tea and coffee."
"Is it indeed? Faith and I always thought it was the whiskey. I drank."
The doctor quietly retired. He was fairly beaten.[20]

Health Care

By April 1864, there were 40,000 soldiers in Union military hospitals, "equal to the entire army of Denmark." Profiles of hospital life revealed pain, suffering, courage and boredom. *What I see from my window* was one such story. "By chance, I occupy a seven by nine foot room in this hospital, which has one window that I call my stereoscope. It overlooks a grass plot and small vegetable and flower garden. Ill with chills and rheumatism, I could see a narrow strip of sky but my weakened eyes denied me satisfaction of reading lying on my back."[21]

Hospital life was portrayed as dull and devoid of excitement.

> We exhaust all reading material, including popular and unpopular novels and newspapers which are hastily devoured each morning and evening. We answer our letters fully and frequently to wives or inamorata's and discuss every topic of conversation until every yarn and stale joke is exhausted. We utter malediction over the uncomfortable wound that brought us here and fault someone, we don't know who, but because we are not home.[22]

Grumblers was defined as "sullen, surly, murmuring bipeds spending their time wishing for something they can't have, or finding fault with that they do have." Exodus described Israelites brought out from Egypt after 400 years of slavery as "incessant grumblers" who remained so even after 40 years of wandering. When Sherman had taken Atlanta, one such *incessant mutterer* complained, "Why didn't he take all of Georgia?" These soldiers were specialists in an organized complaint department called "The Knights of the Quill."[23] Optimists with opposing views urged faith, hope and continued sacrifice on behalf of the government as the best option for victory.

> What a joy to see squads of 20, 50 or 100 who seem to be on deathbed, now able to shoulder the knapsack and musket and with light hearts and determined spirits go forth again to meet the enemies of our country. They cherished fond memories of the faithful nurse, hospital steward and surgeon. Their associations of Hospital life are made so agreeable and ennobling both by the government and by the Christian and other commissions, leaving their mark on the heart of the war veteran who thus appreciates God's goodness and mercy.[24]

Good sanitation was known to be essential for maintaining health. Some wards were immaculate while others had garbage in the corners covered with blankets, overcoats with moldy snacks and drawers needing to be cleaned out. An ex-nurse blamed lazy and incompetent ward masters.

> Men became acclimatized and inured to the fatigues of marching, rough duties and exposure of picket life. The army need be better protected, better clothed, better fed and better in sanitary ways. Health policies are as necessary to a city as water or bread. Devastating epidemics in the South were common. If we have an epidemic, it will come from abroad or be wafted over from our enemies in the south.[25] [Acclimatization worked if soldiers were sent home to recover from malaria, avoiding reinfection, likely to occur if stationed in the South.]

The sin of gluttony was condemned by men of medicine and faith who gave health care tips on personal hygiene, tight clothing and exercise. The tale *A wonderful fat man*, described excessive eating and drinking of potatoes, pies, milk and cream flushed with beer, ale, stout, port, champagne, and rum.

> Life styles have consequences and there are fourteen ways by which people get sick. They eat too fast and irregularly and are awake through the night. They drink too much including poisonous whiskey and other intoxicating liquors. They wear clothes and shoes too tight and too light. They exercise too little and neglect body hygiene. They suffer constant excitement of the mind with borrowed troubles and seek out cheap doctors and quack nostrums for every imaginary ill. They read trashy excitable literature and over-indulge on the subject of politics.[26]

Most nurses were males, but *the right kind of nurse* made a difference. A letter was sent from the Shiloh battlefield highlighting the benefits of the feminine touch.

> The only women we have here are nurses. As a class they manage very well but are not much in the line of attraction. They wear faded down straight from top to bottom ignoring the waist and personifying the appearance of a shirt on a beanpole. The wildest imagination could not induce the divine to admiration. If only they had the slightest idea of how much medicine a sick man needs. Better a full figure with bright sunlight colors rather than dark and somber. Dorothy Dix made a great mistake when she prescribed gaunt females over thirty for sick soldiers. Better a fresh plump little woman with the light of kindness in her eyes and love in her heart. One such woman will do more good than all the doctors and drugs in the Army dispensary. One smile dispels the gloom. I have seen tears raining down soldier's cheek at the touch of those soft hands upon fevered brow and watched his eyes follow them all day long, while health and strength departed their shattered frame.[27]

The Young Ladies Aid Society of Portland, Connecticut, had 15 members all less than 18 years of age, working one year for missionaries and the second for the soldiers. Being of school age, they met at night and sent a letter with $86: "This sum, although is very trifling may help relieve the suffering of our poor soldiers." A grateful response was prompt. "It is most thankfully received for the heart filled work and thoughtfulness of the gift. We of the crutch brigade appreciate your efforts. The rest of us should do our part keeping all states on the right track at the ballot box this fall."[28]

Sacrifice

The role of family and a mother's loving support was central to many stories. The son was dutifully and willingly dispatched to do God's work and be sacrificed.

> "Am I dying doctor? Isn't there any ray of hope?" The feeble hand grasped the arm of the physician making rounds among the sick and wounded in the hospital tent. It was a boyish face, but the Angel of death left its impression; the kindhearted surgeon could only shake his head. "I want to go home once more before I die. Oh, Mother, Oh Mother!" The words were full of agony as tears streaked the boy's face. "My mother taught me how to die, bless God for that!" The New England mother arrived by stagecoach and was offered her son's belongings in silence. "My boy! Oh God help me! Is this all that's left?" She gathered his package of sword and sash coat, buttons and epaulets. He had appeared before her in that same uniform saying, "mother, aren't you proud of your boy? I'm going to fight for the dear old flag, my father's flag and mine. I want to go with your approval and blessing." She placed her trembling hands on his head and whispered through tears. "Go, my son and God are with you." And God was with him as his bible appeared to have been read thoroughly and faithfully. There were pencil lines in each chapter and a packet of letters full of hope. It was a brokenhearted mother who pillowed her head with the treasures of her son.[29]

Five. *The Crutch* 143

A traveler from abroad visiting New York City follows a small urchin into a third floor slum in a squalid neighborhood with filthy doors and prison-like dwellings inhabited by drunkenness, disease and crime. Her grandmother lay on a cot dying, with no food or medicine. There was a cavalry saber gleaming in the light next to her bed. The Good Samaritan gave food and drink to both the child and grandmother who was so pale and trembling she was unable to eat. She had lost her husband and struggled twenty years to raise two sons both enlisting in the war and dying for their country. Her youngest had just become an officer and received that sword when he was killed. "They sent my Willie's sword and bible home. My child, we will never part with them!" The stranger's eyes filled with tears as she died. Her sons were martyrs and welcomed her to an eternal home. The traveler took the orphan by the hand and would minister her wants and needs as protector starting with a soldier's heirloom.[30]

Thousands of mothers suffered pitiless heartaches despite desperate prayer that the pearly gates be left ajar for their loved one to receive salvation and eternal life. "Home," murmured the dying soldier with memory of mother's fond watchful eyes and loving caress. His sisters, brothers and sweetheart stretched out their arms to embrace, in smiles and tears, his return even if in spirit only.

Nostalgia or homesickness was defined as a temporary feeling of morbid depression due to the hardship of field duty or absence of home life. Its treatment was activity, be it making camp improvements, sports or spiritus frumenti.

> A lieutenant finding a home-sick soldier solitary and alone, weeping like a big booby boy, said:
> "What's the matter?"
> "Oh, I wish I was in my father's barn."
> "And what would you do there?"
> "I would go into the house plenty quick!" said the poor fellow.[31]

Disabled

Amputations were a fearful but often life-saving procedure. Stories and poems abound that reflected its fact, folklore, and humor.

> It was a good operation on the poor but jolly soldier who lost his arm in defense of his country and was visited by the Surgeon General who promised him an arm with which he could pick up his hat and write his name. The fellow's early education had been neglected and he could not write. When the distinguished visitor left, the wounded boy burst out in exultation; "Well fellows, I've made money out of this. I am going to have a new arm that can write though I never could with the old one!"[32]

Poetry was a popular literary form, with contributions from prominent and unknown writers.

> The heroic incidence of war has taken a tragic and powerful hold on the heart and imagination of our poets, adding fire to the richness and force of poetry in general. Four years ago, poems were like fairytale stories, tender beautiful scenes in nature with clear faithful eyes. Now they are touched with tragedy, glory, bugle calls and shaded trees. The psalms do not fail the solemn or momentous issues, but comprehend its grandeur and lift us above the hateful spirit of revenge and bravado.[33]

These are odes to those sacrificing life and limb.

> *The Empty Sleeve*[34]
> Till this very hour, I could ne'er believe,
> What a tell-tale thing is an empty sleeve,
> What a weird queer thing is an empty sleeve
>
> It tells in a silent tone to all,
> Of a country's need, of a country's call.

Of a kiss and a tear for a child and a wife,
Of a hurried march for a nation's life.

It tells of a battlefield of gore,
With the sudden clash of the cannons roar—
Of the deadly charge of the bugles note—
Of the gurgling sound in the foeman's throat—
Of the whirring grape of the fiery shell—

Of a scene, which mimic the scenes of hell.
It tells of a myriad wounds and scars—
Of a flag with the glorious Stripes and Stars,
And it points to a time, when that flag shall wave,
O'er land where there breathes no cowering slave.

One proud hurrah for the empty sleeve,
For the one armed man with the empty sleeve.

The Soldier's Elegy, upon his L-E-G[35]
Oh wooden peg! Oh wooden peg!
Thou substitute for flesh and bone—
Thou limb within a forest grown,
Thou mournful semblance of a leg.
I see myself once more a boy,
With all the wonders of a child,
Threading the forests tangled wild,
Roaming the fields with youthful joy.
My eyes behold, look where I may.
Some trusty axe did amputate
The limb of some old giant tree,
To make this wooden limb for me,
And leave me thus to ambulate.
While my poor leg has gone to share,
The mold which makes the small acorn,
That future cripples still unborn
May have an oaken leg to wear.
For since 'twas treason took my leg,
Companion to its whizzing ball,
Tis fitting that on trees I call
To furnish me a counter-peg.
I've moralized you see this much,
Upon the leg "Rebellion" seized,
While on the other now am pleased
To bring this offer to *The Crutch*.

The Invalid Corps[36]
March them out from the hospital wards,
Gather their pale faces into line,
Crutch and bandage and wooden leg;
Wounded heroes. There's work for you.

John with his shattered leg scares the will,
Willie whose arm at Gettysburg fell,
And Harry scarred with rebel shell,
And Frank with his almost sightless eyes.

Gather the invalid, March them out,
The Army needs reinforcements you know;

> True there are plenty of men without,
> But they are the men who oft go not.
>
> True at every corner they stand,
> And talk of the war till the sun sets
> Army, and generals, and government cursed,
> And tell of the way they would have things done.
>
> But never a hand do the cowards raise,
> To strike or labor for truth and right,
> The war has made cripples! They stand and gaze
> And let the cripples resume the fight!

What are the last hours of a brave soldier? Since no one has ever returned from the hereafter, we can only conjecture. A man was shot in the right lung and given a bleak prognosis by the surgeon. Being a Christian soldier, he trusted that "God may support me through the valley and shadow of death when I am ready to go." He and thousands like him sacrificed their lives upon the altar of their country and would ever be held in remembrance. "We shall not forget that to you soldiers we are indebted for the safety and continuance of our noble government"; so ended the Chaplain's benediction.[37]

A most effective medicine was humor without the cost, side-effects or need of prescription. Josh Billings offered his philosophy on burning issues of the day and more often the mundane.[38]

> Dogs as a general thing aint profitable.
>
> Onions are good for bad breath.
>
> Boys ain't apt to turn out well that don't get up till 10 o'clock in the morning.
>
> Ships are called *she,* because they always keep a man on the lookout.

Romance and Marriage

Coping with the fair sex was a challenging proposition, a subject addressed by the editors and correspondents with a manual of practical advice and wishful superstitions. Artemus Ward described consequences of superstition and bachelorhood.

> *Superstitions.* If a young lady finds a four leaf clover and puts it in her hair, the first young man she meets she will marry. If a lady dons a gentleman's hat, it is a sign she wants a kiss. If you swallow a chickens heart whole, the first young man who kisses you, you will marry. If one sits on the table, it is a sign they wish to be married.[39]

> If you want to be a favorite with the girls attend to their wants—that is, give them rides, candy and raisins; talk and laugh about love affairs, and keep on the outside—that is don't commit to anyone in particular, you will be lionized to your hearts content until you become an old bachelor. The more flippant and nonsensical the young man in the company of girls the better. Will he succeed? They prefer the wise men.[40]

> An old bachelor is a poor critter. He does not know the music of laughter from happy children! Their father does not steal spoons from hotels and restaurants, or oats from blind horses but puts coin in the contribution box and fought the British when it mattered at great personal risk. The bachelor is a poor critter who only stays and does not live here. He ought to apologize on behalf of his parents for being here at all. The happy married man dies in good style at home surrounded by his weeping wife and children. The old bachelor doesn't die at all, he sort of runs away like a pollywog tail.[41]

Sermons

As in other hospital newspapers, clergy played a large role, influencing the paper's content, focus and tone. Sermons were given on selfishness, kindness, character, language, and Christian sympathy: "Are we a contented people," "perseverance—you can accomplish almost anything," "what is happiness and whence doth it spring." Man was created to be happy and not to mourn. Benevolence and being courteous was as virtuous as laughter. Seek justice for all. The world would get better when evil was cast off and destroyed by political storms, thus purifying the atmosphere and allowing spiritual health to take hold.

There would be no victory without the great resources and religiosity of the North. Successful commanders knew that there was "no true bravery without a trusting God." A soldier nation had a government that took upon itself to think, believe, and pray for its people. Scripture told the Christian soldier, "a nation shall not lift up sword against nation, and neither shall they learn war anymore. We are convinced that ours is a just and righteous cause and that God will take care that right, truth and justice prevail."[42]

No churchman was more renowned than Henry Ward Beecher, who preached in the hospital chapel.

> Men who have no care or thought for others and are content with looking after their own ease and enjoyment ought to be put in a coffin for their life's work has ended. When God wanted sponges and oysters, he made them and put one on rock and the other in mud. Once he made man, he gave him feet and hands, head, heart and blood and said, "Go to work." If a man says, "I do not want to know any more or do any more, or be any more," he ought to become a mummy. Of all hideous things mummies are the most, and of those the most hideous are running about the streets and talking.[43]

The hospital chaplain stressed that education was more important than rank, wealth, caste and power. "Want of it leaves us helpless slaves to the crafty designs of deceitful men. Who are the real leaders in every department of life? Is it the dreamers or shirking knaves who cheat society out of their living and then demand their dues?"[44] A night school was opened in the commodious mess hall for benefit of patients wanting to improve in reading, writing, and arithmetic, attended by 75 would-be scholars. Lady Nurses from Utica, New York, and the Sanitary Commission acted as teachers, providing materials and refreshments.

Josh Billings humor gave perspective to religious incantations; "yer kant judge a man bi hiz religun any more than her kan judge hiz shurt bi the size ov the kollar and rist-bands."[45] A correspondent took issue with the chaplain's views on how to be a Christian, asking if the war was too great an expenditure for the results achieved? The Chaplain responded that there were many viewpoints. "It is hard to know what is right. For truth seek God not man. Each must account for himself. How can a Christian engage in war and kill when the Bible says it is wrong to kill? David was a warrior. The Jews were commanded to destroy and kill wicked nations who sought to overturn theirs. Know there is but one way and 'let every man be fully persuaded in his own mind.'"[46]

Temperance

The temperance movement was a distinct but vocal minority. A debate at the Lyceum on the "miseries of intemperance" was well attended. The 18-piece band was not allowed to play because contraband whiskey bottles were smuggled on post inside their instruments. In May 1863, a Provost Marshal edict attempted to enforce city-wide prohibition.

> The evils resulting from unrestricted sale of spirituous liquors to soldiers as now practiced are such as to destroy to a great extent military discipline, endanger the peace and good order of the city and camps and barracks in its vicinity and to seriously impair the health and efficiency of the men. All persons residing in the district of Annapolis are positively forbidden to sell or give to any enlisted man in military service spirituous liquors or intoxicating drinks of any kind without the written permission of a medical officer or some commissioned officer attached to the camp.[47]

The great enemy of happiness was despair, and for the clergy there was no greater source than the limitless profanity of the otherwise godly, patriotic soldiers.

> Why is there such an awful degree of profanity everywhere prevailing among our soldiers? You can't take a short train ride without hearing it. Our trip was made hideous by the blasphemies of drunken men and screaming laughter of shameless girls. Perhaps we need separate cars or compartments on trains or different class carriages. The soldiers who do not swear seem to be exceptions. They are gentlemen that endeavor to set a good example and when they have authority use it to keep down this obscenity and brutality. Such men even if they be few, gain greater victories than those of the battle field and are entitled to our respect and honor.[48]

Patriotism

Comparisons of Confederates and Yankees were grist for the propaganda mill. God was on our side, loyalty mattered, we were more industrious, our soldiers were braver and more moral, and sacrifice was gleefully endured and willingly expected. The ordinary foot soldier, mostly volunteer, made the sacrifices patriotism demanded and would endure, no matter the cost.

> The traitors show only expressions of scorn for those who hold labor or live by it. Because of the want of these despised mud-sills [mechanics and engineers] their railroads are in ruins, factories short-handed such as they have, and steamers for all offensive purposes useless. Only in the war riddled south is the voice of labor hushed in the field and the hum of factory replaced by quiet and ruin.[49]

> A rebel letter was picked up in the wilderness by a soldier now in this hospital. "The politicians told us in the beginning of the war to save all our lines and strong cords so as to choke the Yanks. A wounded man at home on furlough receives two pairs of home-made socks but a whole man gets only one pair. I would like a pair of shoes more than that song; we are tired of singing Dixie and we are tired of retreat."

> Market prices in Richmond August 1864 were: flour $250 per barrel, corn $45 a bushel, coffee $35 a pound, port wine $55 a quart.[50]

> With the war ending and after the Yankees left the country, people flocked by scores from all parts of the country, some coming over 100 miles. Every form of vehicle drawn by every form of creature could be seen. Materials left by the Yankees were deposited in wagons and carted off. One lady was found with a rope around the piano, thinking it was a table for her to take. One man carried off $50,000 worth of chandeliers. Steps have been taken to secure all the articles carried off, as well as the offenders. The planners need to be sacked.[51]

> *Demons of the rebellion* Jeff Davis, his cabinet, and rebel Congress, will be pallbearers for: slavery, aristocracy, and inhumanity, state sovereignty, injustice and anarchy. They sit in the flaming car of ignorance, arrogance, and knavery. Jeff Davis and his cabinet have great weights around their necks. Their chief physician, his Satanic Majesty, is the great copperhead serpent and the god of discord.[52]

> How greatly the present war has changed the condition of our country, a nation that had neglected the arts of war. A war forced upon us was for the restoration of the union and those great principles

our fathers struggled to preserve in a revolution. We will fight to the bitter end and secure for the world a Republican Government. After we drop the sword from our grasp, let us turn our minds and hearts to those pursuits that elevate and develop mankind.[53]

Patriotism is dependent on freedom and the country's past for its vigor and inspiration in order to develop the nobler traits of character and hope for the future. Magnanimity, heroism and martyrdom in our national character are the surest proof of the advancement of our national glory. The land that offers the most physical advantages and attractions becomes the home of the widest and deepest patriotism. The magic touch of genius or the threat of traitors is needed to freshen and send blood trilling through the veins and tone the voice to new songs and shouts.[54]

The country is on trial for its life. Rather than turn our money into carpets, pictures, velvets, and popular sin let us convert it into loyalty. Sacrifice cannot be too great seeing the cause and the demand is so great. The man that does not love his country and remains indifferent in the struggle against those who seek her destruction is not worthy of her protection. He should be cast out beyond the pale of all government. To understand *why we fight* watch Michigan's colored regiment march by. Former slaves are defending white men's homes. Rebellion against free institutions must end in its own overthrow.[55]

Almost every man or boy toiling in the field of service for a term of years becomes either better or worse. The change is so great from civil to military life that even those whose life has reached its meridian are affected by it favorably or otherwise. Much has been written about intemperance, dissipation, and demoralization of the Army. The soldier asked himself, "for what am I making the sacrifices and enduring these privations and trials?" There is something in the discipline, the duties and labors of active field service that brings out and develops the sterling qualities of superior manhood that ordinary civil life do not create. The associations and influences of the war are supposed to be injurious. This may be so but not altogether. The rank-and-file of the Army is not demoralized. A hardy majority of the soldiers who come out of this war, though maimed in body will present a character the likes of which has not been seen in our country. Hence the sacrifices and trials of war have been and still are a *blessing* and not a *curse*. Sacrifice by the soldier and his family purifies their souls.[56]

The model soldier is patient, enduring, and good natured and jolly. He likes camp-life, knapsack always ready at a moment's notice, spends all day Sunday cleaning his gun, drinks little on marches thinking it unhealthy, sleeps with boots and cap on, carries pockets full of ammunition, puts up tent and supper cooked in ten minutes after a halt, knows where to find rail fences, always has straw to sleep on, has low opinion of officers, wouldn't do anything for the Colonel if 'twas to save his life, thinks the Major ought to have something to do to prevent him from being lazy, thinks his Captain first rate and helps put up his tent, won't stand any nonsense from the lieutenant, does not like battles any more than others but ready to do his duty, tries to take care of his health, advises new recruits to take care of their health, has reenlisted, sends home all his pay, never spends money at the sutlers, swears some and can't help it, and is willing to sacrifice his life to put down the rebellion. He will vote for Lincoln an honest man or any other man that will put down this rebellion and thinks army contractors and officers with big salaries have kept the war going too long. He is willing to do his duty and hopes Jeff Davis and copperheads go to damnation together.[57]

Politics

On June 9, 1864, the hospital held a mock presidential convention. Soldiers from 16 states voted: 143 for Lincoln, 15 for Grant, 6 for McClellan and 12 abstained. A poll in September showed no change. At the Officers Hospital, the vote was 237 for Lincoln, 32 for McClellan, and 1 for Fremont. At St. John's College Hospital, enlisted men voted Lincoln 435 and McClellan 15. A glimmer of hope was raised in sarcasm for "A great victory—McClellan ahead!" A poll taken at a jail in Wheeling Virginia showed McClellan with 15 votes, Lincoln 6.

Some states sent agents to register and collect votes. Pennsylvania soldiers voted in the hospital's Chapel on the first Tuesday. "It was a most peaceful election with no evidence of greenbacks, whiskey, or ballot box stuffers to buy, persuade or control the election. I loved to see a man who lost one arm in defense of his country has the privilege of voting with others," stated the commissioner from Pennsylvania. "I take pleasure in thanking the surgeons for their hospitality, kindness and attention to the sick and wounded. There is no place better to be cared for then here."[58]

The newspaper that declared no politics would be practiced on its pages ran this editorial on the Democratic candidate for President.

> How sad to see the man we once followed in honorable battle against the enemy of union and liberty is now stooping for sake of position to offer his hand to bloodstained traitors we scorn to touch. The idea of armistice had its origin in a heart of treason and can never find a response among the loyal. Who demands this armistice? Is it the soldiers in the field? No, they spurn the idea of treason and traitors.[59]
>
> They voted as they fought, and they fought nobly like gods." They lived in rain filled rifle pits and trenches unable to sit for his meals, their face, hands, heart, brains and musket all covered with mud. They sleep in mud, eat in mud, watch in mud, fight in mud and shiver in the autumnal wind. They voted with the Chicago platform and its candidate: "Death before dishonor! Fight forever!"[60]

Lincoln

In June 1864, two ladies connected with the hospital called on President Lincoln for presentation of *The Crutch* with complete history of its origin and success. Included was a report on 2,779 federal prisoners, of whom 1,396 were dead. "He seemed very much pleased but did not relate it to any of the many stories he usually tells." Later in the war he visited former prisoners now hospital patients and offered many folksy and funny things. "His speech at the ceremony in honor of the dead at Gettysburg proves that he also says noble and beautiful things. His humor not always dignified did no harm, was neither mean or vindictive but apt and ready, affording him relief from a burdensome load. He was always playful, sometimes grim and sarcastic and adapted his wit to place and occasion with great effect."[61]

The Crutch adopted the names of Lincoln and Johnson as watchwords for liberty and Union. "Lincoln has the confidence of the people and reaches the hearts of the soldier's bitter experience at the hands of traitors ready to strike us. Patriotism of this day is made of sterner stuff than when the war commenced."[62] The paper received a thank you letter for displaying the Stars & Stripes in its windows and honoring ballot-box victory with lights illuminating the names of Lincoln and Johnson in the press room and ladies quarters.

That evening a grand torchlight procession by Union men in Annapolis celebrated the triumph of the Union cause and re-election of Lincoln. In the lead were hospital fire engines drawn by horses decorated with flags and torches. Next rode the provost guard, followed by the medical staff of various hospitals, serenaded by the hospital band. A long line of hospital personnel, the quartermaster department, and ordinary citizens carried torches and signs, followed by a boat on wheels pulled by six horses decorated with flags and torches. "Houses were illuminated along the march with beautiful transparencies and pro-administration mottos. Artillery boomed out with a loud display of pyrotechnics. The entire area was filled with enthusiastic multitudes including many of the fair sex. Resolutions were presented with stirring addresses from several speakers."[63]

Maryland and the national capital were free. The government held portions of every rebellious state. "Copperheads would soon be as harmless and silent as when St. Patrick's drove the snakes and toads from the beautiful emerald isle."[64]

With the end of autumn, thoughts turned to the winter sports of ice skating and snowballing. As per the request of Lincoln, formal Thanksgiving festivities were organized by the Surgeon in charge. A sermon was delivered by the Reverend Love at 11 a.m., followed by a sumptuous dinner at 12 p.m. including turkey, chicken, ham, oysters, pies and potatoes. Supplies were furnished by the Christian Commission and Sanitary Commission, with contributions from New York, Massachusetts, and Pennsylvania. "We lacked for nothing." Walls were draped with flags and portraits of Washington and Lincoln. "Those who opposed the war were quiet or dead. The voice of the North was going on with vigor and earnest determination until every rebel is subdued."[65]

The dome of the capital was scheduled for completion in March 1865. At Lincoln's first inauguration, the grounds had been decorated with piles of masonry, eight million iron castings and blocks of marble awaiting assembly. Despite predictions of failure and decay, construction continued. The dome was raised and crowned; and all this while conquering the rebellion. "The government of the United States has continued to adorn and embellish this Metropolis. The eastern portion of the Senate wing is completed and the House is nearly finished."[66]

Satiric prose about the Confederacy's fall brought smiles in the issue of April 8, 1865.

A Great Funeral will be held April 1865 in Richmond, Virginia caused by a severe attack of the great Union Army and convulsions. The most painful and violent contortions and writhing's a result of the foul spirit of secession. Funeral ceremonies will take place in Charleston, South Carolina on April 14, when a grand procession will be formed through the quarters of the professors of the secession.[67]

Black, funereal margins in *The Crutch* announced the President's death on Good Friday 1865.

A terrible calamity has befallen the country. The nation mourns a man of great uprightness, universal tenderness, and child-like goodness. He was a kind man with gaiety, incorruptible and with indulgence for all. He never recoiled or flinched from fanaticism, despotism or treason. He was sometimes grieved, often worn and exhausted, but never gloomy. God has his own ways manifested sometimes through events by which the horror and gloom of today is cleared by the dawning tomorrow. Our times are both tragic and thrilling, but we must believe that right will triumph and shadows be rolled away preparing a future of peace.

A hospital ceremony was performed under Union blue skies. Colonel Chamberlain and his young daughter unfurled the flag raised by two one-armed volunteers, surrounded by the 213th Pennsylvania Volunteers standing at attention in a semicircle. A flash of artillery signaled the hospital brass band to play the "Star Spangled Banner." The chapel was draped in mourning and its windows darkened. Following the chaplain's prayer, the glee club sang "Battle Cry of Freedom." A large assemblage with many ladies and officers was graced by speeches from Surgeon Stewart and Colonel Chamberlain, culminating with nine cheers for General Grant.

Prisoners of War

It was Christmas Sunday morning in Annapolis. A token of remembrance was left under each plate from the amiable and devoted nursing director, Miss Hall. Most of the

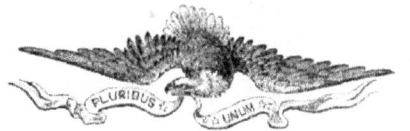

THE CRUTCH.

VOL. II.   U. S. A. GENERAL HOSPITAL, DIV. NO. 1, ANNAPOLIS, MD., SATURDAY, APRIL 22, 1865.   NO. 68.

The Crutch. Issue following Lincoln assassination (Maryland State Archives).

600 patients were returning prisoners whose response to the banquet and gala was childlike glee. "Their long confinement nearly accomplished the traitors' goal, that they return with crippled emaciated bodies, some imbecilic in mind, to be of no further use as soldiers."[68] Their dinner consisted of turkeys, chicken pie custard, port, vegetables, pickles, pies, hickory nuts and cranberry sauce. The building was decorated with evergreens, flags and pictures.

On this Sabbath all efforts were made to provide comfort and joy for the patients. "Death had done its work in the field at full speed. Hundreds have been received for medical care, having escaped the barbarous treatment of the 'chivalrous' South. If men are dying all around us, we must not forget that they are also living all around us. Cheery comfort and encouragement is the duty of all who labor to relieve them."[69]

The return of Union prisoners struck a nerve in a public thought inured to the horrors of war. Soldiers' descriptions of treatment and living conditions as confederate prisoners were excoriating. In Annapolis, returned prisoners got the best possible Christmas gift.

> Our hospital is the best thing we have seen yet born of military necessity. The poor crippled soldiers still lying in tents can look out upon soothing and beautiful water and perhaps forget their sufferings. The Richmond victims [returned POWs] can approach water's edge and breathe the pure air of Heaven. We think that they appreciate liberty as few of us can who know little of the trial of a long imprisonment. The difference is as great as between hell and heaven.[70]

By February 1864 discussions about retaliation for the consequences of Libby prison and Belle Isle appeared in print.

> Medicines as well as provisions are not as plentiful as they are among us. This is beyond dispute. We know the desperate condition in this respect in every part of the rebel territory. It is better to err on the side of mercy but mercy is never exercised at the expense of justice. Every act of the rebel government showing barbarous and fiendish hatred to Union soldiers should be met with like treatment towards their soldiers held as prisoners.[71]

A quarterly report on federal prisoners from January through March 1864 noted 50 percent mortality. The causes of death were chronic diarrhea 708, pneumonia 244, typhoid fever 69, and debility 42. "This is sufficient proof that our statements in regard to the treatment of federal prisoners have not been exaggerated. Attention is particularly called to the total and percentage of deaths. It may be pleasant for the copperheads to contemplate the remarkable amount of humanity prevailing among their southern brethren."[72]

In one week in April 1864, 125 prisoners were paroled and exchanged. Some asked to return to their regiment, requiring approval from a hospital medical officer. Many were paper-thin and not recovered from effects of long imprisonment, yet some claimed an intense desire to return to their regiments. "They have a grudge against the rebels for certain courtesies shown them while in Richmond which bear heavily upon them. Depend upon it; these boys will never come to Annapolis again as paroled prisoners, their faces will first bite the dust. We wish you God speed, boys."[73]

In May 1864, the *Harper's Weekly* front page showed lithographs of photos taken at this hospital showing cadaveric soldiers with gaunt faces and with protruding bones covered with skin but without underlying muscle or fat. For those who believed in Southern honor and chivalry, those pictures were devastating. "No further proofs of rebel inhumanity were necessary. Those who would sign a peace treaty with these barbarians would need to hang their head in shame."

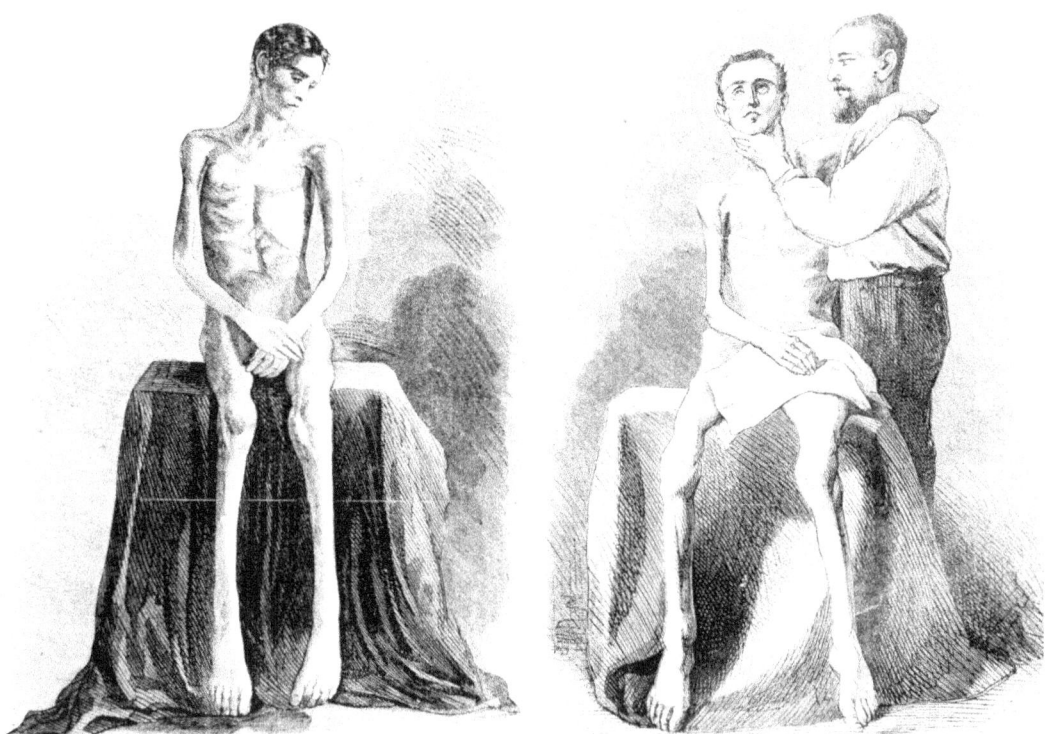

"Rebel Cruelty—Our Starved Soldiers." An engraving from a photograph taken at Division I U.S. Army General Hospital, Annapolis, Maryland. *Harper's Weekly,* June 18, 1864.

Dr. Ellerslie Wallace reported that of 100 "bad" cases brought over the past six weeks, 30 had since died, including the two pictured on the front page of *Harper's Weekly*. Was their appearance due to starvation or disease? Chief of staff Vanderkieft ascribed their deaths to "the effects of neglect and cruel treatment at the hands of the enemy." Twenty-two-year-old Private W. M. Smith of Kentucky was captured in September 1863 and transferred to Belle Isle, where his rubberized blanket was taken, exposing him to the elements. He survived smallpox, leaving him with chronic diarrhea. His face was shriveled, almost ape-like with seams and wrinkles in folds. He asked for a copy of his photo to send home to his mother. Twenty-year-old Private J. Brosilers of Indiana was captured December 1863, imprisoned and exposed to the elements also at Belle Isle. His diet was starvation followed by chronic diarrhea, and he arrived in Annapolis March 1864, weighing less than half his original weight. The surgeon described a third soldier, a prisoner for seven months, whose forearm was so thin, it was transparent when held up to the sunlight. He was unable to change his position in bed without assistance. Upon admission, he received a teaspoon of milk every 15 minutes but it was all he could hold without vomiting. He died one month later.[74]

The daily ration of these men was corn bread five inches long, four inches wide and one and a half inches thick. They received two ounces of meat three times a week. Those with diarrhea received bean soup described as "coarse, dark, ill-tasting and repulsive." Due to bad and deficient food "their stomachs gave out," followed by indigestion, nausea, weakness and diarrhea often complicated with pneumonia. "So they suffer and die or return to the care of those for whom country, honor and them-selves have been sorely afflicted."[75]

Charges of cruel treatment including starvation were reported by the hospital newspaper as "palpable proofs of rebel brutality. This indictment should awaken righteous wrath against inhuman cruelties by the enemy to prisoners in Libby, Belle Isle and Andersonville prisons."

> By August 1864, there were long rows of beds with pale faces and glazed eyes staring at death. Their hands stretched out to invisible figures in delirium, to the hand of mother or sister or wife. There were long nights of vigil for the fevered brow, whispering through trembling lips words of cheer to encourage hope and to endure pain. The light of the new sunrise could not resuscitate the newly departed. Sights and sounds like these are compiled and echo in the chambers of hospital life. "I want to be with the boys in the Regiment, before I go to my mother." Once so eager for battle now weary of the march of life, by the roadside he falls and is gone, where his feet once tread on enemy soil. He was a prisoner on Belle Isle taken ill from exposure and want of food for months and months. His life waned and finally ended from a fearful hacking cough and unearthly luster of black eyes. He came back to die. "If I could only go home—I want to see Grandpa and Granny; I'll die and never see them again!" These were homesick tears.[76]

Two thousand eight hundred Union prisoners were transported from Savannah, Georgia, on a ship flying a flag of truce. *The Crutch* ran an extra edition on December 10, 1864, just to list patients admitted.

> The largest funeral, known in any hospital was witnessed here Tuesday last. At 10 a.m. thirteen ambulances held forty-three bodies of paroled men, many of whom had died on their passage here, drew up in line before the Chapel and was saluted by the hospital band with muffled drums, playing a solemn dirge. Tributes were delivered before a silent awestruck crowd.[77]

One of the patients described being stripped of hat, boots and most of his clothing.

> They took my money and possessions including family relics. I was forced to sleep on open ground without blanket and then marched 200 miles with little to eat. Deserters were taken out and shot along with civilians whose property was taken. Fifty prisoners were placed in filthy and crowded boxcars. No blankets were offered and many perished from cold and hunger. Scores were swept away by fevers, smallpox and other diseases. Some of the men had their arms amputated but it did not save their lives. Upon release, I weighed 108 pounds.[78]

In March 1865, returning prisoners arrived daily for two weeks. "Their conditions were a most pitiable one, starvation, wants of clothing and every convenience to secure cleanliness and refuge from cold and heat. Many have frozen feet. Hundreds were carried in as mere skeletons from the dock to the hospital."[79]

Doug Cole was the son of a Presbyterian minister from Michigan who was long a prisoner in Andersonville, Macon and other rebel camps. He attempted to escape in September 1864, but was recaptured. His diary told of the cruelties, hardships and privations. He lived only two weeks after hospital admission.

> It is more than the tongue can express. I have seen suffering and disease in most all forms and had not the power to alleviate the misery of one single sufferer. Over 3,000 have died since I've been here, which would be one sixth of the prisoners. Do our authorities know that thousands live with just hope day-to-day, threadbare and naked hoping for release? Do they know hundreds give up all hope and get discouraged and just lie down and die? I have not heard from my family in five months. I believe the day will come when the bonds of prisoners will be broken and the oppressed go free. There will be warm greetings from my parents, brothers and friends. Let me have patience—the patience of hope, and all will be well. I was so sick and weak with diarrhea and fever on the train from Andersonville.[80]

One hundred seventy paroled prisoners arrived under a flag of truce by steamer in the first week of April 1865, in a "low and wretched condition," and several died. Eight were officers and 100 were sent to the division hospital. Some had been prisoners for days but most for months. Spring season at the hospital seemed to work magic in restoring health and maintaining life. Lilac, crocus and magnolia were finishing their bloom, to be followed by violets, buttercups, and tulips. "Newly arrived were bluebirds, blackbirds, martins and swallows providing boys in blue lying in the grass a pretty picture with a bright promise of peace written on their radiant faces."[81]

"Some precautionary measures were taken that week by the Post Commandant against any sudden surprise from prowling rebels. The guards were stationed with guns ready to pepper the rascals. They have been seizing vessels in the bay and murdering citizens, not many miles off; it is wise to be on the lookout."[82] With the war ending, some wanted to preserve Libby Prison as monuments of the infamy of the rebel leaders. "We should maintain the discipline of these prisons and give rebel inmates the same rations given our unfortunate prisoners. Let the accommodations for sleeping be the same and that prisoners looking out the window be shot. Let those prisoners who object to northern prison camps be allowed to taste Libby. After the rebellion is subdued, let's burn them to the ground as final retribution."[83]

Ulysses S. Grant

Among the hospital's celebrated visitors was General Grant. He was on his way to Washington but stopped and received a hero's welcome by the surgeon in charge and an 18-piece hospital band. A biographical piece in the newspaper described Grant's spare but efficient and egalitarian field mess hall. "All is for use and economy of trouble and space." Dishes were plain, and camp cots, often without mattresses, served as beds. No wine or liquor was permitted for him or others. His clothes were threadbare, mostly flannel not linen. He dealt only with severe issues and not frivolities. He did not swear and rarely laughed, though he had a grim humor. An aide told the story of a meeting with a quartermaster sporting shined boots, immaculate attire and a fancy salute. Grant took him for a walk in the muddiest places until the boots were mud-covered and both men were soaked to the skin. His point was made.[84]

When Grant met Lee at Appomattox Courthouse to sign the surrender treaty, roses were in bud, violets and daffodils were in bloom, trees were green, and the air was still and silent. At 2 p.m. Sunday afternoon, Lee arrived first, followed minutes later by General Grant, accompanied only by Colonel Parker Chief of the Six Nations, a man of color. Lee was stooped a bit, wearing a dress suit in gray. Grant wore the same suit he wore in the field, without a sword, and offered parole for Confederate officers and their men. Officers could retain their side-arms and those who owned horses could take them home for spring plowing. Arms were stacked and 25,000 rations provided for the rebel army. He adhered to Lincoln's admonition to "let 'em up slowly" and avoid humiliating terms. The rebels were Americans citizens of a restored United States, not a degraded one. A parable about the rehabilitation of a captured Confederate parrot makes the point.

> A rebel parrot lost its owner at the Battle of Chickamauga. He was handsome enough but lacked an amiable disposition. He shouted "polys a soldier, polys worn her teeth off." When General Butler's name was read aloud from a newspaper article, the parrot replied: "Butler's a boot! Old Abe's a scare-

crow! Little Mac's a slow coach! Hurrah for Jefferson Davis!" Our parrot was a rebel and a most violent one. Attempts at conversion by singing union songs and locking her in the closet failed. She explored great holes in the chair, recovered stolen food from our plates, hairpins from our hair, and strings from our shoes and was as much a nuisance as a pet can be. She was a released prisoner of war taken into the house after falling and declining to go back to the hospital. The Union soldier treated the bird as if he was a nurse. He had picked the bird up previously in the battlefield, and thus became acquainted with her politics making her take the oath of allegiance. She vowed to shed her last feather in the Union cause, saying "old Abe's an honest man, honest man! He makes greenbacks! Polys a greenback!"[85]

The peace rainbow was darkened by a memoriam. One of the hospital's own, Miss Walker, who had for two years with quick wit delighted, nursed and generally cared for suffering soldiers, died of typhus fever after a short illness. "It was touching to see the soldier boys carrying the coffin of her who had been so good to them in their hours of pain."

The newspaper's Valedictory statement reiterated the goal of making its columns "open to the literary venture of the soldier, patriot and poet, each of whom has left some proof of his cherished love of liberty in law. We thank them for the precious legacies, borne of sunny imaginations. We remember the suffering and terror of that experience of which you gave burning evidence. A white cloud sailing out of the South, a breath of fragrance, a glimpse of the stainless blue of sky or sea, shall recall the hidden charm of life in the hospital."[86]

Six

Hammond Gazette

Key elements for a military hospital were well-drained soil for a septic system and a bountiful water supply. The one hospital that violated these principles and suffered the consequences was located at Point Lookout, Maryland. The Hammond U.S. Army General Hospital was built at the southern tip of a saber-toothed peninsula jutting south of Baltimore, anchored by a lighthouse and bounded on the west by the Potomac River and on the east Chesapeake Bay. This was a major route for British war ships during the War of 1812, providing a lookout for military activity, but failed to forestall the burning and sacking of America's capital city.

It was 90 miles south of Baltimore and 60 miles southeast of Washington, reachable by boat but not a standard destination for ships. There were arrivals and departures of steamers daily, delivering patients, supplies and newspapers. It was a flat plain with poor drainage, few shade trees, little grass and even less to recommend as a construction site. Summer sea breezes were modestly helpful in dispelling the sun's heat and the glare of the sandy beach. The outside of buildings were whitewashed with yellow in order to reflect summer heat.

Facing Chesapeake Bay was a small, two-story hotel and a series of cottages extending along the coast to the north. To accommodate 1,400 patients, 16 one-story pavilions with ridge ventilation were arranged like the spokes of a wheel, separated by 30 feet and connected with a two-story administration building. Eleven Wards were labeled A through K. Separate quarters were built for nuns, officers, guards, and contrabands. There was a baggage house, quartermaster offices, reading room and library, various kitchens and dining rooms and bakery, chapel, dead house, ice house, guard house, commissary building, stables, and printing office. The new replacement bakery turned out 20,000 loaves a day. The central axis of this wheel was a kitchen, laundry, guardhouse, knapsack room and water storage facility. The laundry was eventually partitioned into a washroom, drawing room, ironing room and engine room. Construction started in the summer of 1862 and took over a year to complete, though some parts were never finished.

The wards were 175' × 25' with 14 feet to the eaves and 18 inches from dirt to floor, holding 50 beds per ward. Roofs were covered with felt and coal tar sprinkled with white sand to reflect heat. Multiple windows encouraged ventilation and exposure to sunlight. There was a 16-inch-wide gap the whole length of the roof's central ridge with an overriding roof three feet wide.

A large water tank was built but "inflow and distributing pipes were late being installed and didn't work particularly well" despite the presence of a steam-engine and force-pump. It was elevated on a platform over a bathroom fitted with eight tubs designed

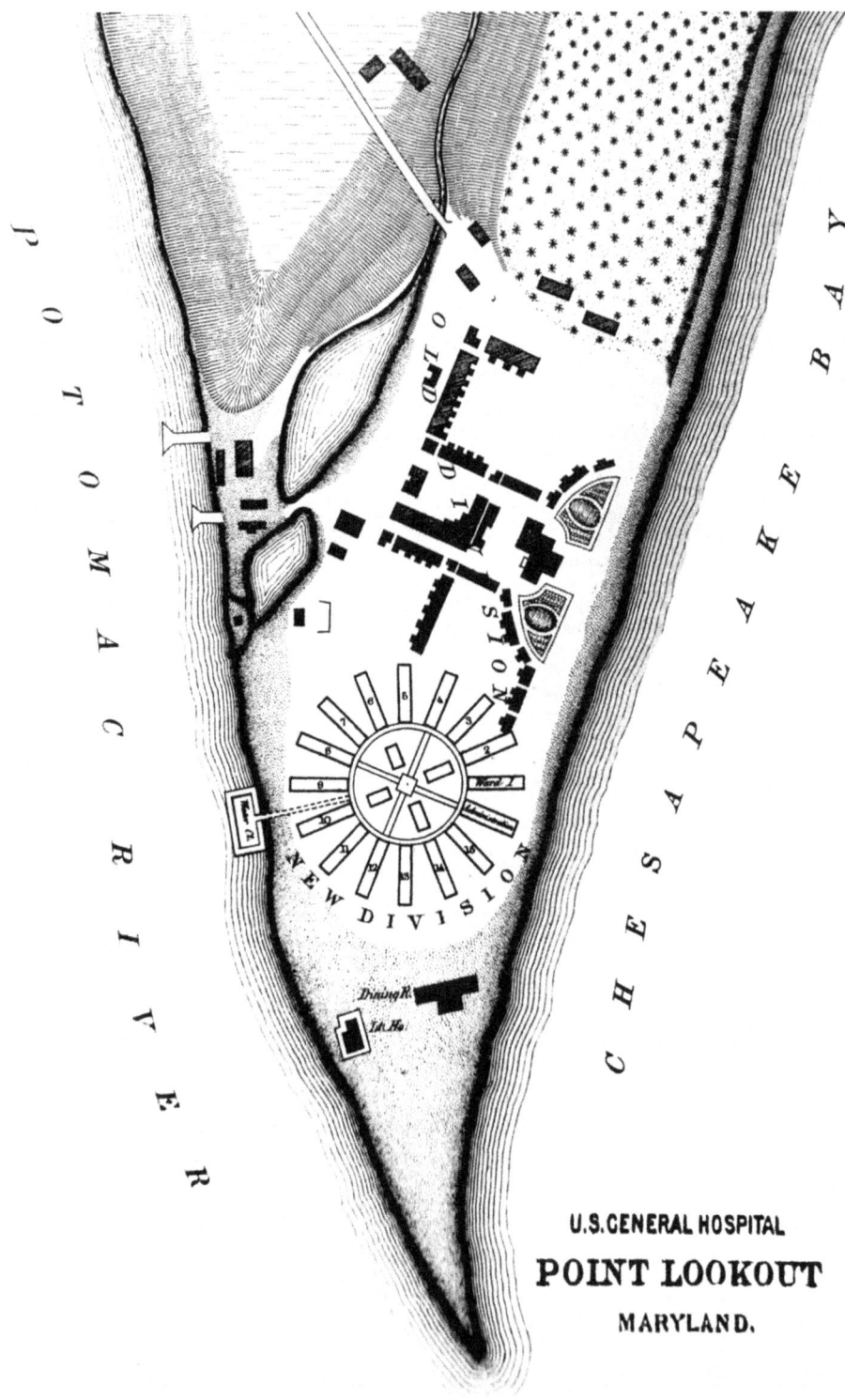

Hammond U.S. Army General Hospital. Point Lookout, Maryland. *Medical and Surgical History of the War of Rebellion.* Part III, Vol. 1. Pg. 943.

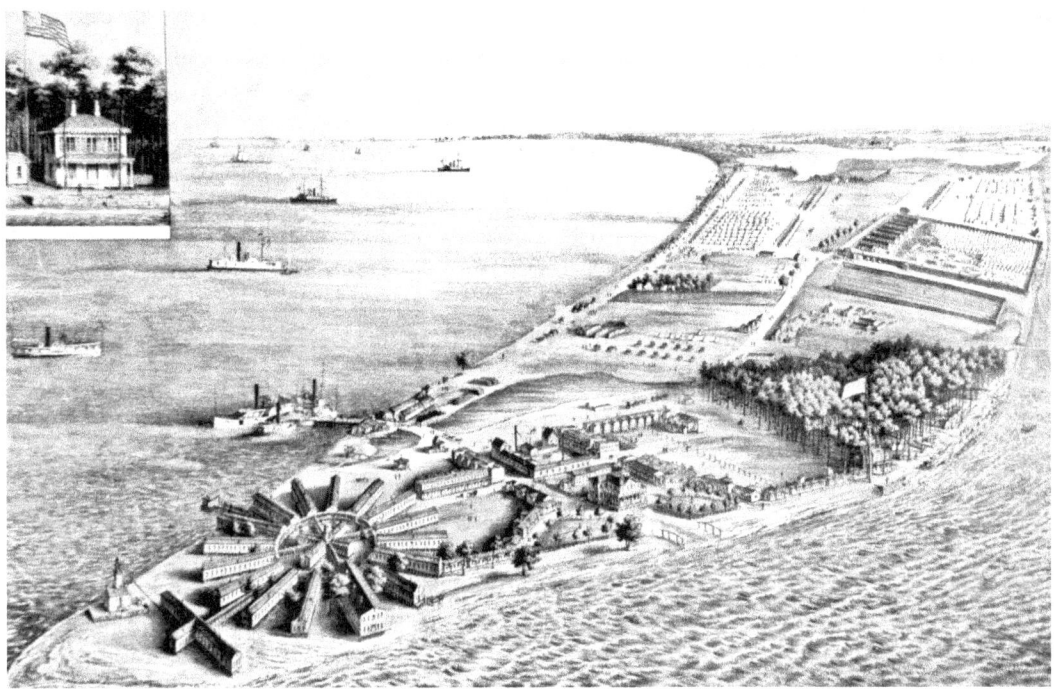

Hammond U.S. Army General Hospital. Chromolithograph (author's collection).

to supply hot and cold water. Patients were exposed in a room too dark and too wet from leaks. The Chapel was 85' × 24' × 20' with an elevated stage and sat 400.[1]

A stone's throw from the hospital was the largest of the Confederate prisoner of war camps, located on 40 acres and surrounded by a fourteen foot fence. Their black guards worked day and night shifts and lived in local barracks. They could be as brutal as white guards in Southern camps, some having no sympathy for former masters while others showed acts of kindness. From 1862–1865, 50,000 Confederate prisoners lived in tents with no heat and a polluted water supply. There were 3,384 known dead, buried in mass graves. The camp's 6.6 percent mortality rate would have been less than half the death rate of the battlefield and one-fourth of Andersonville or Elmira, New York.

Today Point Lookout is a state park with glistening summer beaches conducive to swimming, fishing, bird-watching, kayaking, sailing and camping. Paranormal groups have studied sounds thought to be wandering ghosts of Confederate souls still suffering from the torments of prison camp. Much of the former hospital site is now under water.

On July 20, 1864, Secretary of War Edward Stanton defined proper military hospital construction using as source reference a textbook written by the Surgeon General he had removed from office by courts martial. No water was available from a nearby town, spring or reservoir, and collected rain water was an unreliable source. The main supply was seven wells each 12 feet deep, but "the water often caused irritation of the bowels in newcomers."[2] Drainage was poor, the water brackish, and sewers inadequate. Sinks were built over the Potomac River on which the free ends of the Western pavilions abutted. Having thousands of nearby prisoners with similar sanitary facilities, connecting ponds and a common aquifer was "prone to cause diarrhea."

The quality of water was determined by its looks: if you could see through it, it was considered potable. Water filtration by canvas bag removed sticks and gravel but not organisms whose existence was unknown. Satisfactory disposal of excreta from hospital wards required a reliable water supply and an effective septic system. The leading cause of death in the Civil War was diarrhea-dysentery. Inspectors at Point Lookout noted the "water supplied was not of good quality."[3] An outbreak of disease prompted General E. Hines to issue new orders on April 13, 1864.

> There will be no horses within 150 yards of buildings. Proper sinks and urinals will be constructed over water [the Potomac River] and its use mandatory day or night, to be enforced by both Regimental and Hospital Guards. All trenches now used as sinks are to be filled up and covered with clean gravel. All other cottages and buildings are to be thoroughly cleaned of all litter and filth and placed in barrels or boxes and removed daily. All buildings are to be policed and kept clear of garbage, filth and animals. No offal, slop or litter of any kind is to be dumped upon ground or pond but put into barrels and boxes and removed daily. Dumps, prisoner of war camps, and slaughter houses are to be cleaned out and policed daily. Carcasses of all horse and other animals are to be buried or burned. The above regulations will be enforced by inspector general and field officer of the day.[4]

The *Hammond Gazette* was a small sheet newspaper published on hospital grounds every Tuesday with the byline "for the benefit of the sick and wounded at Hammond General Hospital."[5] Each issue listed those admitted, furloughed, deserted, transferred, returned to duty, died or discharged from the service. Names of the hospital's medical officers were posted with assigned wards. The price was five cents a copy or for three months 50 cents "in advance." It ran from November 1862 through June 1865. Thirteen copies were located for review from February 10, 1863, through August 29, 1864.

To raise funds, lithographs of Point Lookout were sold at $1.50 each. Printing of ballots, broadsides, military orders, and envelopes with hospital addresses helped cover expenses. Favorable press coverage was expected for those providing generous printing jobs. General Benjamin Butler, expert in attracting cash or gold, gave his agent Casimir Bohn of Fort Monroe, Virginia, exclusive right to import and sell within the department daily and weekly newspapers so "parties so interested in this shall be aware." Military authorities allowed regulators to protect this right by imposing fees to sell papers outside the hospital.[6]

Copies were exchanged with the *Baltimore Daily Clipper*, the *Hospital Friend* of the Continental Hospital of Baltimore, and *The Soldiers' Journal*. The latter was called a "small army paper published at Camp distribution outside Alexandria Virginia, printed on excellent paper and from clear type making a fine appearance and promises to win a name for itself among the journals of the larger size. Long may they be afloat."[7]

Waverly Magazine and the *Boston Medical and Surgical Journal* [New England Journal of Medicine] were also exchanged and made available to all in the hospital reading room. Whether from larceny or selfishness, leaving an issue for others to read was not a priority for some and was reason for the chaplain's complaint to the "powers that be." "Just a few hours after these papers are placed they are stolen. The mischief is done by those who are disposed to evil and do not care whether others have the benefit of these papers or not."[8]

Advertisements

Advertisements were an important source of revenue but because of location there were few local businesses. J. Hobson Company was on campus and sold "a large assort-

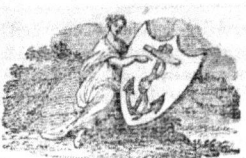

Logo of *Hammond Gazette* (personal collection).

ment of the latest stationery and have a supply of tobacco and cigars of better quality and cheaper than can be obtained elsewhere on the Point. We sell at least 10 percent cheaper than any other place in the vicinity thus making it your interest to give us a call." Bay oysters were a desirable feature on any menu, especially the brand new Union Oyster Saloon. The Sanitary Commission ran its voluminous ads about their many offices located throughout the Union, including an aid to locate soldiers. The Directory of Hospitals was open from 8 a.m. to 8 p.m. and open to "any with a friend in the Army, members of Congress, soldier aid societies, or clergy."

Northern states needed "colored troops" to fill its black regiments and had agents recruiting in Philadelphia, Baltimore, Annapolis, Alexandria, and Washington. An ad requested "sound" men, between 20 and 45, bound or free to be enlisted and mustered into the U.S. service. Free men would get a $400 bounty in Maryland, and if resident of Baltimore an additional $200. Slaves received $100 from the state, his master another $100 and if loyal another $300 from the U.S. government.[9] Those sent to Northern states to satisfy quotas dealt with profiteering agents who mostly kept the bounty, leaving little for the black recruits, a practice legal in some states though a violation of federal laws. In Connecticut the state provost marshal was tried and convicted of fee-splitting with agents denying black soldiers their rightful bonus money. It was overturned by Secretary Stanton thanks to the interference of Governor William Buckingham, who pointed out that what was illegal by federal law was in fact legal by Connecticut law. The provost, a Buckingham appointee, was returned to his post instead of jail.

Stories included the effects of summer drought on Maryland's vegetable farmers rescued by "providential" rain, battles fought by successful generals, and failures of the confederates. Fictional stories referencing actual events offered entertaining and sometimes informative interludes for its readers. An elderly "lady" presided as hostess of a large house with "darkies" and a number of pretty girls, three allegedly her "daughters" provide companionship for Generals with gleaming epaulets, dangling swords, voluminous handkerchiefs and boots with spurs. No civilians were about. Slaves played piano, banjo and violin for waltzing and feasting in a South "supposedly starving." A Confederate militia man attacks Union officers at the party but is subdued, tried and shot the next day. After that episode, only the other big houses in the area got favors from the army, not the one with the widow and three daughters.[10]

Surgeon General Hammond

It was not surprising that the hospital namesake would be vehemently defended if necessary. William Hammond was 11 years an assistant army surgeon who despite being stationed in frontier posts published medical experiments and observations, winning him national awards. Peacetime in the army meant no promotions, and being recently married caused him to resign and become University professor in Maryland, where his family had been early founders. Appointment at age 33 as Surgeon General reversed the seniority system, enforcing the modernization of the antiquated medical corps. In so doing, he created and then antagonized unforgiving enemies. Initially there was firm support from the eastern establishment, including the McClellan family and the American Medical Association. A letter to the editor about his grand new program came from a Washington source: "We have an excellent Surgeon General. We shall achieve great things." In Hammond's time of need, he stood alone, few coming to his defense. Opposition to his programs came from the Department of War and physicians from western states, as this editorial reply from the *Gazette* indicates.

> *A grunt from Cincinnati.* There is a fine suggestion of pork packing pigheadedness in the following paragraph: "Surgeon General Hammond has just received a report from the regular medical profession of Cincinnati Ohio. The report is disrespectful and strongly condemns the Surgeon General's prohibition of the use of calomel striking it from the medical supply table. They recommended removing Hammond which would "meet the approbation of the profession, be of advantage to our soldiers, and a credit to the government."[11]

> We deny the capacity of the "regular medical profession of Cincinnati Ohio" to pass judgment upon propriety or use of calomel in Army hospital practice. The only malady in which their medicos have ever had any experience is measles peculiar to swine districts. They know nothing about the ills which the soldier is liable, such as bombshells, bullets and bayonets. Their ideas are limited to calomel and saltpeter both in connection with pigs. We would not allow them to cut off a leg even for $50 as every cut would produce a pork chop. The bacon of the pig may be saved by the Cincinnati practitioner, the bacon of the soldier never. To bristle up is natural enough for Cincinnati practitioners, but if he *must* grunt all the way to Washington let him grunt like a well-bred animal of the pure Berkshire breed, instead of giving vent to a "disrespectful" *honk*.[12]

One of the complications of calomel [mercury] treatments was gangrene of the maxillary cavities. Hammond rounding in New York and Washington hospitals saw the devastating complication and the heroic attempts to reconstruct by Gurdon Buck, the first American plastic surgeon. Calomel or "blue mass" was used for a wide variety of ailments, but its adverse side effects led him to ban its use from the U.S. Pharmacopeia along with tartar emetic [antimony], another vile compound whose ingestion offered no known benefit to mankind. Since many experienced physicians routinely used these chemicals, a national protest was launched, putting Hammond on the defensive and leaving him a general whose orders were ignored.

Antagonisms from bypassed senior medical officers, personality conflicts with his boss, Secretary Stanton, and failure to support the administration policies in an election year led to his courts martial and dismissal, just 14 months after his appointment, on trumped-up charges before a rigged jury. No medical officer sat in judgment, and some witnesses were men he had previously helped convict of bribery and real estate fraud. Instead of leaving town with pride and pension intact, he demanded a trial, which took five months. His self-published, 61-page booklet detailing his innocence did not prevent a guilty verdict, forcing him to move to New York City in the summer of 1864 and start a new career as one of America's first neurologists. He was denied a pension, which brought pain in old age when his finances collapsed. Attempts to get Congress to reverse the trials' verdict and get a pension failed.

The Armory Square Hospital in Washington was pro-administration with no allegiance to Hammond and was viciously gleeful at his downfall in August and September 1864.

> William Hammond convicted at court-martial January through June 1864 on charges of defrauding the government out of large amounts of money in contracts with several parties for flannels, medical supplies and hospital stores. He was dismissed from the service with no pension, and disqualified from holding any office of honor, or profit or trust under the government of the United States. President Lincoln approved the sentence. We don't know that a more severe punishment could have been inflicted on such a man. If so, it should have been resorted to. An old patient said, "Put them on a special diet for 30 days and allow him nothing but the deep extract he contracted for and had supplied for hospital use." "Maybe 15 days would be enough." The crime he was convicted of is a most flagrant one cheating sick and suffering men out of what was indispensable to save life, to their medicine, wholesome diet and good stimulants. The crime he was convicted of is "far more flagrant than that was of the murderer of the first modern Abel. Cain slew one not hundreds."[13]

> *The Boston Transcript* showed similar sentiments. "The District attorney filed a suit against the late official for $450,000 defrauded out of the government. The court-martial, the Judge Advocate, and the President all believe Hammond guilty of these enormous offenses compared with which the wickedness of the common highway robber or the poisoner is light. Yet he is only dismissed and disgraced. Is this justice? Is this common sense? Death or imprisonment for life would in military law be held the only proper punishment for such gigantic crimes."

> We at the *Armory Gazette* feel the sentence is very light when we consider the crime: "Purchase of inferior medical supplies and stores, compromising health and comfort and jeopardizing lives of sick and wounded soldiers suffering in hospitals and upon the battlefields."[14]

Sermons

Sermons emphasized honor, duty and sacrifice. Truth and justice opposed ignorance and prejudice. The war was punishment for the sins of its citizens. It was God's will that slavery be abolished, and patriotic citizens were to act as His instrument.

> Fault finding because of the government's slow progress in putting down the rebellion is giving aid and comfort to the traitors and hindering and impeding our side. It encourages our enemies. Is it not treason to encourage the enemy? It is a time of stern war where fate of humanity and civilization is at stake. Let us do our duty by patience and endurance.[15]

The truth is, no political party is essential to the well-being of our republic and there are good and bad men in all parties. But the effect of party zeal and prejudices is to lead people to support their rulers right or wrong on the ground that they must defer to their party. The spirit of patriotism is not yet extinguished in many hearts and that opposition and trial has refined it like gold in the fire. We are fighting in obedience to the ordinance of God who has made us a nation and in the end will sustain us and render us more prosperous, happier, purer and more glorious than ever before. War is to purge us from our sins and political corruptions and remove scales of ignorance and prejudice from the southern masses. There should be no debating with the south and reunification only without slavery.[16]

By March 1863, the exigencies of war demanded even more sacrifice. The following sermon on the good fight promised eternal joy and salvation for the righteous consummation of God's will.

Why wish to live?[17]
Why wish to live? To battle, struggle on:
Gasping, panting, reeling through life's storm
With bleeding hearts, and hope a battered shred.
Which ne'er distrust the slumbering silent dead?
Hopes of the future! Painted from the past
When all was bright, and ere the die was cast.

Prepare to die! And when life's setting sun
Warns you that its sands are nearly run,
Be strong in mind, resigned and strong at heart,
And know that soul and body shall forever part;
And calmly say, as you await the tide,
"Thy will, oh God be done-not mine!"

Sacrifice

The volunteers would continue to make whatever sacrifice was required, but the source of willing, able-bodied men was running out. Those who had already served were offered bounty to re-enlist, but a draft was needed to fill the gap.

"Say what's to be done with this window dear Jack; the wind rushes in it every crack!"
Replied Jack, "I know little of carpenter craft, but I think my dear wife you will have to go through the very same process the rest of us do, that is—you must list, or submit to the *draft*!"[18]

English papers were astonished at the resilience and strength of this undisciplined volunteer army and the attraction to American shores. European wars were about geography, aristocracies and nationalism, not individual human rights.

The war has created something great which will survive the war. The United States were once only material for a great power, but now they are one. British Conservatives oppose the Union [one man one vote]. Ireland the bright recruiting ground is being depleted of its hardy peasantry at 10,000 souls per month by emigration to this country.[19]

The telegraph allowed prompt dispersal of news. The first week of July 1863 was the most momentous of the war, followed world-wide. "The Army of the Potomac has made some rapid movements under its new head reaching the town of Gettysburg on Wednesday. We regret to learn that Major General John Reynolds was mortally wounded and has since died. Brigadier General Paul was killed in the same engagement. Rumors of the death of General Lee abound." General Meade's dispatches from the field were soon published for all to see, along with related news items.

The enemy attacked us at 4 p.m. of this date [July 3, 1863] and after one of the severest contests of the war was repulsed at all points. We have suffered considerably in killed and wounded and have taken a large number of prisoners. General Longstreet and A.P. Hill's forces were much injured yesterday and many general officers killed. We thus far have 1,600 prisoners.[20]

Remaining in hospital are 1,124. Eight patients return to duty. 145 patients arrived on the steamer *George Washington* from Baltimore. The steamer *Balloon* brought 175 more from the same place. The steamer *Belvidere* arrived Saturday bringing 480 also from the same place.[21]

On the same date, another momentous battle took place in Vicksburg, Mississippi. A victorious outcome was prematurely but correctly announced by the Union press. "It turns out the workman of the Navy yard were deceived this morning by a false report on the fall of Vicksburg. There is no truth in the report whatever."

The enemy seemed on the run on all fronts with the end in sight the summer of 1863. "*The New York Times* predicted an attack on Richmond lead by Generals Dix and Keys who were moving with a heavy force to a city finally within reach."[22]

Politics

The Democratic Party Convention in Chicago during the summer of 1864 had planks that were anathema to the Lincoln administration, the *Gazette's* editorial board and its readers. This included opposition to the Emancipation Proclamation, thought unconstitutional, opposition to blacks as soldiers, arbitrary arrests, suppression of speech and press, loyalty oaths, and proclamation of martial law. Lincoln asked the rebels to lay down their arms, return their allegiance and submit to the laws of the land. The war would cease and states would be restored with the right to determine their institutions, minus slavery.

Lincoln and Copperheads

The commander-in-chief was a frequent visitor of military hospitals. There was no shortage of literature concerning the soldiers' favorite.

President Lincoln was asked for a pass to Richmond. "I would be happy to oblige you if my passes were respected; but the fact is sir I have written the past two years passes for 250,000 men to go to Richmond and not one has got there yet."[23]

Why is the president like an owl in the daytime? Because he's a blinkin.' (Abe Lincoln).

LINCOLN: "A henchman eh? I thought you are a native of New York. You speak English well for a henchman Mr. Wood. I wish I could speak Hench as well as you do English."
WOOD: "There is a cry for peace. Our poor lambs of New York have been terribly cut up by this foul and unnatural war. Thousands of them are fertilizing the soil by mingling their dust with it. Pandora's box is wide open."
LINCOLN: "Why doesn't she then keep it shut? Shut it down and sit on it. I think you are an agent in Pandora's interest."
WOOD: "When are you going to put your foot down on this fratricidal, destructive and wasteful war?"
LINCOLN: "That's been said before. Is your mission to obtain the use of my foot for quashing the noblest effort made by a great nation to keep itself intact?"
Wood proposed a truce, believing the promise and motives of the noble fire eaters of the South, as do his followers.

LINCOLN: "Why don't you go and live with the religious fire eaters of the South? You shall have a free pass over the lines. I gave one to Vallandigham. Sic Semper Copperheadibus!"
WOOD: "I find I am not making any impression on you with regard to the movement for peace. It is fearful to see a human being at your time of life addicted to wallowing in [blood], Mr. Lincoln."
LINCOLN: "I am."
WOOD: "Perhaps, I am boring you with my presence, Mr. Lincoln."
LINCOLN: "You are."[24]

Wood, a leading copperhead, became mayor of New York and a Congressman whose biting tongue made him a favorite antagonist and target.

A large and enthusiastic Peace Democrat meeting was held at Cooper Institute in New York under the auspices of the notorious Fernando Wood. Extremely violent and denunciatory speeches on and resolutions against the Administration and the war were made and passed. Mr. Wood gave evidence that Lincoln was extremely rotten and corrupt at the heart. His views were the same as Vallandigham. At a meeting in the White House Congressman Wood was offered a glass of wine—a decanter of mushroom ketchup known as his favorite tipple. He protested to any who still listened: "My speech concerned peace on earth and goodwill. We peace Democrats are but shorn lambs, standing on a hilltop and bleating for a tempered wind. I am but a poor henchman of the peace apostles and a humble henchman at that."[25]

Copperheads did not receive favorable hospital press. The *Gazette* defined them as chronic complainers treated with rebuke by the Union soldier. "A professional growler about the war criticizes everybody including Generals whom he says are blockheads and blunderers."[26] National election results demonstrated that the growlers opposed to the administration had their comeuppance, in this satirical piece.

This war has done one thing at least. It has developed more military generals in any other war in history. There are men in every village in the north with their feet cocked upon the stove, cigar in their mouth, a gin cocktail in hand who will fight a better battle in ten minutes than ever afforded by Caesar or Napoleon. I have no doubt there are those in this room who can capture Vicksburg or Charleston while a man is trying on his cravat, marching into Richmond in forty seconds and putting down the rebellion in half an hour. Halleck and Hooker are good enough as far as they go, but they have no military genius. To find that quality you must come North and mix among the bar room and fireside heroes.[27]

Immigrants

Foreign minorities were considered fair literary game. Unlike other papers, there were few satirical articles about blacks, perhaps because many served guard duty at the nearby Confederate prison camp. The *Gazette* noted that their pay was three dollars less at $10 a month but the rations, clothing and equipment were equal to their white counterpart. They joked that "old timed abolitionists had become negro-insurrectionists," in supporting arming the blacks.

An Irishman on trial pleaded not guilty. The state called Mr. Furkisson as witness.
"Do I understand your honor that Mr. Furkisson is to be a witness against me? Well then your honor I plade guilty sur an' yer honor plaise, not because I am guilty for I'm as innocent as yer honors suckling baby but must on account of saving Mr. Furkisson's soul."[28]

Pat's evasive answer—Patrick O'Neil was in the service of Father Conley. The priest was expecting a visit from a Protestant minister whom he wished not to see, asking Patrick to make it so.
"Make some excuse and send him away."
"What shall I tell him? Would you have me tell a lie, your reverence?"

"No, but get rid of him. *An evasive answer* will do."
Father Conley retired to his library and Patrick went about his business.
"Well Patrick, did the minister call to see me today?"
"Yes sir."
"Did you get rid of him?"
"I did."
"Did he ask if I was in?"
"He did."
"What answer did you give?"
"I gave him an *evasive answer*. He asked was ye in, and I asked him was his grandmother a monkey."[29]

Lo. The poor refugee. A Jew named Barnstine and his wife were arrested a few miles from here hailing from Richmond claiming they had been robbed before leaving Virginia. While searching the person of Mr. Barnstine, they found a secret belt with several hundred dollars in silver and gold. In the ladies petticoat were six gold watches with setting of diamonds, valuable rings, thousands in bank notes both confederate and greenbacks, watch chains and other articles of jewelry. They have been held for further examination.[30]

Terrorism

For decades the South had warned of a slave insurrection, while the North feared attacks by terrorist agents bent on kidnapping free men of color that would escalate to general mayhem and destruction after hostilities began. To boost morale, both sides resorted to calls for increasing violence as a way to victory. The *Gazette* often reported the incendiary remarks allegedly emanating from the Palmetto states.

> The *Richmond Whig* recommends a plan to burn all major northern cities. Millions of dollars would lie in ashes in New York, Boston, Philadelphia, Chicago, Pittsburg and Washington. There are daring men in Canada, Morgan's militia and other commands who have escaped Yankee dungeons and would rejoice at an opportunity of doing something that would make all Yankees howl with anguish and consternation. Under the circumstances this is justifiable, legitimate and right. If confederate government rejects this project there are private citizens who can carry it out. Enough money would raise the right men for the job. Canada would make an excellent jumping off point.[31]

One example of a terrorist attack was the murder of Surgeon Fairchild in Texas. He had an escort of 26 men who were attacked by 50. The Doctor and nine others left behind were found "mutilated, castrated, and faces beaten in with butt of rifles. The Doctor was shot through the head and shoulders." A witness stated that he informed the assailants of the doctor's status and that he was on a mission to treat others.

A piece labeled *Murderous assault* described two Hammond Hospital attendants on a Sunday afternoon while visiting the pines being attacked by "drunken natives of secession views. One soldier was severely beaten and the other shot through the head." Maryland had Southern sympathies, and rebel prisoners escaping to friendly environs remained a possibility.

The flow of captured rebels accelerated with the activities of General Grant and the Army of the Potomac in the spring of 1864. A steamer arrived from Petersburg with 175 prisoners, another with 50 from Baltimore and 400 rebel officers from Belle Plain, with a total of 1,300 needing placement. "At the rate they are pouring in we shall soon have the 'pride of the south' on Point Lookout. General Grant must have struck the back bone of the rebellion such a heavy blow that it will take a better doctor than Jeff Davis to heal the wounds."[32] Steamers also brought 204 wounded from Sheridan's front in just one day. Dealing with mass casualties, many with no prior medical treatment, became an ordinary occurrence for military hospitals.

Freedom of Press

In several hospitals "corruption" charges were filed against medical chiefs of staff who were summarily arrested and then released. Arresting editors and reporters without charge, closing newspaper offices and destroying presses was a feature of this era. Negative criticisms of a local officer's treatment of soldiers produced forceful retaliation. Rough treatment of ordinary soldiers, often immigrant, such as forced sitting on a wooden horse, was demeaning and counter-productive. Freedom of the press required eternal vigilance, lest it vanish and along with it other precious rights.

> *Outrage upon the press.* On Tuesday night we were suddenly aroused from sleep and found a man with a drawn saber at the front door. We escaped and called some friends. The vandals smashed in windows, sashes and panes, upset the whole printing office and then knocked over all the type. It is nothing less than house breaking and robbery. What is the cause of this outrage? As faithful chroniclers of the times, we have in the past mentioned the acts of Major Brown and his command confining strictly to facts. We would be pleased to devote our small columns merely for entertaining the patient and suffering soldiers for whom the paper is printed. We confine ourselves strictly to facts and indulge in no personalities to which objection could be taken, excepting by those to whom the truth is unpalatable. We bear no ill against the guard here as a body. We were first called upon to publish an account of the illegal arrest of the surgeon in charge of the hospital and his forcible ejection from quarters by Major Brown. This clearly unjustifiable act accompanied by personal indignity to Dr. Wagner was described by the highest officer of our department as "gross usurpation of authority." He is innocent until proven guilty in this unjust action.[33]
>
> In addition we were compelled to mention operations against the contraband and in our last issue that of the dining room to make allusion to the degrading punishment of "bucking and gagging" against which General Winfield Scott once issued an order. We know that the outrage on Tuesday night was due to our columns and was committed by soldiers of the guard without doubt. One of them conferred with another days ago prophesizing the press should be "smashed." We understand it was intended as a "warning." That means if it is not palatable to a few men here we shall further suffer and that freedom of the press is threatened. We solemnly warn them we shall defend our rights at the expense of life and respectively call attention of the commanding officer to this necessity. Soldiers of the New York Battalion not yet fortunate to meet our country's enemies have only to show their "most gallant" exploit in a night attack on two unarmed fellow soldiers and destruction of a little paper published for the amusement of a few hundred sick soldiers. You are waging war against the very men you were sent to protect. Do you know that General Schenck, the energetic head of this department recently imprisoned an editor for uttering disloyal sentiments? Do you think he will countenance the destruction of the only loyal paper in this county? We shall fearlessly continue to do our duty as impartial journalists![34]

In the next edition of the paper, a calming voice was heard. "Your squabbles with Major Brown have been really entertaining."[35]

The surgeon in charge had under his command the quartermaster, 13 assistant surgeons, one chaplain, two medical cadets, two hospital stewards, one chief steward and three assistants. Reveille was at 5 a.m., breakfast at 6 a.m., fatigue call at 6:30 a.m., surgeons call at 8 a.m., daily inspection at 10 a.m., dinner at noon, fatigue call at 1 p.m., supper at 6 p.m., tattoo at 9 p.m., and taps at 9:30 p.m. Church call was every Sunday at 10:30 a.m. This schedule was similar to others in the federal hospital system. By December 1864, there were 1,400 beds of which 450 were occupied.

Romance and Marriage

Women masquerading as male soldiers was worthy of report. A Long Island girl named Fanny Wilson, while visiting her relatives in Indiana, met a lad from New Jersey and promptly fell in love. She and another woman enlisted in this regiment just to be near their romantic interests. They marched, drilled and provided nursing care for the sick and wounded while disguised. They were discovered to be women and promptly discharged, but undaunted repeated their adventure.[36]

A constant topic for young men with a pulse was young women. How did one find true love and what secrets needed revealing? What follows were the soldiers' and humorists' conclusions on kissing, courting, marriage, intemperance and infidelity.

> A jealous woman cannot be cured either by word or deed. She resembles a kettle-drum which of all instruments is the most difficult to tune and keep that way.
>
> It is just as sensible a move to undertake to get married without courting as to attempt to succeed in business without advertising.
>
> An old topper was advising a youngster to get married "because then you'll have somebody to pull off yer boots when you get home drunk."

On Kissing

When a Cape Cod girl is kissed she says, "What are you about?"
NANTUCKET: "Sheer off or I'll split your mainsail with a typhoon!"
BOSTON: "I think you should be ashamed."
ALBANY: "I reckon it's my turn now," and gives him a box on the ear that he won't forget for a month.
LOUISIANA: She smiles, blushes deeply and says nothing.
PENNSYLVANIA: She puts on her bonnet and says "I am astonished at the assurance Jedidiah, and for this indignity I'll sew thee up."
Western ladies are so fond of kissing that when saluted on one cheek they instantly present the other.
JERSEY GIRL: "Now Josh your better hugging a body."
PHOENIXVILLE: "I dare you to do that again."
POTTSTOWN: "O hush."
BRISTOL: "I'll tell your mother."
MAINE: "I sweow ef I don't tell my marm."[37]

In a Chicago Tribune "wants" column:

This is leap year. I'll wait no longer and here I am. 21 years old, healthy, prepossessing, medium size, full chest, educated, prudent, large sparkling eyes, and long black flowing hair and as full of fun as a chestnut full of meat, born to make some man happy, and want a home. Does anybody want me?

Josh Billings on romance and marriage.

Tha tell me that females are so scarce in the far western kuntry that a grat menny married wimmin are already engaged to the sekund and third husbands.

I hev finally kum to the konklusion that a good, reliable set ov bowels is worth more tu a man than eny quantity ov branes or wives.

Squire Crane, Justice of the peace in Missouri knew less of law and legal forms than about killing bears. His first marriage ceremony went thusly.

"Miss Susan Roots, do you love that 'ar man?"

"Nothin' shorter!" she laughed.

"And you John Kennon, do you take Sue for better and worser?"

"Sartin' as shootin'," said John while chucking Sue under the chin.

"Then you both, individually and collectively do promise to love, honor and obey each other world without end? If that be the case know all men by those present, that this 'ere twain aforesaid is hereby made bone of one bone, and flesh of one flesh; and furthermore, may *the Lord have mercy upon their souls!* Amen!"[38]

A wife's cure for a bad habit. A newly married wife living in New Orleans found her other half coming home frequently late at night in a state of "oblivious forgetfulness." As usual he arrived at midnight staggered into the bedchamber and fell asleep. She procured a large darning needle threaded it with twine and sewed him into the blanket. About 10 a.m. the neighborhood was startled by distressing cries and rushed in to rescue supposing murder was being committed. He was bound as tightly as a bale of cotton in the blanket of his own bed. As they tried to extricate him in rushed his wife; "Cut not a thread! I did it. He shall lie there till he makes a solemn promise never to come home drunk again." He declared he would keep better hours and drink less rum. In the future, if he is disposed to take a little too much she can just say "take care Sir, or I'll sew you up."[39]

"I like to tend weddings," said Mrs. Parrington. "I like to see young people come together with the promise to love cherish and honor each other. But it is a solemn thing—is matrimony—a very solemn thing where the minister comes into the chancery with his vestments on and goes through the ceremony of making them man and wife. It should be husband and wife for it isn't every husband that turns out to be a man. I declare I never shall forget when Paul put the nuptial ring on my finger and said with my goods I thee endow. He used to keep a dry good store then and I thought he was going to give me the whole there was in it. I was young and simple and didn't know till afterwards that it only meant one calico dress a year. It is a lovely sight to see young people 'plight the trough' as the song says and coming up to consume their vows."[40]

The case of Joe Stanberry. Mrs. Esther Stanberry was draining a bucket of water from the hydrant when she saw an old basket suspended from the knob of her front door. She saw something move and found a piece of paper addressed to her husband.

To Joe Stanberry—"Sir I send you the baby which you will please take care and bring upright so that it may turn out better than you it's daddy. Who would think such a staid old spindle shanks could be such a tearing down center! The Child is yours, you may swear to that. Look at it—it is Joe Stanberry all over. You deceived me shamefully letting on to be a widower; but do a father's part by the young one and I'll forgive you. Yours heartbroken, Nancy. P.S. don't let that sharp nose wife of your see this letter. Win her over first with some kind of story about the baby."

Mr. Stanberry was eating his supper quietly as the storm began to brew. His wife's voice called out "Stanberry, come up here you villain, here is a mess for you! Don't you want to see Nancy the heartbroken?" shouted Mrs. Stanberry. "Nancy! What Nancy's that?" said the sly old rogue with well feigned perplexity. "Nancy is the mother of the baby that's been hung up at your door. You look mighty innocent so just read that letter and look in the basket. It won't bite; it's got no teeth poor thing. You'll know it for as your hussy says, it's just like you all over."

The room was soon full of spectators anxious to witness the unwrapping of the baby. As rag after rag was unwrapped the movements increased vigorously. Mrs. Stanberry said, "it is full of the devil already and that shows it's his. You will soon see it is like him and everything."

Out jumped a big tomcat![41]

Dr. Esmarch and U.S. Military Hospitals

Hammond U.S. Army General Hospital found its way into European medical literature thanks to Dr. Friedrich Esmarch. He was one of Europe's finest military surgeons of the nineteenth century, having written landmark books on the treatment of gunshot wounds. The German government projected a prolonged and costly war for the late 1860s and recruited him, then age 45, as superintendent of a department of surgery in Berlin, with the goal of planning the most modern of military hospitals. This culminated in a manual detailing a state of the art medical facility with 4,500 beds. He included a chapter replete with drawings and lithographs of eight U.S. Military Hospitals of the Civil War, later published in the MSHWR. Thanks to the American experience which included Point Lookout, he was able to detail the latest advances in sanitation, ventilation, barracks construction and design.[42]

Seven

The Cartridge Box

York County, Pennsylvania, was one of the richest farming regions in the Union, a cornucopia of abundance and a tempting target for the bedraggled, shoeless and famished Army of Northern Virginia. Confederate goals were to capture the capital of a Union state, replenish a depleted army, and rest a war-weary Virginia soil. If successful, recognition by European powers might follow that would break the blockade of Southern shipping. Three quarters of York's tax payers were German and the rest Dutch. Local resident and hospital surgeon A. R. Blair called them "Dutch cheese and sour kraut."[1] Some had relatives in North Carolina and Georgia and sympathies for secessionists. The local paper, the *York Gazette*, was the voice of the Democratic Party, representing the local majority sentiment, and described Philadelphia as a hot bed of abolitionists. Lincoln carried Pennsylvania by 20,000 votes in 1864 but lost here; the *Gazette* lamented, "four years more of such a rogue! Can the country survive it? Is there any hope?"[2]

One of the 18 hospitals built in the Department of Pennsylvania was in York. Just south of the center of downtown was Penn Common, an elevated, grassy spot with shade trees and access to clean water and a railroad. Initially it was a training camp for cavalry and raw recruits, housed in wooden, one-story barracks. Eight buildings, 125 by 28 feet, were converted to 14 hospital wards by installing more windows and roof slots for ventilation, water proofing the leaky roof, and whitewashing both inside and out. The 14th ward was reserved for Native Americans and blacks. Infirmaries, operating rooms, offices, laundries, stables, library, chapel and mortuary were added. Buildings could accommodate up to 1,000 patients with movable bunks every six feet. There was a post office, printing press, cabinet and carpentry shop, tin shop, bakeshop, wash house, kitchen and dead house.

On July 1, 1862, 19 patients were admitted to the just-opened military hospital. Proximity to major battle fields meant many a sudden influx of large numbers of patients. After the Battle of Antietam in September 17, 1862, hundreds were admitted, and after Gettysburg a few thousand. By the spring of 1864, they had admitted 4,704, returned to duty 2,080, and discharged 715, with 88 deaths. In May of 1864, 100 tents were added for the arrival of 1,500 sick and wounded. On just one day in June 1864, there were 763 admissions "with mostly hand and arm injuries" transferred from Baltimore and Washington.[3] As of December 17, 1864, the hospital had a bed capacity of 1,600 and held 1,003 patients.

Rainfall was plenty that season, prompting hospital gardens to flourish with flowers and vegetables, much to the benefit of the convalescents. They ate in three shifts, sometimes 800 at a time. To reduce the need for servers, a horizontal dumb waiter with ropes and pulleys moved food along tables in small, train-like cars. On Thanksgiving 1864, 125 turkeys of "huge dimension" were delivered, cooked and sliced. The convalescents ate well, having a varied menu which included fresh vegetable soup, mince mutton pot pie, pork and beans, boiled cabbage and potatoes, Irish stew, and roast beef with mashed potatoes.

Regardless of sympathies, the locals provided total support for the volunteers. Mass casualties received assistance from "liberal and patriotic ladies" and civilian contract surgeons. The response to a request for one rocking chair was a large wagon filled with many. A Ladies Soldier Aid Society was organized under the guidance of Mrs. Rachel Miles, providing bandages, baked bread, nursing and clerical care. They offered untiring devotion in regular visits to wards, bringing comfort and consolation to the sufferers and earning undying gratitude. Nearby Bedford sent dried and canned fruit. The patriotic ladies of Lancaster sent the hospital chaplain one large box with lint, bandages and old linen. Reading sent four barrels of lint and bandages. Ladies from Brooklyn, New York, sent wine, blackberry brandy, jellies, farina cakes, and dried fruits. From the Christian Commission came shirts, drawers, slippers, bandages and reading material.[4]

The Cartridge Box was printed and published on site every Saturday for five cents each and ran from March 5, 1864, through April 22, 1865. Its logo was "going to hunt snakes," meaning two-legged reptiles. Their goal was to improve soldiers' welfare, provide a sounding board to reflect and share experiences, and educate minds and souls. Volunteers needed and deserved their own voice.

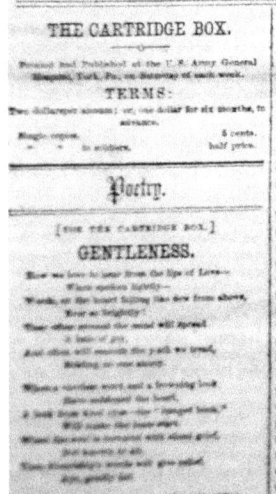

The Cartridge Box. York U.S. Army General Hospital, York, Pennsylvania (from the collection of the York County Heritage Trust, York, Pennsylvania).

Our object is to promote the best interests of our sick and wounded companions, to cheer them during their sufferings, to afford them a medium of interchange of thought and sentiment, and to relieve the monotony of hospital life. We ask our friends to lend us their assistance and furnish such communications that will be of interest, pleasure and profit to use. Give them medium to express their thoughts and opinions on subjects now agitating the country. They had ten months prior written a preamble and resolutions expressing their opinions on national affairs and no one would publish it.[5]

As for name: we would rather fight until the last man is slain than yield to southern tyranny: though we are at present unfit to take the field and hurl the contents of our trusty cartridge boxes against armed rebellion. We endeavor to make a vigorous use of this cartridge box and arm it with such missiles as the God of nature has given us for the benefit of such rebels that are too cowardly to fight.[6]

We would not apologize for sentiments unbiased by party prejudice that sound harshly upon copperhead antagonists. It is as laudable to oppose traitors in the north as to fight their more worthy brothers in the south.[7]

A principal object was to enlarge the hospital's library and establish a reading room for the benefit of the soldiers. Give them books to read, sermons to heed, and not be a cheerleader for the administration. By 1864 the hospital library had Shakespeare's complete works, an 11-volume series by Barnes and his notes on the New Testament, and tomes on *Napoleon and His Marshalls*. A sponsor donated New York dailies and books such as *Trout's Commentary on Popery*, *The Refugees*, and *Incidents of the War*. The Reverend Street sent Abbott's *Life of Napoleon* and Kitto's *Daily Bible Illustrations*. Other tomes were *The Life of General Scott*, *Life of John Quincy Adams*, *Everyday Scripture Readings* and Lord Byron's complete poetical work.[8] The editor was disappointed with the last item, claiming "It will excite warriors to an unbecomingly sentimental state of mind that will be aggravated by his poetry." The Sanitary commission donated 50 books and 250 magazines to an ultimate 1,800-volume collection which included 80 weekly newspapers. They exchanged with two hospital newspapers, *Armory Square Hospital Gazette* and *The Soldiers' Journal*.

The Library was open daily except Sundays from 10 a.m. to midnight. Mail arrived at 9:30 a.m. and 3:30 p.m. and was sent at 7 a.m. and Noon. Prompt delivery of mail was central to morale. To ensure safe delivery, envelopes were sold embossed with "Soldier's Letter. U.S. Army General Hospital at YORK, PENN'A." These morale builders required just a three-cent stamp that could be paid by the letter's recipient.

No one knows the amount of good a letter does to the soldier. It buoys up his spirits when he feels lowly and keeps him from temptations and sin. All mothers and sisters should write to their sons and brothers in the army.[9]

Never was such a letter writing army as ours. We call upon the ones at home to write and write often. If no answer is received write again and keep on doing so until you get a reply. Be cheerful; breathe confidence in the will of divine providence. Do not tell them you feel sad and can't enjoy yourself and dread to see casualty lists. He needs words of encouragement to help him in stern duties. Tell of little incidents around you no matter how small.[10]

In 1865 the hospital library was moved to the newly renovated chapel and reading room, the eastern end holding desks and appliances for writing letters. The west end of the chapel became a school room where a Yale College graduate taught courses on elementary rules and the classics, including one in German that was perfectly suited for this population. English commercial education was taught, including bookkeeping by single and double entry, stenography and telegraphing. The medical staff felt that "cheerful occupation was a valuable auxiliary in treatment." Divine services were held Sunday

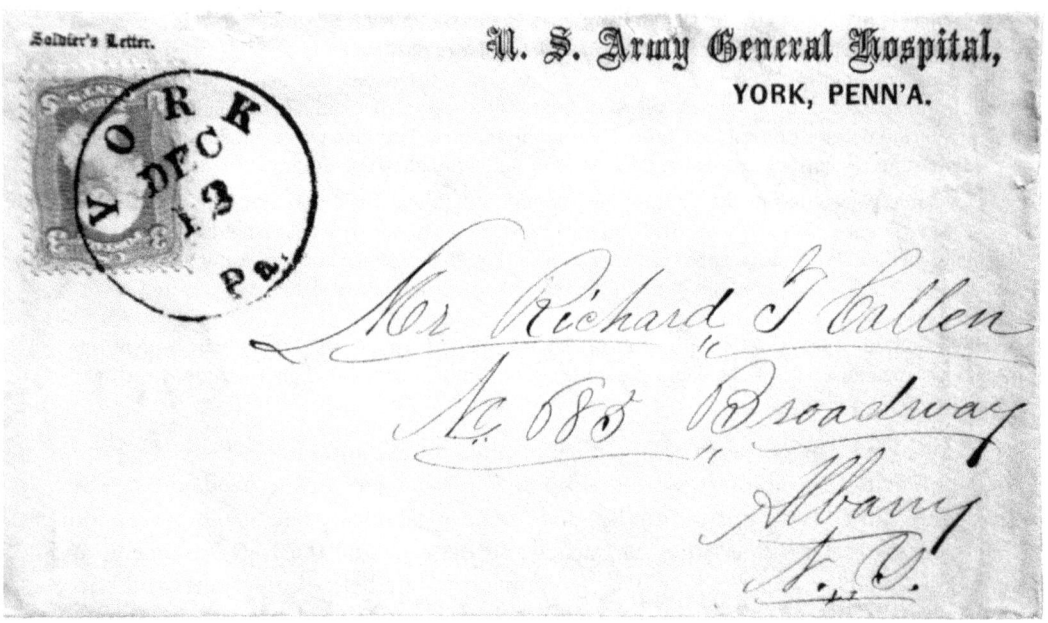

"Soldier's Letter" from York U.S. Army General Hospital, York, Pennsylvania. The 3 cent postage was paid by the recipient of the letter rather than the hospital patient (personal collection).

morning and evening and Tuesday evening. The Union Literary Society met Saturday evenings.[11]

The Cartridge Box was widely circulated in both town and hospital, but a plea for more subscribers was continuous to maintain its main source of funding. William Nelson from Massachusetts was known as "Judge," the foreman of the printing office. He brought with him skills as an accomplished civilian compositor with neatness and style.[12] "Readers will note the paper has been enlarged and appearance better. We are the exponent of true Union sentiment and correct principles and yet some Union men are not subscribing. We need more subscribers to better the library."[13]

    Nov. 12, 1864: "Many of our subscribers have not sent payment for six months and still complain because paper was not regular in coming."
    Dec. 10, 1864: "Attention subscribers-send money.
    Dec. 31, 1864: "Subscribers in arrears need forward amount due or paper will be discontinued."

Correspondents were given appropriate "hints" on getting published. Use good ink on good paper, use ample margins, number pages, and write in plain bold. Use no observations not to appear in print, underscore for italics, get proper names right, check every word for spelling and correctness, and send no private letters to the editor not meant to be published.[14]

Advice on how to write was on point. "Use your own language not foreign. Be simple and unaffected but honest. Use short words not long. Write as you would speak. Speak as you think. Be what you say. After you have written an article take your pen and strike out half the words and you will be surprised to see how much stronger it is."[15] The editor noted that the immensely popular Charles Dickens made more from his readings than from his "copyrighted" books.

There were three editors for the run of this paper, all enlisted men "subject to orders

Seven. *The Cartridge Box*   175

and might at any time be ordered to other scenes and pursuits."[16] They were dedicated to whoever was surgeon in charge and his corps of assistants. Charles McElroy from nearby Lancaster served the first eight months and was the most erudite and skillful writer. He was an "unyielding supporter of principles of truth and justice" and continued to contribute after his discharge on subjects ranging from death and religion to politics. His valedictory noted that "most of the editorials were written when others were in bed. Our personal sacrifices were not in vain as our paper became a favorite with the public. Our main object was to furnish a register of the names of officers and patients who arrived, furloughed, returned to duty, deserted or died."[17]

He thanked local and distant citizens for prompt and ready aid of money and supplies. After his three years in service, a new and younger editor was due. He was a patient of surgeon Dr. Henry Bowen and felt indebted to him for "life and comparative health which we now enjoy. When we were placed under his care we were terribly broken down and debilitated, the mere shadow and wreck of our former selves with little hope of continued life. To the soldiers, I hope your country will reward your services with tears of thanksgiving and gratitude and your children and your children's children will rise up in praise and you will be blessed."[18]

A model editor was defined as "a walking cyclopedia of knowledge and a locomotive for every-bodies beliefs. He must be both changing and unchangeable in his principles. He must never be convicted for his opinions and yet be ready to embrace every principle or issue propounded to him. The world is the most shameful, unreasonable, old rascal of a tyrant that ever sat upon a throne."[19]

The mythology of the printers "devils" was grist for the writing mills. Being a "ladies man" was a goal not always reached. As the story went, one such gentleman and his lady love were taking an evening stroll and while walking along and chatting about topics of the day, she suddenly caught his hand and with radiant smile asked, "Do you know why I cannot get religion?" "No," he said. She answered, "I do not my dear, because I love the 'devil.'"[20]

Local and general news was a constant feature with reporting on a wide spectrum of activities covered during the life of the paper.

>Four letters of General Washington written in 1783 in favor of union of states sold at auction in London for $90.56.
>A lock of Washington's hair sold at Philadelphia fair for $20.
>The smallest pony in Ohio is 20 inches high and weighs 21 lbs.
>There were snow squalls at Mount Washington, September 7, 1864.
>A young lady in western Canada while playing with her lover shot him dead with a loaded gun.
>The world will come to an end in 1865 when according to Professor Neumeier of Munich, a comet will rim earth.
>More than 79,000 shrubs and trees were planted in New York's Central Park last year. The carriage drive is 80 miles and walks 20 miles.
>Parisian women are dying their dogs the colors of their dresses.
>Robert Lincoln, son of the president, has left for the front to report to General Grant to be assigned to his staff.
>Over 700,000 persons enter London every morning on business and leave in evening. Over 500,000 are foot passengers.
>Six miners died in Minersville Pennsylvania from a blast.
>Since news of Lincoln's election, there has been large escalation of desertion to our lines from the rebel army.
>Army pies are so terribly tough that the soldiers call them leather pies. A recent amputee of Grant's

army passing a stand selling pies by an old woman said, "I say old lady, are those pies sewed or pegged?"

General Grant has ordered all embalmers of the dead to leave the Army of the Potomac.

The latest gift presented to Mrs. Grant is a fine piano valued at $1,200 in a rosewood case. It will form part of the furniture in her Philadelphia mansion.

Mrs. Samuel Colt of Hartford Connecticut owns a quarter of a mile of glass houses. She has already tomatoes, peas, string beans, radishes and lettuce fully ripe and peaches and grapes far advanced towards perfection.

On Thursday evenings, the Union Literary Society had formal presentations. The first was by chief hospital steward Cheney; "Does the soldier obey his officer more through love than fear?" decided in the affirmative.[21] Other subjects included evil versus good, do animals reason, the cause and results of the present rebellion, the demands of the present hour, and how Romans, Jews, Greeks, Egyptians and Persians sat at dinner feasts. Hospital Steward J. M. Johnston led the debate: resolved that we are indebted more to man than woman for our character as a nation. Their pro-war discussions were often summarized and published in the paper.

Sermons

The original Chapel was initially a patient ward but was enlarged and refurbished in 1865 to accommodate daily meetings and provide room for a growing library and reading room. The building was 173 feet long and 20 feet wide with 40 windows. It was well ventilated with a movable stage for readings and music. As soon as convalescents became fit for duty of any kind, they were employed. "Want of occupation is one of the predisposing causes of disease; our surgeon in charge fully understands and has made improvements and changes."[22] The new chapel was dedicated on a Sunday afternoon with 1,000 attendees, of whom 275 were from the Ladies Society. The Hospital band played, a choir sang, and an opening prayer by the chaplain gave thanks to the new chief of staff, Dr. Mintzer. The convalescent band gave concerts, including German operas, in a newly built pavilion on Wednesday, Thursday and Friday evenings and played every morning at guard mounting.

Summaries of the Sunday sermon, aphorisms and short stories on war, religion, sacrifice, behavior and love made weekly appearances in print.

> Sorrow can never wholly fill the heart that is occupied with others welfare. Constant melancholy is rebellion.
>
> Tart words make no friends. A spoonful of honey will catch more flies than a gallon of vinegar.
>
> Is there no place for pity in a place where death and carnage reigns? There is as humanity perseveres.
>
> It is easier to set up a new religion than to invent a new sin.
>
> It is strange that men should hate each other for the love of God.
>
> Repentance is the key that unlocks the gate where sin keeps man a prisoner. Charity may gush forth from the hardest heart, like silver water from the rock. Most men hate all lies which they don't utter themselves.
>
> There are more sorrows of women than of men, just as in heaven there are more eclipses of the moon than of the sun.
>
> *Maxims for young men*[23]
>
> 1. The world estimates men by their success in life, success is evidence of superiority.
> 2. Never assume responsibility you can avoid consistent with your duty to yourself and others.

3. Base all action upon principle of right. Preserve integrity of character.
4. Self-interest will warp judgment. Look to your duty when your interest is concerned.
5. Never make money at expense of your reputation.
6. Be neither extravagant or niggardly. Cultivate generous feeling
7. Say little, think much and do more.
8. Balance expenses. Ready money is a friend in need.
9. Keep clear of law even if you gain your case you are generally a loser.
10. Neither lender nor borrower be.
11. Wine drinking and smoking cigars are bad habits. They impair the mind and pocket and lead to a waste of time
12. Never relate your misfortunes and never grieve over what you cannot prevent.

The Sanitary and Christian Commission provided materials for both body and soul. Weekly sermons and services were available for those interested. Twenty-five vigilantes against profanity and alcohol were busy at work on the hospital's sixth ward, forming an association prohibiting both. "A profane man should be avoided being desperately wicked and debased, destitute of all moral and gentlemanly principle and an unfit companion. The offenders are sinful brothers in crime with indecent habits, bad breeding, and no self-respect."[24] They grudgingly admitted that intemperance and profanity were features widely present in the army and society in general. A petition "resolved we will not drink any intoxicating drinks unless ordered by proper medical authority and that in case we break this resolution to pay seven cents into the treasury. We believe the habit of using intoxicating liquors or profane language a great sin against our Creator and degrading to ourselves. Resolve that we will do all in our power to suppress these evils."[25]

A temperance story involved two men in a boarding house who came home drunk, fell into the same bed only to find an invader alongside, and attempted to kick the villain out. The two hapless drunks found themselves tangled on the floor jousting until fatigue rendered them unconscious. The real invader was the now empty liquor bottle. The drunkard spent his life digging his own grave of eternal hopelessness. The drunkard left his home in despair and would never enter the kingdom of heaven: "turn ye from your evil ways, for ye will die alone."[26]

Another vice to be condemned was the pernicious use of profanity in the hospital. "It is a calamity and sadly to be lamented the taking of the name of God in vain. We must meet it decisively but in a kind and pleasant manner otherwise we shall fail in our object. It is a vice and a sin and the worst kind of sin. It is contagious and requires moral courage to stop. We must stop one of the worst practices in the world. Some have promised the writer to stop and have done so."[27]

Completing the trinity of vice and in need of prohibition was tobacco, smoked or chewed. It was reliably reported that "a tobacco chewer spits 525 gallons in 25 years with a ton and a half of weed."[28] It was known to make women feint and become ill. It was reported that a man who smoked in bed on his wedding night was sarcastically informed by his bride that "no gentleman ever lighted his cigar with the torch of Hymen."[29] [God of marriage] The Ministers declared this habit impertinent, deplorable, inexcusable and disgusting.

The ill consequence of human behavior was attributed to God's will. You have sinned, now suffer and repent. Slavery was a sin, an illness self-inflicted. Only through righteousness and faithful following of the Lord's words would the disease be cured. With the surrender at Appomattox Court House, the conviction that God was on the side of the Union was consecrated.

God in his infinite wisdom has decreed the downfall of the rebellion. His power has strengthened us. His favor alone has given us victory. To Him belong all the praise and all the glory. Our executive authorities, our officers, our armies have only been instruments in His hands to aid in the great work of regeneration which has been wrought. Liberty has triumphed over oppression, right over wrong and slavery abolished. It has freed both slaves and masters. It has relieved the people of the south from the terrorism of one of the vilest and most oppressive military despotism ever to disgrace the earth. Free government has been vindicated.[30]

The ills of slavery were a common topic, and whipping fellow man or woman had no defense in this satiric piece.

A man was imprisoned two days and sentenced to pay a fine of $50 in Cincinnati for whipping his wife. This is another glaring instance of the tyranny toward which the whole country is hastening under the influence of Lincoln's hateful administration. It is a pretty state of affairs when a man can't whip his own wife without such a fuss being made about it.[31]

A foreboding sermon in March 1865 described the danger of the isolated young male stewing in poisoned juices, a plague on society. Such a creature might take the life of a grand and generous leader.

Men who isolate themselves from society and have no near and dear family ties are the most uncomfortable of human beings. Happiness was born a twin. We are gregarious and not intended to march single file. The man who cares for nobody and for whom nobody cares has nothing to live for, nor take the trouble of keeping soul and body together. You must have a heap of embers to make a glowing fire. Scatter them apart and the fire becomes dim and cold. Groups of lives are needed for mutual encouragement, confidence and support. If you wish to live the life of a man and not a fungus be social, brotherly, charitable, sympathetic, and labor earnestly for the good of your kind.[32]

The cardinal sins included greed and taking advantage of fellow man. The sutler sold goods not otherwise available such as pies, candies and whiskey. They served a purpose in difficult times. What follows was a morality play with the transgressor facing just punishment.

All paymasters look alike and draw a crowd-chubby and jolly. Israel Pennyworth was the sutler, a shrewd, tight fisted and hard hearted rascal and the only one in five miles. Buy or not buy, the price remained the same and no limit to customers. Avaricious wretch was his name. He extended credit exceeding the soldier's salary meaning always being on the hook. He is contemptible and should be tarred and feathered. Israel Pennyworth clutched the money with a metallic chuckle and snapping fingers extending his bony hand while demanding his toll. They all owed him something. He had preserved meats, honey, cider, sugar and a thousand things almost necessary to existence in environs where fevers and other diseases were so prevalent. One day they were attacked by rebels and the sutler shot through the head. While counting his money, a bullet pierced his brain. He was buried last and not a word of pity was pronounced as the damp clods were heaped upon his remains.[33]

Ads

The last page contained advertisements with contributions from town shops: dry goods, hardware, military clothing, boots, shoes, photo gallery, musical instruments and sheet music. A druggist sold "fresh" drugs and medicines with dye stuffs, spices, perfumery, and coal oil. Physician prescriptions were compounded with care and at the shortest notice.

At $13 a month salary, price mattered. "Soldiers attention! Cheap book store. Lowest rates on anything and everything in books and stationery. Liberal discount for our gallant soldiers."[34]

Saloons provided shave, hair-cut, and shampoo with the best of styles for hair and whiskers. Tobacconists offered chewing and smoking tobacco, pipes, cigars of the finest quality and snuff. Restaurant menus had oysters in the shell, roasted, stewed or fried with "all kinds of fancy drinks at all times and all kinds of game."[35] A constant feature was how to obtain well-earned pension and bounties and "all with claims upon government" for widows, mothers, fathers, minor children, or dependent sisters. There were no charges by agents until a claim was collected.

Romance and Marriage

Adam was as similar as he was different from Eve. The differences were no small matter to the readers of *The Cartridge Box*.

> Men are made in the image of God. Gentlemen are manufactured by tailors, barbers and bootjacks. Woman is the last and most perfect work of God. Ladies are the productions of silk worms, milliners and dressmakers.[36]
>
> The faces of soldiers coming out of an engagement and those of young women getting into one, are generally powdered.[37]

Advice on picking a wife ranged from beauty is only skin deep, dance hall moments don't last, and the quiet ones often work out the best. If that failed, there was always bachelorhood.

> *The Bachelor Song*[38]
> It is better to love than fall moping,
> Alone on the pathway of life.
> It is better to keep on hoping,
> Some day you will meet with a wife.
> And although it is ten years creep over us,
> And steal our good looks away
> We will never let dirty time floor us,
> But still remain festive and gay.

There was keen interest in how to choose a mate. "When bent on matrimony look more than skin deep for beauty, dive farther than the pocket for work and search beyond the good humor of the moment: remember it is not always the most agreeable partner at a ball who forms the most amiable partner for life. Virtue like some flowers blooms best in the shade."[39]

The year 1864 was a leap year, which by tradition meant bachelors expected to be asked by the ladies. The mechanics and mythology of kissing were outlined in a poem, *The Parting Kiss*. A handsome man promised to love a maiden forever and never deceive or roam. Upon leaving he gently touched her hand but forgot to give her a parting kiss, giving away his real intentions. "Kisses are precious as frankincense and myrrh, but when they are poured out loosely and in any night air and bestowed on any reckless mite who may step up, it is to say the least a great waster of treasure."[40]

> The way to victory is outlined with this advice. "A woman wins an old man by listening to him—a young man by talking to him."[41]
>
> "What did you come here for?" inquired Miss Harriet Rakestraw of a bachelor friend who made her a call when the rest of the folks were out.

"I only dropped in to borrow some matches," he meekly replied.

"Matches! That's a likely story."

"Why don't you make a match for yourself? I know what you came for," exclaimed the delighted Miss Harriet, as she pushed the old bachelor into a corner.

"You came to kiss and hug me almost to death, but you shan't unless you are the sternest, and—strongest—and—the—Lord—knows—you—are!"[42]

Advice to the love worn comes in these *Maxims for husbands*.[43]
1. Laugh heartily at finding all buttons off your shirt as usual.
2. Say boys will be boys when the children empty water jugs into your boots.
3. When accidently cut self-shaving recite Shakespeare or sing harmony and do not curse.
4. If breakfast is not ready chuckle and grin.

If a woman wants to keep her husband at home, let her send him to the top of the house and take away the ladder.

The venerable lady of a celebrated physician one day casting her eye out of the window observed her husband in the funeral procession of one of his patients of which she exclaimed, "I do wish my husband would keep away from such processions, it appears too much like a tailor carrying his work home."[44]

An old Dutch inn keeper had his third wife and was asked his view of matrimony.

Vell you see de first time I marries for love and that wash goot.

Den I marries for beauty and that was wash goot too, about as goot as de first.

But dis time I marries for monish and dis is petter den both.[45]

The humorist Artemus Ward had fixed views on the fair sex. "Yu ma differ as much as you please about the stile of a young ladys figger but if she has 40,000 pounds, the figure is about as near rite as you will get it."[46]

Humor

Josh Billings was a popular satirist with soldiers. His aphorisms and stories spiced up many issues.[47]

Woman will confess her sins but never confess her faults.
Woomans inflooence iz powerful especially when she wants ennything.
Conshense in only another name for truth.
Moral swashun consists in asking a man to do what he ought to do without asking and then begging his pardon.
Music hath cords to sooth a savage but I wud rather tri a revolver on him fust.
A man wants to bekum a rascal may be beter built to be a fool.
It always seemed to me that a left handed fiddler must play the tune backwards.
Men aint apt tew git kicked out ov good society for being ritch.
Don't mistake arrogance for wisdom. Menny people have thought they wuz wize when thay was only windy.
There is only one advantage in going to the devil and that iz the road is easy and you are sure to git there.

Animals served as metaphor for a slew of topics ranging from the draft to loyalty.

My dorg is mixed breed, I tied him to a post and he nearly hung hisself horizontally so I released him and then plac'd him in a boording skool.[48]

Cats is adikted to a wild state. Haint got affeckshun, nor vurtue of enny kind. Thay will skratch their best friends and wont ketch mice unless they are hungry. Dogs make better sausages. Thay hard to kill, old maids like 'em because cats never marry.[49]

I have offen been tole tha best is to take a bull by the horns, but I think in many instance I should prefer the tail hold.[50]

A hoss dont kno his strength and a skunk does nuther.[51]

The draft was no laughing matter except for Billings, who knew evasion was best accomplished with absent teeth, parent dependency or being in jail for a felony.

> Widow wimmin and their only son is zempt if widow husband has already sarved 2 years and iz willing to go agin. If a man runs away with his draft he would not stand the draft agin. Xemps are those drafted into stait prizzen for trying to git onest living bi supporting 2 wives at onst. Also allo nusepaper correspondents and fools in general. No substitute if less than three or more than ten feet high; must know how to chew tebaker, drink poor whiskee and not afeered of the itch nor rebels. Moral charakter aint required as government furnishes that and rashuns. No person can be drafted twice in two different places without his consent. All men have right to be drafted onst. I don't think even a rit of habeas corpus could deprive a man of this blessed privilege.[52]

A local correspondent gave his list of the top four ways of *How to avoid the draft*.[53]

1. Get lodged in jail for lengthy charge. The Provost Marshall does not want jail birds.
2. Eat camphor and get fits.
3. Partake a quart or more of whisky daily and become a confirmed sot.
4. Should these fail the next best thing is to enlist.

Dr. Sam Wiltbank served on an examining board for men claiming exemptions. One recruit had a dentist remove all his upper teeth for $5, then claimed he could not masticate, chew hardtack or bite off a powder cartridge to fire a musket. He was denied exemption and ruled fit for cavalry or artillery service.[54] The absence of teeth was the most common cause of exemption from the draft. The teeth were viewed as a window into the health of a prospective soldier.

Humorist Petroleum V. Nasby sometimes masqueraded as pastor of the Church of the Noo Dispensashen who Waileth Muchly about an experiment that did not work, namely doing unto others as you would have them do unto you.

> Mankind is the moste perverse and onreasonable of the human family. Wile they may assent two a princapole they never will put it into practis if it goes hard onto em as indivijules. (He lectures on divinity of slavery and why some races are inferior and arrives at a neighbor's house demanding their furniture since being inferior they were naturally his slaves. He would sell their children and make the lady his concubine. He is charged with stealing property and does a 30 day jail term.) How kin we establish Demekratick institooshuns wen the Cortz wunt recognize the lawys of nacher? The ecksperment, for the presnt, hez the apperentz ov a faleyer.[55]

Irish and Blacks

Anecdotes using Irish or blacks as foil were common.

> A son if Erin was hired to cut ice and was asked if he could work a cross cut saw. "I could entirely." He went with a co-laborer to the center of pond noting a saw with both handles still in their place. The verdant son drew a cent from his pocket, saying to his companion "Now Johnnie fair play, head or tail who goes below."[56]

> A Hibernian was reprimanded by an officer for whistling in the ranks while going on duty. Just as the officer spoke one of the enemy's bullets came whistling over. Pat said "there goes a boy on duty and be jabbers hear how he whistles!"[57]

> Two Irishmen in smart engagement were firing their artillery gun in quick succession when one

noted it was very hot. "Mike, the cannon is getting hot, we'd better stop firing a little." "Devil a bit," replied Mike. "Just dip the cartridges in the river afore yee load, and kap it cool."[58]

"See here mister," said an Irish lad of seven summers who was treed by a dog. "If you don't take that dog away, I'll eat up all your nice apples."[59]

How a copperhead was shaved.[60]

A frequenter of a barber shop came for a shave to remove his beard. The barber was an African and he was duly shaved.

"How much is it?"

"Fifteen cents, boss."

"Why I thought you shaved for ten cents at this shop?"

"Dat ars de averages at," was the reply.

"Ten cents is de price of a shave in dis shop. You come in and read de news of Sheridan victry and your face got six inches longer den when you cam in. If your face was likit was afore you read dat news, ten cents was de price. When you read about de defeat of Early den your faced stretched down about four inches more. Dats what makes it wuff fifteen cents for de shave."

The customer could not restrain a grin though he was a copperhead and the hit was made by a "nigger." He laid down the fee and walked out.

Governor Oglesby of Illinois from Kentucky spoke on what was to become of the Negro. "He can labor, he can learn, he can fight, improve and aspire and if after we shall have tried for as long to make him a useful freeman as we have a useless slave there will be time enough left to solve this persistent question."[61]

Evacuating the Disabled

The first surgeon in charge was 35-year-old Henry Palmer, with a staff of four assistant surgeons and three hospital stewards. He was born in New York, the ancestor of English and Scottish Puritans and a graduate of Albany Medical School. He began medical practice in 1856 in Janesville, Wisconsin, his wife's hometown, becoming surgeon for the 7th Wisconsin Infantry and later the Iron Brigade. He stressed cleanliness, exercise and activity for the convalescents while organizing patients into a fighting force that drilled each day on hospital ground.

On June 28, 1863, acerbic General Jubal Early and 6,000 dust-covered Confederates arrived in York, population 8,600. A self-appointed, five-man defense committee offered no resistance (for a town that had no defense) if person and property were left intact. They did not view this as dishonor but rather respect for hearth, real estate, and avoidance of needless death and destruction. The rebels commandeered the York Court House and Penn Common with demands for large amounts of bread, sugar, coffee, molasses, meat, hats, socks, 2,000 pairs of shoes, and $100,000 else the town be sacked despite General Lee's order that no such thing occur. All items were fully provided except a discounted $28,600, all the cash allegedly available from local banks. That Sunday well-dressed York citizens attended church while Confederate soldiers departed 25 miles to the west and their destiny at Gettysburg.[62]

Dr. Palmer, anticipating this invasion, sent all those patients who could travel 20 miles east beyond the Susquehanna River to Columbia, allowing himself and five non-transportable patients to be taken prisoner. He then escaped and found his way to Gettysburg to treat casualties.

After the rebels left, workers cleaned the military hospital, left in disarray. Pictures on the wall had been destroyed. Market houses where invaders slept were crawling with lice and other bugs, requiring rooms and houses to be hosed down. In only two and a half hours, townspeople carried enough supplies to Central market to fill 40 wagons for the battle at Gettysburg: bread cakes, hams, fruit, clothing, blankets, bandages and hospital supplies.

Mary Fisher, wife of a proud and independent judge, went to Gettysburg as a nurse, taking with her dozens of bottles of imported liquor and fine whiskey. She described seeing hundreds of maimed soldiers, some lying on the ground, some under trees, others half buried in mud. Doctors claimed her brandy saved more lives than their instruments and medicine combined.[63]

Surgeon Palmer came back to York, preparing the military hospital for massive casualties. Trainloads of wounded men from Gettysburg began arriving along with 75 men with gunshot fractures of the femur who did surprisingly well. Transportation was difficult as railroad agents required payment and their cars had no water, lanterns or straw. Palmer refused to treat any rebels, perhaps related to his recent experience forcing 25 casualties from a North Carolina regiment to receive medical treatment in a town hall by locals.

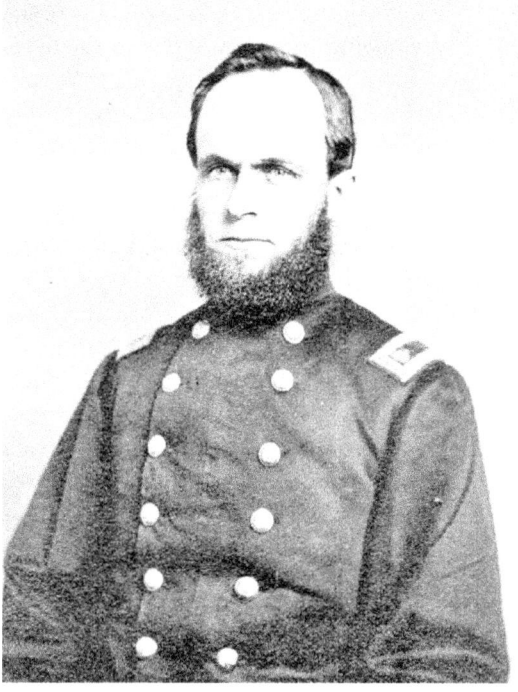

Henry Palmer (1827–1895), Chief of Staff, York U.S. Army General Hospital, 1862–1864, York, Pennsylvania (from the collection of the York County Heritage Trust, York, Pennsylvania).

By summer of 1864, in response to increasing casualties from battles in the Shenandoah, the number of assistant surgeons ballooned to 14 and hospital stewards to six. Palmer's five-year-old daughter Kittie died after a lingering illness of three weeks. She was buried in York at Prospect Hill Cemetery and transferred to Wisconsin after the war.[64] By August, Palmer had a non-descript illness thought related to uninterrupted duties for over two years. "He is a man of untiring energy and industry and has worn himself out for the time being. Respite from labor and healthful exercise and recreation abroad will restore him to increased strength and re-establish health and vitality. The government cannot afford to lose the services of such a man."[65]

He was replaced by Dr. St. John W. Mintzer, "a good natured surgeon," who planned to fix eyesore grounds and change the chapel into an enlarged library and reading room. The paper's editor noted that the change in chief of staff was not officially witnessed. The hospital library thanked Palmer for $519 of new books from Lippincott of Philadelphia meant for soldier improvement and self-culture. Before going on a 60-day furlough, he had photos taken of officers and detail men and posted a letter giving thanks "for faithful and energetic manner that duties were performed. The duties have been laborious and many times unpleasant, but promptness and cheerfulness which every order has been obeyed, your hearty cooperation towards the comfort of sick and wounded entitled you to the confidence and esteem of those under your care and thanks of the surgeon in charge."[66]

Before leaving, he had to reimburse the federal government for soldiers' petty larceny. Government property was the ultimate responsibility of the surgeon in charge. Several gross of knives, forks and spoons were removed from wards and mess rooms by patients transferred, discharged or returned to duty. In addition, a large quantity of clothing was being sold by soldiers to private citizens.[67]

Palmer visited the hospital briefly in November 1864, before becoming medical inspector of the Eighth Army Corps headquartered in Baltimore. "He could have resumed his old position here or accept the transfer and chose the latter as best suited to the present condition of his health. We will miss him in the daily rounds. He is a man of rare talent, an able surgeon and stern and rigid disciplinarian."[68]

Mintzer was Surgeon of the 26th Pennsylvania Volunteers, promoted to brigade surgeon followed by hospital duty in Philadelphia. He began his tenure in York the summer of 1864, providing watermelons at his expense. The paper described him as able and efficient, a kind-hearted surgeon, a warm friend and genial companion. He tempered justice with mercy and dealt with patients more like a brother than a commander. Executive officer and Surgeon Blair gave him a glowing review.

> He is universally beloved, being kind, generous and loose in discipline. I am much more frequently surgeon in charge than executive officer by reason of his frequent trips of pleasure to Philadelphia. The indefatigable industry and energy of the doctor has made decisive improvement in the prisonlike barracks and most grounds. In front of our office and extending to the end of the 5th ward, the grounds have been handsomely laid out and planted with trees and flowers. Dr. Palmer has been here since and twice looked at the improvements in silence offering no compliments. I think he must have felt some sight degree of shame, as he had been here 2½ years without paying any regards to the proper comfort and improvement of the general condition of men. You may well remember his cry "economy and men to duty."[69]

At first it was thought Palmer would resume his post. "It will be a painful necessity with Dr. Mintzer who has done so well. He has received golden opinions and a fully sustained reputation gained elsewhere. He is a popular young surgeon, a universal favorite with the men, having been here for three months. He is kind and courteous and has planned and is now engaged in carrying out many improvements in the buildings and hospital grounds."[70] Statistics were published in the hospital paper comparing six months of Palmer versus Mintzer, showing a slight decrease in mortality and a drop in desertions of one-third.

Hospital improvements included a fountain with goldfish in a flower garden walled by brick, an elevated pavilion surrounded by plants for the band, a new laundry and sewer system, and water hydrants for fires. At the camp's entrance was a six-pounder and flag pole, and a gilded eagle accented the administration headquarters. All buildings were painted bright white, and the 200-foot-long chapel pea green. Even gymnastic appliances for athletic exercises were installed. Water pipes went to all wards, where water had been hand carried before, and 1,100 feet of new barracks were erected. Financial costs were small as all labor was done by convalescent patients.[71]

On July 1864, Dr. Charles Woodward, acting assistant surgeon, was a surprised participant in an award ceremony witnessed by a large number of soldiers in the mess room. He received a fine case of surgical instruments purchased by patients of the tenth ward as "a mark of respect and esteem for him as a gentleman and physician." Chief Steward Cheney presided, noting he was a careful and attentive surgeon, with a kind heart and warm sympathy for the sick and suffering.[72] Four months later it was announced that he had married Miss Eliza Templeman, they were off on a short wedding, and he would resume his position on return.

In April 1865, Dr. James O'Neil, acting assistant surgeon for 6th ward, was given a case of surgical instrument for "respect and esteem as gentleman and appreciation of his skill as a surgeon. The gift was a surprise."[73]

A month later clerks and attendants gave executive officer Dr. Blair an "elegantly chaste tea service of plate engraved by clerks, attendants and convalescents as token of love and respect." The presentation was in the chapel and many patients were present. "The doctor was thankful for gift and that men were going home and hoped they received due deference from fellow citizens."[74]

The staff took great pride in the hospital's low mortality rate despite "some cases being hopeless when arrived. Care and attention of our efficient officers and attendants are unremitting, greatly aided by patriotic ladies. May God bless the ladies of the borough of York."[75]

One health issue that seemed insurmountable was the growing nuisance of rats. "Hospital barracks despite large number of terriers and tom cats seem troubled with rats. They shelter under planks and buildings, in sinks, drainages and out houses especially at night. Hundreds peep out from holes with impudent defiance. The boys are murdering them in great numbers yet they seem to increase and multiply. We need extermination skills."[76] A news item noted that rat catching was a fine art in Paris. "A college professor caught 2,500 in 18 months. Their skins are sewed to make "kid" gloves."

On Soldiers

A soldier in a winter Kentucky camp said his motto was "United we sleep; divided we freeze."

The character of soldiers varied: some were dissipated and profane, immune to the efforts of the Chaplain and others. In Indianapolis, bounty jumpers marched in a dress parade where over 100 were lashed to a long rope, with a Herculean African leading the column through the main streets ringing a bell. "Notwithstanding the low estimation in which soldiers are held by some, there are others who know and esteem them, who vindicate and protect their integrity, their honor and their rights. Among these noble vindicators may be found the patriotic ladies to whom thousands of our boys are indebted."[77]

How soldiers felt in battle was discussed by those with experience. "None of us had any idea that such a terrible shadow was rising up in our midst."[78] There was no eagerness for the fray or desire to meet with a surgeon for limb removal. A soldier's notion of immortality existed only in those without experience. It was the second confrontation with battle that determined eagerness to rush forward or to quickly seek cover.

War stories written by its participants were delivered in a section of the paper called *touching incidents of the war*. A 21-year-old lieutenant from Rhode Island sustained a gunshot wound to the foot at Mechanicsburg one week before arriving at York Army Hospital. An amputation was performed which became infected. He telegraphed home that he was doing well. He had served his three-year service but now faced additional surgeries, which failed. His pulse became feeble and the prognosis foreboding. His mother arrived at midnight and in darkness glided to his side. The sleeping boy opened his eyes and said, "that feels like my mother's hand; is she beside me? Turn up the gas and let me see my mother." They met in joyful, sobbing embrace.

When death drew near he was told they could only make him comfortable. He looked death in the face too many times to be afraid now and died as gallantly as any, with his grieving mother at his side.[79] Infected wounds often ended badly.

> A soldier saying goodbye to his family could bring tears from the hardest stone amidst trepidation and fear for the future.
> *The soldier and his mother*[80]
> "Well boys we are off to war."
> "Won't we give 'em fits, eh."
> "Maybe we won't."

Just as the soldiers were to depart, an old woman pushed her way through the crowd and stood before a man. His eyes dropped and his face flushed as he lifted his finger which he shook with a twirl. "Now mother, mother you promised me that you wouldn't come out didn't ye. Now you promised me. When I said good bye I told you I didn't want you to come out here and unman me and here you've done it. I wish you hadn't."

The old woman put her hands on his high shoulder as tears streamed down her check.

"Oh Jack; don't scold your poor old mother. You are all I have and I didn't come to unman you. I have come to say God bless ye Jack, god bless ye!"

The big fellow drew a sleeve over his face and bringing down his arm with a vexed emphasis tried to defy his emotions then faced the men.

"Hang it boys, she is my mother you know."

He will be a brave man in the field, a noble true fellow. Men who have a true appreciation of their country's causes love as much their homes and families. [This story is repeated in all wars by sons and mothers whose hail and farewell offers the prayer, "until we meet again."]

> *On the horrors of war.* The once green and bounteous landscape turned muddy brown, desecrated with heaps of mangled and slain and piles of limbs. Mutilated horses shrieked in pain, soldiers in the same predicament. "Shovels made shallow graves as surgeons toiled with blood stained hands and clothing made crimson by their trade while the roar of muskets and cannon boomed. We are at home in church, markets booming, labor plentiful, money available, our innocence escaped and guilt unpunished. The great estates have been emptied surrounded by bloody fields as the avenging angel poured out his vial of wrath upon the land. The last measure of retribution has yet to fall."[81]

As in other communities, prisoner exchange in the spring of 1864 was of great interest. "Rebel brutality" headlined reports of crowded prisons with filthy water and few rebel surgeons, protesting the pitiable conditions of their patients but in vain. Hunger, cold, vermin, madness and death oozed malevolence in all its horrible forms.

As cadaveric prisoners returned, blame was sought for "rebel cruelty and why this wholesale slaughter by starvation? It was done not from necessity but from sinister motives. Sherman's men are living witnesses of the abundancy of the confederacy. Was it to enfeeble men, to make then wholly unfit for a long time or at least for active service and consign them to hospital graves." Families mourned those who "sleep and know no waking beneath sods as murdered victims demanding revenge. I was hungry and ye fed me not, naked and ye clothed me not, sick and in prison and ye visited me not."[82]

"VET"[83]

Vet. Vet. What does it mean?
Upon your soldiers faded coat.
His hand is hard and rough and brown
From scarf along his throat
It means my child that rugged hand
Has wielded musket long and well
Has sent the iron thunder home
And tuned the song of screeching shell
It means that steady staunch and true
He fairly won that ragged scar
While dad and I sat safely home
And read the news about the war
What wonder if the name is me?
And yonder strangely lingers yet
The eye that has looked straight at Death
His image you may soon not forget
He serves the guns in rifle pit
To sleep beneath the silent sky
To dream of heaven and wake to war
To see a comrade drop and die
And this my child is what it says
That little word of just threes
Go clasp his hand and give him thanks
For battles fought for you and me

The ancient and venerable General Winfield Scott was appointed president of a bureau for employing disabled and discharged soldiers and sailors in New York and Boston to deal with a burgeoning and long-term problem.

The Invalid Corps[84]
Have you never hear of the invalid corps?
Composed of old soldiers whose place in the war
Is but little understood except tis to guard
Public buildings and stores, which some think dreadful hard.
How sweet look the girls on the veterans of war,
Although there's an arm gone or a leg,
Unfit for the field they still do their duty.
And still stand firm as granite.
And though we are all cripples our hearts beat as strong
With love to our country as those who belong
To the army of Meade, Grant and Sherman
Will stick to the blue of the Invalid Corps.

Politics

While the paper opposed the extreme dogma of abolitionists, it did support the administration and its efforts to crush the rebellion and break up the slave oligarchy. Their goals were forthright concerning the demon of succession. As for copperheads: "we would want those fungi of human humanity to beware of the bluecoat and brass buttons in the approaching presidential campaign. The most venomous reptile is not cobra, asp, viper, whip snake, moccasin, or rattlesnake. It is the copperhead. They denounced the war as tyrannical and despotic and like Judas committed the unpardonable sin."[85] But redemption was near. "The vilest sinner may return. There is a fountain open for them where they can wash and be clean."[86] Members of the Democratic Party who were "aiders and abettors of those in arms against the government" needed to show signs of loyalty and be repentant if they desired to feed at the public crib.

Copperheads were traitors. "We have in our midst a loathing venomous reptile half-brother, the southern rattlesnake who under cloak of loyalty makes ready to strike its fangs deep into the fiery heart's blood of the nation; and thus make a grand effort to destroy this union."[87] *The Cartridge Box* held fast to no compromise, no slavery and no Confederacy.

Not all hospital patients were supporters of this sentiment. A letter to the editor defended their right to a different point of view. "You ought not to construe differences of opinion as disloyalty." The editor's reply was unequivocal. "One must by actions and speech support the constitutional authorities in bringing us out of our difficulties, or we are nothing more than a sympathizer with treason and ought not to be looked up as a man worthy of the title of an American citizen."[88] A favorite villain was former Governor of Ohio, and now on the run, Vallandigham, who was "worse than thief or murderer."

George McClellan, at five feet three inches and former head of the Army of the Potomac, was no longer a soldier favorite. "It took McClellan nine days to write his letter of acceptance (for the presidential nomination) about the time it takes a pup to get his eyes open."[89] They conveniently made a list for those *who go for McClellan*.[90]

1. Vallandigham, the traitor
2. Notorious copperheads
3. Those clamoring for peace and disgraceful submission to traitors
4. Every rebel general, colonel, captain
5. All who say abolitionists started the war
6. All officers dishonorably dismissed from army
7. Deserters
8. Those voting against law allowing soldiers to vote

Many soldiers were furloughed home to vote in the Presidential election in November 1864. Straw ballots at York hospital showed Lincoln 1,240 versus McClellan 368.[91] St. Alban, Vermont, the scene of a recent rebel raid from Canada, voted 608 for Lincoln and 223 for McClellan. All the border towns gave strong Lincoln majorities. Their heroes wore blue and won real victories on real battlefields. York County gave McClellan a 3,225 majority, which was an even larger opposition margin than in 1860.

> This rebellion was gotten up by men notorious for their unprincipled lives. It has not a particle of right or justice in it. The secret of all their claims was to establish slavery upon a firmer basis. The slavery question, the cause of all our troubles is the vital doctrine that the south labors for and is the eminently proper one for us to fight against in order to subjugate our enemies.[92]
>
> A Connecticut man living in Atlanta sought counsel with General Sherman to avoid being destroyed by his invading army. Civilians were given twelve days to leave. He owned a block of stores, plantation and a foundry that made shot and shells for confederates.
>
> "You have been making shot and shell to destroy your country. Do you still claim favor on account of being a northern man? I will make an exception in your case. You shall go south tomorrow at sunrise."
>
> "But general can't I go north?"
>
> "No sir, too many of your class are there already!"[93]
>
> A rebel correspondent says that the destruction of property by fire during Sherman's march through Georgia was caused entirely by outsiders and never done under the inspection of any officer.[94]

Lincoln

President Lincoln was being lectured to by a moral philosopher who noted differences of undercurrents in the Black Sea and the Atlantic and Pacific Oceans. After a tedious dissertation, Lincoln replied, "That don't remind me of any story I ever hear of."[95]

An old farmer from the west who knew Lincoln slapped the president on his back. "Well old hoss, how are you?" Abe said, "So I'm an old hoss am I? What kind of a hoss pray? "Why an old draft hoss to be sure."[96]

He dismissed a party of hungry place seekers who wearied him and exhausted his patience. They reminded him of the schoolmaster who asked his pupil to read the third chapter of Daniel. The boy started but when came to Shadrach, Meshach and Abednego, he stumbled. He tried again and failed. A flogging failed to stimulate his memory. Relenting, the master told the boy to read the preceding chapter and let the present go. He did so and getting to the last verse said, "why here are those rascally fellows again."[97]

> While making rounds in hospital, he was accompanied by a young lady who asked a soldier the location of his wound.
> "Where were you hit?"
> "At Antietam."
> "But where did the bullet strike you?"
> "At Antietam."
> "Where did it hit you?"
> "At Antietam."
> The President took her hands in his and said in his most impressive style, "My dear girl the ball that hit him would not have injured you."[98]

Sojourner Truth called on Lincoln to thank him for what he had done for her people. She told him he was the only president who had done anything for them. Mr. Lincoln replied, "And the only one who had such opportunity."[99]

On answering the many press attacks on Lincoln, an officer suggested he set them right. "Oh no! At least not now. If I were to try to read, much less answer all the attacks made on me, this shop might as well be closed for any other business. I do the very best I know how and I mean to keep doing so until the end. If the end brings me out all right, what is said about me won't amount to anything. If the end brings me out wrong, ten angels swearing I was right would make no difference."[100]

By May 1864, it was clear to these editors that Providence had provided a "man of steel" as pilot for the ship of state, watching with an eagle eye to bring her safely through the breakers. It was a painfully prophetic request: "May he live to see the end of his great work and receive the heartfelt thanks of a grateful and Christian people. We have in our midst a loathing venomous reptile half-brother, the southern rattle snake who under cloak of loyalty makes ready to strike its fangs deep into the fiery heart's blood of the nation and destroy this union."[101]

On April 6, 1865, after Lee's surrender, a crowd of convalescents and other celebrating York residents walked through town to ensure American flags, 50 of which were supplied by Dr. Mintzer, were displayed from all houses as a sign of loyalty. Rocks were thrown and windows broken at the Courthouse as Judge Fisher declined the honor and would not be dictated to by a mob including drunks calling him a copperhead and traitor.

Days later a catastrophic assassination shocked America. Shouts of joy for victory turned to cries of mourning and sorrow. "The evil fire of treachery and treason killed the South's best friend. His simplicity of character, un-ostentatious manners, even handed justice and magnanimity showed too much mercy for those who showed none."[102]

Why did this evil happen and who was to blame? Father Abraham became an American Moses who freed the multitude of slaves by inflicting plagues on the Confederate pharaoh but would not cross the Jordan River into the Promised Land. Lincoln attributed the war to God's punishment for the sin of slavery. Mortal man did not have the capacity to understand the grand scheme unfolding. The principals of freedom and justice transcended one man and need be carried out for generations to follow. Removal of a great leader was another punishment for an unrepentant flock.

Lincoln would have pardoned all. Would his successor be as merciful? At chapel service, Surgeon Mintzer spoke with glowing terms on the life and character of Lincoln. He referred to punishing rebels, confiscating their property and giving it to enlisted men.

The town paper quoted the *New York Herald* suggesting that Lincoln was a dictator; "the latest instance of the liability of tyrants to be an assassin's weapon." Rebel sympathizers who were in charge of the court house of York County did not drape for mourning.

Everybody except copperheads was downhearted and no emblems of mourning were displayed so that patients and guard of the hospital took up the matter. On Sunday at 9 a.m., Dr. Mintzer led twenty hospital convalescents and officers to the astonishment and chagrin of many, quietly and decorously festooned and draped in a proper manner the main entrance, building columns and cupola, at their own expense and risk. No one interfered and some applauded.[103]

A funeral train heavily draped with flags and emblems of mourning arrived in York on a Friday evening and remained for ten minutes. People let their feelings run and for a while buried forgotten prejudices and animosities. Guns were fired. "Our brass band under Dr. Mintzer united with citizens in forming a procession and marched to the depot station to keep back the crowd. Not a word was spoken. Crippled and wounded soldiers, old men and women, and fair maidens brushed away tears. 'He was crucified for us' said an aged colored man as the shrill whistle sounded and the scene ended. The train left-never to be forgotten."[104] A man in Philadelphia distributed to people on the streets slips of muslin saying "Pardon died with Abraham Lincoln."[105]

Valedictory and Closure

What will be done with our hospital? The *Cartridge Box* considered the possibility of the hospital closing unlikely. York County had an outstanding military hospital in an agricultural center with good water and rail connections. There was no rent to pay, and the buildings were well kept, recently refurbished with excellent grounds and good management. Those advocating closure were "notorious sympathizers of the rebellion who never had any special love or affection for Union soldiers."[106] The *York Gazette* noted, "now that the war is over there will probably be no occasion for the continuance of this hospital for any great length of time." In May orders came from Washington to discharge all those who did not require treatment.

"And still they come" was the headline for the week of May 20, 1865, with the arrival of over 400 patients. Their regiments may have mustered out but many of their soldiers were still trying to get home without paycheck and railroads demanding payment for a seat.

Some began refusing orders, often those with criminal tendencies. A hospital riot was quelled by guards and officers who sustained serious though non-fatal injuries. New orders demanded that "any soldier guilty of insubordination or mutiny is to be placed in irons."[107] Rowdies would not be tolerated.

> We have been infested with a species of characters with vulgar parlance that prowl in squads, and congregate in dens of outlaws, vagrants, and vagabonds. They are too lazy to work, attack travelers, countryman, farmers, wounded and sick soldiers. They favor assault and battery, gambling, burglary and pick-pocketing. Some local citizens are afraid to go out at night as life and property are no longer safe. We need to protect soldiers from ruthless and merciless criminal mob who assault without provocation.[108]

On the week ending June 24, 1865, 556 mustered out, leaving 456 inpatients. The newspaper was financially supported by the hospital fund, and delinquent newspaper subscribers were asked to pay up. On July 8, 1865, the band played its last concert. Hospital supplies went to the children's home in York founded for those orphaned by war. They would "educate and board poor white orphans and other friendless, destitute or vagrant white children under the age of 12."

The editor noted that soldiers were

> well cared for here, in a quiet and comfortable ward, by tender surgeons and faithful attendants. Faces of ministering angels relieved his suffering, his solitude and loneliness. Reader, do you ever pause to consider that you too are going home? Your term of enlistment is about ended. Have you been a poor soldier that skulked and straggled in the hour of duty and trial? Loved ones await your familiar face and your placement on the muster roll while nervously complain that others are released and not you.[109]

The last editor wrote a valedictory thanking Surgeon Minzter, whose actions "greatly improved the soldier experience" over the past eight months. He suggested making the facility a home for disabled soldiers. The statistics covering hospital life from June 27, 1862, through July 8, 1865, follow.[110]

Admitted	14,253
Transferred	1,348
RTD	7,549
Discharged for disability	1,120
Furloughed	3,788
Died	193
Remaining in hospital	328

The mortality rate of 1.3 percent compared well with other facilities. Today the Commons is a city park with basketball courts and a playground for youngsters. A 61-foot tall Victory soldier and sailor monument made of Vermont marble is surrounded by life-size bronze figures and depictions of experiences commemorating their Civil War legacy. Ten percent of York County volunteered for the Union army and ten percent of those failed to return alive. Thirty-six hometown boys are buried at nearby Prospect Hill Cemetery, overseen by a Union soldier of granite.

Eight

Knight Hospital Record

New Haven was the hub of rail and water transportation, making it the best location in Connecticut for a hospital complex. On a 12-acre site just off the harbor sat the Connecticut State Hospital, built in 1830 for the indigent and itinerant seamen. It seemed no expense was spared this fortress-like building covered with 70 large windows and mahogany window sills.[1] It became the anchor of a health care complex funded and regulated by the federal government. The land was rented from the state for $1,000 a year and its buildings declared federal property, thus enabling physicians to be paid as contract surgeons. For each hospital bed filled, the federal government paid $3.50 a week covering all costs as a primarily single-payer universal health care system. The state legislature contributed as did individual donors, volunteers, and a generous, wealthy governor, William Buckingham. Providing health care for citizens was for the first time a federal responsibility.

A city within a city was created with a library holding 800 books, magazines and newspapers.[2] The chapel was non-denominational, serviced by two ministers who also ran the library and post office. The hospital was named after Jonathon Knight, the first professor of anatomy of the Yale Department of Medicine, later the chief of surgery for 26 years and the first President of the American Medical Association.[3] His junior partner and fellow Yale graduate was Pliny Adams Jewett, destined to become chief of the new hospital's medical staff composed of Yale medical professors and students, regular army medical officers and physicians in private practice.

On May 20, 1862, following the Battle of Fair Oaks, a steamship deposited 260 sick and wounded soldiers at this new army hospital to be housed in newly erected tents. They were replaced by the standard one-story pavilion buildings filled in rows of 60 to 100 beds separated by a small table and chair, with a card indicating bed number, name of patient, date of admission and diagnosis.

The *Knight Hospital Record* began publication on October 5, 1864, issued every Wednesday through 12 July 1865. It was affordable at $1.50 a year, also sold at city news stands and shops. Its goal was "to place before the reader's news gathered from any source, such as incidents of battles, march and bivouac from eye witnesses. Hospital events and news items would be of interest to their friends, family and the public at large."[4] It would be a "welcome visitor" to the bedsides of the sick and wounded, in their Connecticut homesteads, and in camp, fortress and picket duty. "Patients will receive the best of treatment and no soldier will find any fault in the hands of the surgeons in this Hospital."[5]

Submissions came from hospital wards, battlefields and literary salons. Articles of interest were reprinted from other Northern and Southern newspapers, as well as the foreign press. Copies were sought by Connecticut soldiers stationed in the Southern battlefields. The workings of the hospital were described, including construction of the 1,000-bed hospital, and the details of how, when, and why patients were treated and transported from the battlefield. The most up-to-date status of Connecticut soldiers, sick or wounded, alive or dead, could be found in this publication. For the three years of hospital existence, there were 9,547 admissions, 3,000 returned to duty, 2,317 furloughed, 1,500 discharged, 206 deaths and 453 desertions.[6]

Details of hospital daily life were described from reveille to Surgeon Call. Hospital supplies and food consumed were listed in detail in *The Outfit* and *What is consumed in a Hospital*.

Notions of a "gloomy and forbidding" atmosphere were dismissed. "Nearly everyone is briskly employed all day; everything goes on systematically and like clock-work and that everything possible is done to make the brave boys who have lost health or limbs or been wounded in their country' service as comfortable as possible."[7]

Library

The Hospital Library was created from civilian donations and contained religious and scientific works, novels, and an assortment of non-fiction works. There was a gaggle of newspapers from New York, Hartford, Boston, New Haven and London. Other hospital newspapers were also displayed. "Old books are read so often, some now are unfit to read," declared the librarian. The books most sought after were "novels and adventure stories that appealed to soldiers." Library hours were 1 to 3 p.m. daily except Sunday. The reading room, filled with newspapers and magazines, was open daily from 9 a.m. to noon and 2 to 6 p.m.

Mail

The importance of mail was stressed in editorials and letters to the editor. The phrase "write me" was included in most soldiers' letters of this or any war. Health is discussed as were current events, the quality and quantity of food, and inquiries about goings on back home. But always came the plea "write me" and do not forget me, and reminded family and friends to do the same. In the first week of December 1864, the Knight Hospital post office processed 1,000 letters. "Printers devil" urged the fair sex not to forget paying postage on their letters as soldiers often had no stamps or pay.

Advertisements

For sale were the same items as in other hospital newspapers. Inexpensive coats, pants, boots and shoes were made expressly for soldiers' wear. How to obtain photographic portraits, bounties and pensions was prominently displayed.

Proprietary medicines were popular, there being no government regulation of drugs or much else. One hundred proof alcohol, opium, and cocaine were frequent ingredients in over-the-counter products. A notice in the *Record* gave soldierly medical advice for sore feet.

> An excellent composition for anointing the feet of soldiers during long marches: "Take equal parts of gum camphor, olive oil and pure beeswax, and mix them together, warm, until they are united and become a salve. At night wash the feet well, dry them, and then apply this salve, and put on clean stockings and sleep with them on. The next day the feet will be in excellent condition for marching."[8]

Sure-fire remedies for tuberculosis, rheumatism and the common cold were readily available. *A Cold in the head* cautioned that "doctors pills are death on bills, which does not change that time will fly, the nose will run and sneeze trumpeting will prevail. Is consumptions dreary cough better than the misery and headache of the hard disease that mortal flesh is heir such as a bad cold?"[9]

The Sanitary Commission and the Army distributed pamphlets outlining what the soldier could do to maintain his own health. "Preserving the Health of the Soldier" recommended that ground selected for encampment be dry and elevated, and that appropriate latrines be built and maintained. Fresh foods and vegetables were essential for success along with vaccination, regular exercise and weekly bathing. The *Record* made its views known on the virtues of being outdoors.

> *On sleeping out of doors.* How mistaken our mothers were when they warned us against exposure to night air, and sleeping in damp clothing and going with wet feet! Judging from a two years' experience of almost constant field services, I conclude that these things are wholesome and restorative. It is sleeping inside of walls that ought to properly be called exposure, and demands vigorous vitality; I have a screed to deliver some day on this subject to a misguided and house-poisoned public.[10]

> *Sleeping with open Windows.* A letter in the *London Times* says there is no doubt of the beneficial effect to health of sleeping with windows open in opposition to the old notion of the noxious quality of night air; "Beware the vile contagion of the night." Health and prolonged life are enhanced by sleeping with open windows. Early exercise in open air is the best of medicine.[11]

The extraordinary hardships of battlefield evacuation were described in *how a wounded soldier gets home.*

> In three or four days you reach the welcome quarters of a General Hospital where sleep is on a mattress. Efficient nurses perform a thorough washing of the bloody and dirty volunteers. By rail a bed of straw in box car is anticipated. By ship the worst are below decks, helpless in intense agony and suffering. Stretched out on cots the entire lengths of long cabins are hundreds of helpless forms, with intense agony and suffering. The attendants move silently and specter like from bed to bed. No day light is admitted, just attendants with dimly burning lamps casting feeble rays on whitened ghastly scenes. Few words are spoken. Finally you arrive at the dock and now reside in a hospital until your wounds heal.[12]

The assistant surgeon rendered initial treatment at the battle site. Doctors became specialized in amputation surgery, becoming expert in *how* to operate and more importantly *when*. The *Record* published cost and availability factors for the amputee's prosthesis and names of like patients for further information. "Hospital Notice: soldiers who have lost an arm and who wish to get one can see Edward Riecker in Ward Four."

Stories and poems both serious and humorous centered on amputations.

> *An off-hand joke.* A sturdy sergeant of one of Massachusetts regiments was obliged to have his hand amputated. The surgeon offered to administer chloroform as usual, but the veteran refused saying: "If the cutting was to be done on him, he wanted to see it." He placed his arm on the table and submitted to the operation without a sign of pain except for firm setting of the teeth. The operator he looked at his victim with admiration and remarked. "You ought to have been a surgeon." "I was the next thing

to one before I enlisted," said the hero. "What was that," asked the doctor. "A butcher," replied the sergeant with a grim smile, which despite the circumstances, communicated itself to the bystanders.[13]

Justifiable superlative. 'Tree mend us!' exclaimed the amputated young hero, calling for his wooden leg after the first glorious battle.

Sometimes it was necessary to sacrifice a limb to save a life, but never a life to save a limb. This medical metaphor explained the need for union. Profound sacrifices were required, in this instance a patriot's right arm.

Goodbye, old arm
A wounded hero was lying on the amputating table under chloroform. They cut off his strong right arm and cast it still bleeding upon the pile of human limbs then laid him on a couch. He woke and missed his arm. With his left he lifted the cloth and cried, "Where's my arm? Get my arm! I want to see it once more, my strong right arm." He took hold of the cold clammy fingers and looking steadfast said "Goodbye, old arm. We have been a long time together. We must part now.

Good-bye old arm. You'll never fire another carbine, nor swing another saber for the Government," and the tears rolled down his cheeks. He said to those around him "Understand, I don't regret its loss. It has been torn from my body that not one state should be torn from this glorious Union.[14]

The poem *Song* reveled in the honor, fame and glory naturally bestowed on the nation's volunteers: free and brave men who "fill up the bowl," and preserved and protected freedom, motivated by love of country and the will to be "savior of our nation." This required a "manly bearing" as they "put it through" against men of treason so others could be free and God's work be done.

Women in America had three things in common with slaves: they could not vote, own property or sign a legal contract. Nonetheless their contributions and sacrifices filled the starry firmament. The nation needed to pay attention to their energy, nobility, and quiet heroism. *Women and the war* declared, "the patriotic fire has blown nowhere with a brighter and steadier radiance than among the women of our country. The nation must take notice of their energetic and persistent devotion along with such earnest, benevolent, and modest countenance." Flocks of Florence Nightingales cheerfully left happy homes for distant hospitals to care for the sick and wounded volunteers. A debt of gratitude was owed noble women who stood by in the darkest hours.

Romance and Marriage

Prayer and the love of a woman could bring salvation for what seemed hopeless. A young girl living in the Western frontier received a letter each week from her soldier love but was too poor for writing materials to respond, but love found a way and they happily re-united.

The following were stories, morality tales and jokes concerning romance, the fair sex, heartaches and consequences.

A woman in England has just been tried for having five husbands. She said her experience was trial enough.

An order to undertaker from an afflicted widower:
"Sur; my waif is ded, and Wants to be berried to morro. At wunoklok. U nose wair to dig the hole-bi the side of my too uther waifs-Let it be deep."

The Sayings of Josh Billings, humorist and journalist, added seasoning for the hospital funny bone.[15]

> Adam invented luv at first sight, one of the greatest labor saving machines the world ever saw.
>
> I suppose the reason wi wimmen are so fast talkers, iz because they don't have tew stop tew spit on their hands.
>
> I hav heard a greater deel ced about broken hearts and there may be a few of them but mi experience is that next tew the gizzard the harte is the tuffest peace of meat in the whole critter.
>
> There is nothing in this life that will open the pores of a man so mutch as tu fall in luv; it makes him az fluent as a tin wissel, as limber as a boys watch chain, as perlite as a danzing master, his heart as full with sunshine as a hay field and there aint any more guile in him that there is in a stick of merlasses candy.
>
> There is "one cold, blue, lean kiss that always makes him shiver to see. Two persons (ov female purswashun) who have witness a grate many younger and more pulpy dazs, meet in some publick place, and not having saw each uther for 24 ours, they kiss immediately; then tha tork about the weather, and the young man who preached yesterday, and tha kiss immediately, and they blush and laff at what tha sa tew each other, and kiss agin immediately. This kind ov kissing alwus puts me in mind ov two old flints stricking tew start a fire."[16]

A bashful youth was paying his addresses to a gay lass of the country, who had long despaired of bringing things to a crisis. He called one day when she was at home alone. After settling the merits of the weather, Miss said, looking silly into his face:
"I dreamed of you last night."
"Did you? Why now!"
"Yes, I dreamed that you kissed me."
"Why now! What did you dream that your mother said?"
"Oh, I dreamed she wasn't at home."
A light dawned on the youth's intellect, and directly something was heard to crack—perhaps his whip, and perhaps not, but in about a month they were married.

> *How to propose.* A party of ladies and gentlemen were laughing over the supposed awkwardness attending a declaration of love, when a gentleman remarked that if ever he offered himself he would do it in a collected and business-like manner.
>
> Miss S ----, I have been two years looking for a wife. I am in receipt of about three hundred a year, which is on the increase. Of all the ladies of my acquaintance, I admire you the most; indeed I love you, and would gladly make you my wife.
>
> Miss S ---- replies. "You flatter me by your preference. I refer you to my father."
>
> The gentleman exclaimed "Bravo!"
>
> They were married soon after. Wasn't that a modest way of "coming to the point and a lady like method of taking a man at his word?"

The process of dating was explored in *At Dorchester*. A maiden's angelic face promised much, was so near and yet so far. Ladies fair with soft blue eyes, golden hair, and orbs the color of raven's wing, kept any man's heart fluttering. The devilish hand moved the innermost heart with an unrequited love extinguishable only by death.

The search for a soul mate brought up the age-old question as to what kind of gal would be best. Did the "orbs of Dorchester" match the importance of a kind soul and gentle touch? A more earthly approach was *I'm Not Particular*, recommending being humble and easy to please. The writer's wish list included youth with winning grace, pleasing face, rosy health, and untold wealth, someone who could kiss and squeeze without smothering, please! On the negative side were several cautions; "not scolds, fat or stately, and not 'too good,' dreadful bashful or rude." Job applicants needed to be flexible to his moods and know he was not particular.

In *Delusion*, the maidens were fair, fresh, and sweet with glowing charms and winning smiles. Caution was prescribed for *The Dangerous Maiden*, a radiant beauty with seashell-pink lips, violet eyes, and hair black as the night. Beware, as her power enthralled, beguiled and bewildered and could plunge thee in woe! The fear of rejection and inexperience in finding a mate was the subject of *The Sensitive Man*. The shy and self-effacing young man envied the happily married and yearned for the same.

In *The Old Maid's Lament,* the struggle to catch a beau seemed doomed by foolish and shallow men. Their young smiling faces, bewhiskered and often bewildered, left the maiden with an aching heart, disappointment and unfulfilled dreams of bliss. The only consolation might be a warm, ungrateful cat. Why did men chase young girls when the older were steady and the rents so much less?[17] The readership's response to this poem was so sharp that a parody was published four weeks later, *The Old Bachelor's Lament*.[18] It appeared that winsome beauties, with dainty face and figure and cunning feet, were just as foolish as their male counterparts. Youthful ardor trapped in a dreary attic while spying on promenading lassies, not surprisingly got a cold shoulder or no look at all. Seeking love as if stalking prey would bring no smile but irksome trepidation and a dull, eventless life. His only company would be man's best friend (his two hounds) and a cigar. No wonder none ever would be his wife! His mature outside was 40-plus and becoming less handsome, but with a heart still warm and a pulse most youthful. Desire and hope kept the home fires burning until time ran out.

In December 1864, a Social Hop was held in Smith's Hall with music provided by the Thomas Quadrille Band, costing 50 cents, and a Grand Masquerade Ball in Exchange Hall. Advertisements for such social gatherings were displayed in the *Record* and memorialized in *Home from the Hop*. A captain from the hospital convalescing from a saber thrust met an old flame but parted without an embrace. Wounds of the flesh or psyche did not always heal leaving scars unseen.

The Union Soldiers Glee Club was formed by six hospital clerks, giving free concerts at 8 p.m. in the gaily decorated Chapel. Solo and chorus group performances were aided by fife or drum. When weather permitted they performed atop the observatory of the State Hospital building, which allowed the entire camp to hear. The drama critic remarked, "we have passed many pleasant hours in their company listening too many of their choice selections. Unfortunately they are awaiting discharges and soon will be gone."

Blacks

Some Northerners were strict abolitionists. The majority favored maintaining the Union and abolishing slavery but reflected the predominant belief in racial inequality.

- A former slave in Alabama finds himself guarding his previous master who objects.

"My own slave can never stand guard over me, it's a damned outraged; no gentleman would submit to it. Listen, Sambo."

"You hush, dar; I'se done one talking to you now. Hush rebel!" was the Negro's emphatic command, bringing down his musket to a charge bayonet position, by way of enforcing silence. The nabob was now a slave, his once valued Negro the master: and think you, as he sank back upon a blanket, in horror and shame that night, that he believed human bondage was a divine institution, ordained by God?

- A contraband recently inquired a volunteer:

"Can you tell me why it is that Massa Burnside found that it took five Northerners to whip one southerner."

"No," replied the solider, "why is it?"

"Why sir, it takes four Northerners to catch one Southerner—he run so fast—and it takes the other Northerner to whip him!"

Pretty good for a Contraband.

- *An Intelligent contraband.*

The colored contraband known as the "intelligent contraband" was enlisted and in Cincinnati when a merchant doing business was confronted by a bayonet held by one of our American brethren of African descent.

- "What hab you got dar?" said the sable warrior pointing to the suspicious valise.

"Three dirty shirts, four pairs of socks, a comb and a bottle of Hiawatha," was the reply.

"What am your permit to bring dem articles into Kentucky?" demanded the vigilant sentry.

He took from his pocket a promissory note for $130 and handed it to the intelligent contraband who after regarding the document upside down with a profound attention returned it saying "All correct; you may pass."

- A contraband called Tom was asked about the idea of the South arming slaves. "I heard of right smart talk. Bout half de colored men thank dey would run directly over to the Yankees wid the arms in their hands and toder half think dey would jiss stand an' fire a few volleys to de rear fust'for they run, dat's all the difference."

- At the siege of Nashville, Confederate soldiers under General Stedman were captured by a colored brigade and would not surrender to a "damn nigger." "Bery sorry, massa," said Sambo, bringing his piece to a ready, "but we's in a great hurry and hain't got no time to send for a white man." He was afraid his father would kill him if he knew had surrendered to a nigger.

- In a border state, a Captain Davidson had cut the ears off a Negro and sewed them together using them for barter for whiskey. He offered the ears as "Lincoln skins" to pay for the drinks. "Well, take your change out of that." They had called union paper money, Lincoln skins. The ears were substituted for the same. Surely, such a fiend incarnate should be hunted from the earth like a wolf or a mad dog.

- Wendell Phillips, a strict abolitionist minister, tells the story about George Washington. He had traveled a long distance and was looking for a rest, coming across a camp with the black servant of another general. The servant gives him a buffalo robe to lie down in. Washington curls up and falls asleep. He awakens a few hours later and sees the servant shivering in cold. He says, "come here, there is room for two under this skin. Today the American flag is broad enough to cover black and white equal together."

- After the fall of Richmond, nearly every Negro is now seen with a cigar in his mouth. Last week it would have cost him fifteen lashes on his back to indulge in that luxury. New masters make new manners.

Irish

The Irish were the latest immigrant group, coming to America to escape starvation from the potato famine on the Emerald Isle.

A lawyer is disgusted at seeing a couple of Irishmen looking at a six-sided building, which he was occupying, shouted out.

"What do you stand thus for, like a pair of blockheads, gazing at my office? Do you think it a church?"
One answered, "I was thinking so till the devil poked his head out of the windy."

Obeying orders
A certain general in the army supposed his favorite horse was dead ordered an Irishman to go and skin him.
"What! Is Silver Tail dead?" asked Pat.
"What's that to you? Do as you're told" replied the officer.
Pat went about his business and returned two hours later.
"Well Pat where have you been to all this time?"
"Skinning the horse, yer honor."
"Does it take two hours to do such an operation?'
"No yer honor, but it tuck half an hour to catch him."
"Catch him! Was he alive?'
"Yes yer honor and you know I could not skin him alive."
"Skin him alive! Did you kill him?"
"To be sure I did; you know I must obey orders without asking any questions."

General Grant and Irishman
A rollicking Irish soldier was trudging along a road to Petersburg with a pig on a string behind him, when General Grant overtook him.
"Where did you steal that pig you plundering rascal?" said Grant.
"What pig general," exclaimed Pat.
"Why that pig behind you on your string, you rascal."
"Well then I protest," looking behind him and acting as if he had not seen the beast before. "It is scandalous in this wicked world to see how ready folks are to take away on honest boy's character. Some blackguard, wanting to get me into trouble, has tied the baste to my cartridge box."

An Irishman was told that a certain person had eaten ten saucers of ice cream whereupon Patrick shook his head. "So you don't believe him?" With a shrewd nod Pat answered, "I believe in the crame but not in the saucers."

An Irishman was asked to furnish proof of his marriage, and he took off his hat. "Here is me marriage certificate. That' Judy's mark."

An English schoolmaster to his Hibernian pupil, "Dennis my boy, I fear I shall make nothing of you; you have no application." The quick-witted lad then replied, "isn't it myself that's always told there's no occasion for it? Don't I see every day in the newspapers that 'no Irish need apply, at all?"

Examples of the dry humor of the time follow:

A prickly and innovative editor heads his list of births, marriages, and death as; "hatched, matched, and dispatched."
Down east they put a fellow in jail for swindling. The audacious chap had dried snow and sold it for salt.

Comments on human nature by Josh Billings follow:

The only wa tu git yure rights is tu demand them.

He who can hold awl he gits, kan most generally git more.

There are a great multitude of individuals who are like blind mules, anxious enough to kick, but kant tell whare.

Don't never parade yure good luck, nor yure bad luck, before men; the first sight will make them think less ov yu, and the second will make them think more of themselves.

Patriotism

The American Revolution was a common reference point, a great victory offering hope and inspiration in the creation of a republican democracy. The theme of bravery was extolled in the Battle of Ticonderoga, where the courage and boldness of Ethan Allen and the Green Mountain Boys ensured that Americans would prevail. In another Revolutionary tale, a British spy swallowed a silver ball containing secret information. His deception was proven by persistent Americans who ingeniously made him throw up evidence, then hanged him as a "traitor."

A life-threatening avalanche was overcome and all survived due to heroic efforts and self-sacrificing teamwork. Individualism was extolled by a six-foot, four-inch Texas Ranger who galloped through a hundred Comanche Indians, escaping into a forest as sanctuary. Despite being outnumbered, the forces of good managed to triumph over evil thanks to bravery, skill and daring.

Patriots left a home with wife and children for peace and love of country. Under freedom's banner, "manly bearing" brought honor, fame and glory. Men bled, defending the rights of others, creating their own orphans and widows. Immune to golden treasure, ease and pleasure, they were imbued with love of country requiring sacrifice at a steep price.

The Volunteer, brave and undaunted, mustered in to face the venomous bite of the vile copperhead and defend and protect freedom's light against all such traitors. Hospital editorials defined traitors as not necessarily limited to the Confederacy but to the Democratic Party in the North as well. Peace at any price was marked the call of traitors!

The stars and stripes was freedom's banner, sometimes torn and tattered but always inspiring the hearts and minds of its countrymen. *GOD SAVE THE FLAG* identified a banner washed in the blood of the brave, much as the burning bush of Moses was seen only by the faithful and never consumed by its fire. False prophets sought its fall along with the freedom and justice it represents. God blessed this flag only and its defenders.

The Draft

Camp Rendezvous, just outside New Haven, housed raw recruits kept under watch for bounty jumpers deserting. The substitutes were "men of almost every nation under heaven, speaking in so many different tongues that even the learned blacksmith would be puzzled to hold conversation with them." A series of articles offered a detailed account of the problems encountered, similar to the camp of recruits near Augur Hospital outside of Alexandria.

The recruits were from Vermont, Rhode Island and Connecticut and were kept in a converted carriage factory.

> The men were placed before an enrolling board and while stripped and thoroughly examined by an experienced surgeon put through a variety of motions inspecting limbs, ears, eyes, chest. They were then dispatched to the quartermaster who provided uniform, blanket, haversack, canteen, tin cup, plate and bounty. Numerous dodges and ingenious devices on part of substitute brokers made the business of procuring recruits notorious and lucrative. They evinced much skill in covering up defects. Once mustered in, they could ask for medical discharge and pension for an undeclared preexisting or imaginary disability. Some enlist out of necessity and laudable motives. Among them are numerous foreigners, recently arrived and not subject to the draft.[19]

Buildings were surrounded by a 14-foot fence with perimeter guards. Some recruits ran singly or in a stampede, while others tried escape through tunnels.

> They threw away knapsacks and overcoats while scattering in various direction pursued by several officers and an NCO. Revolvers were used to some extent accounting for two wounded; one through the chest though not mortal. If the officers in command would make a severe and summary example of a few we think the crime would speedily go out of fashion. Many of the fugitive rascals were captured. John Stannard, a convalescent guard was "badly bruised about the face while attempting to stop a substitute who had escaped from Conscription Camp. The substitute did his best to get away but fell into the hands of 'Uncle Sam's boys' who are not to be trifled with, and who don't believe letting bounty jumpers escape, surrendered and was marched back to camp."[20]

Duty of the North and why the war is not over placed blame on overestimating the number of Union soldiers and underestimating the Confederates. The quality of some soldiers was called into question. Volunteers required little monetary encouragement, and the majority of new recruits were foreigners "without the same interest in this strife as those who are native." A substitute could be purchased for $300 but might desert at the first opportunity. "If the North trusts its hordes of hireling, there must be feeling of shame and humiliation witnessing a body of recruits under strong escort of soldiers with loaded muskets and fixed bayonets. They are not needed if our young men had the true spirit. There are thousands who could join the army without great sacrifice or inconvenience that patriotism or duty requires; otherwise the South will win."

Politics

The chilling rebel yell pierced the stillness, hailing not victory over Grant or Sherman but the Chicago nomination of diminutive General George McClellan, who had yet to gain a victory on battlefield or election booth. "Strength through Yankee treason" might save the South yet.

Man's best friend in *The Dog and the Copperhead* was mean, sinful, and untendered evil sitting on its hindquarters, able only to bark at the Freedom Train thundering by whose holy mission was to gladden each disloyal heart. The copperhead could only lie flat on his back and bark incessant grumblings since all knew he had no bite.

The soldier's newspaper contained many references to the political adversaries of the Lincoln administration.

> *Then and now.*
> Six months ago dialogue between a returning soldier and a copperhead ran thus.
> SOLDIER: Sir I have just returned from fighting for my country. I am wounded sick and sore. I am naked and hungry. Will you please give me something to eat?

COPPERHEAD: No, not even a mouthful. Clear out or I'll set my dog on you. I won't have a d—-d abolition soldier around my premises.
SOLDIER: Sir I am a loyal man, and have bled for my country's freedom.
COPPERHEAD: You are Abe Lincoln's hireling, fighting like a fool in this nigger war.
SOLDIER: Have you no sympathy for those who spill their blood to put down treason?
COPPERHEAD: Sympathy! I wish every d—d soldier from the North might be shot dead in battle today!
Six months later.
COPPERHEAD: Well, John we have licked old Lee and got him and his army of seventy thousand! Now we will have the good old Union again.
SOLDIER: Union! Do you go for Union?
COPPERHEAD: Certainly. I always did. No man rejoices more sincerely than we democrats at the success of our army!
SOLDIER: You lying hypocritical old traitor. Ain't you ashamed of yourself? You are ten times more rebel than Lee or Jeff Davis and now do you expect your copperhead party can deceive honest men who know how to read. Run to Niagara Falls, get on the British side and consult your friends.[21]

The *Charleston Mercury* was said to have given a harsh review of their army, reproduced in the *Record*. "The troops are a herd of stragglers and outlaws, under the command of imbeciles. The path we are now traveling is straight to destruction. The results of the next six months will bring the confederacy to the ground or will reinstate it in power. Without reform we are doomed."[22]

In an ode to *Nursery Rhymes Humpty Dumpty*, Jeff Davis and the Confederacy had a great fall, tumbling down while breaking their crown, and could not be put back together again. Sentiment against the Southern leaders was unabated.

Ensign Stebbings, was asked what he would do with a captured Jeff Davis. "Sir, I would have him dressed in garments made of the American flag from hat to boots, and marched the length of the country for one year whistling Hail Columbia, and if he wavered in the least, I would hang him high as Haman."

Jeff Davis is a base and unprincipled instigator of the great rebellion, notorious rebel chief, robber, murderer, assassin, who was captured in petticoats. He fled to Florida with stolen gold desperate in attempts to ruin the country. He assassinates murders and still he fails. He steals from his own deluded followers starving as they be and flees the country. Of course he will be hanged. If Booth deserved mutilation and an unknown grave, Jefferson Davis merits no better fate provided his punishment is commensurate with his crime.[23]

The beggars in Richmond do not ask for pennies. Their petition is put thus—"Will you give me five dollars to buy a loaf of bread?"

A Confession.—A rebel private, who deserted at Southwest Creek, North Carolina, says on the night of Hoke's bloody assault and repulse, he was on duty as sentry, when he overheard the following conversations between General Hill and Col. Beard:
Hill—"Colonel, what shall we do?"
Beard—"Retreat to Tennessee, from there to Texas, and from Texas to Hell. So far as the privates are concerned, if they had half sense, they would desert and go home."
Hill—"True, every word of it."
Our rebel informant tells us that he took Gen. Hill's advice, and before morning had put the above suggestions into practice.

A Richmond editor says Grant's army is so largely made up of "the riff raff of creation" that it is no honor for the rebels to defeat it. That is probably the reason they don't.

On October 5, 1864, a hospital poll on each of nine wards favored Lincoln with 515 votes and McClellan 202, reflecting the national mood.

An Army letter says 60,000 men were furloughed to go home and vote. Most furloughs are now expired. A fine soldier of a New York regiment was seduced into desertion by his wife. His mother lived in Canada and had not been seen for three years. Taking his wife with him he made a visit and was persuaded by mother and wife to desert. There are some such cases where respectable men desert the service through the influence of their wives and relations at home. There are of course numerous bad men in the army who seize upon every opportunity to leave the service.[24]

Nearly 500 soldiers have been furloughed from this Hospital within the past few days for the purpose of voting in the coming election.[25]

Messrs. H. Lynde Harrison and Alvin Meade, the Commissioners to receive soldier votes for the Department of the East, will be in New York City through the present week, until election day, for the purpose of receiving the votes of any men who may be unable to vote in the State on election day. One or the other of them may be found at any time at the Irving House, on 12 Street, near Broadway.[26]

An editorial declared the coming presidential convention "conceived in wisdom, nourished by the blood of heroes and martyrs and prospered by heaven would be given over to the tender mercies of domestic traitors and foreign enemies." The Democratic platform was peace at any price with submission to the demands of rebels. The *Record* described the President of the Democratic Convention as a "foreigner and agent of a foreign Banking House whose only concern for this country is to make as much money as possible out of it." Their leaders were Congressman Vallandingham, a "convicted and banished traitor," Senator Pendleton, a "recreant who voted against all appropriations of men wanted for defense," and Seymour, who "recognizes and addresses armed murderers and incendiaries as his friends and whose agents were on trial for stupendous frauds intended to cheat soldier of their votes." The record of Fernando Wood opposed all that was honest and true. "They stamp their own infamy on high reputations of America with such foul slander that the war has been a failure. Thousands of brave men have poured out their blood like water and offered up their lives in every battle field." The Lincoln administration's principles were Union now and forever and the prohibition of slavery everywhere.[27]

"Can anyone tell the difference between the Copperheads and Rebels? A victory gained by the 'Peace party' at home greatly encourages the rebels and dispirits the Union soldiers. Let the election set upon a grand and overwhelming Union majority at home and the news be born upon their exultant shouts across to the rebel army lines. A glorious and lasting peace will be secured by Union victory. The days of the Rebellion are numbered."[28]

The *Record* reported a pre-election Grand Union Procession of 10,000 people in New Haven, exceeded only by a demonstration in New York City. Among the participants were 131 hospital patients, 75 discharged soldiers, and 110 men from the Conscript Camp. A stone was thrown by "McClellan brats," hitting a soldier just above eye, while another sustained a wrist laceration. A transparency carried by soldiers read, "Bullets for our enemies in the field, and ballots for our enemies at home." The editorial expressed the "hope there will be plenty of the latter for them on the 8th day of November."[29]

New Haven County gave a majority of 921 votes to George McClellan and Hartford County a nine-vote majority to Lincoln. Out of 85,443 votes cast statewide, Lincoln lead by 2,427.

Military Leaders

The exploits and personal lives of the "peacemakers" were of great interest. The quiet courage shown by the enlisted man was reflected in the honesty and forthrightness of Ulysses Grant. He was a humble man with a quiet and modest simplicity, a young yet manly bearing and unbounded confidence of the troops and in himself.

While strolling in Philadelphia, he was spotted by a soldier arousing a cheering, enthusiastic crowd, forcing him to take refuge in the Mayor's office. He and his family were revered, though not so much by his father, who once described his teenage son as "useless" rather than Ulysses because of his lack of business sense. Grant spoke plainly and with reticence. At a reception for the General in Chicago, General Sherman said he was "always ready, always willing, and always proud to honor my old commander. I was willing to do anything he asked me to do, and I know he never wished me to make a speech." The crowd shouted, "Order him to speak, general." Grant replied, "I never ask a soldier to do anything which I cannot do myself."[30]

Comparisons between Lee and Grant were inevitable. Lee violated the oath required to enter West Point to support and defend the Constitution. Grant compelled the surrender of three Confederate armies at Fort Donelson, Vicksburg and Appomattox. Lee compelled none. Even handwriting was fair game. Lee was "bold and stiff, letters large and distinct, bearing heavily upon the pen and abbreviated many words." Grant was not so bold or distinct, letters not large or erect but legible and striking. He was full of energy and action. "Great men write poor hands." [Grant's memoirs are considered one of the best ever written and include the finest description of how the Mexican War inevitably led to the Civil War.] General Winfield Scott was in his mid-seventies, weighing over 300 pounds as the first chief of the Union army, and sent Grant a copy of his autobiography with an inscription, "From the oldest to the ablest general in the world."

Victory converted Grant's recklessness to bravery, obstinacy to gallantry, and butchery to military genius. The *London Star* editorial of April 1865 celebrated the triumph of being on the right side of history.

> When Lee fought and piled up victims in defense of slavery, he was a hero. When Grant fought and with prodigious effort won victories for freedom, he was a butcher who knew neither military strategy nor was swayed by the feeling of our common humanity. Grant is considered pertinacious or obstinate but not called a military genius or gallant or magnificent of qualities.

His will power was accented in *General Grant and the Pony*. Many fairs had a pony with a monkey on its back, offering rides to those who could hold on. A strapping fellow was easily thrown, thus compelling others to try. A much smaller boy named Ulysses S. Grant [born Hiram Ulysses Grant] took the reins and tucked his heels close behind the shoulder blades of the pony, locking his hands around its neck. Before the cheering crowd, the pony reared high and ran the rink at great speed but could not throw young Ulysses. He "fought it out on that line," much as in taking Richmond and Vicksburg, unwavering to a proper, final conclusion.[31]

Grant was quoted on all matters, whether accurately or not did not matter as nothing detracted from the public's great admiration. Unlike most celebrities, he owned his accomplishments, a shining light in the firmament, a man who had earned his stars. Modest, generous and magnanimous was his nature, reflected in his understanding of his commander-in-chief's wishes for the same as post-war policy. Arms, artillery and public property would be parked, stacked and turned over to officers appointed by Grant. Officers could keep sidearms, private horses and baggage. Those officers and men who went home would not be disturbed by U.S. authorities so long as they observed their parole and laws in force where they resided.

He spoke and wrote plainly and clearly. "When the war is over I am going to give up cigars."[32] He died of cancer of the pharynx in 1885, perhaps caused by chronic smoking and thus self-inflicted much like the wars he fought.

The editorial on Wednesday, April 5, 1865, recalled the virtual invincibility of Lee's army with "dashing and impetuous charges. These butternut soldiers threw themselves into battle reckless and savage abandon buttressed with confidence of success and great pride," but all for naught. At long last, a headline trumpeted, "Richmond has fallen!" "Man's inhumanity to man" was over and wounds could begin to heal.

THE UNION FOREVER!
HURAH! HURAH! HURAH!
GLORIOUS SURRENDER OF LEE'S ARMY!
VICTORY! VICTORY! VICTORY!
ALL HONOR TO GENERAL GRANT AND THE BRAVE GENERALS AND SOLDIERS UNDER HIM.
UNION! ONE FLAG! ONE COUNTRY!

Soon again will be heard the sounds of peaceful industry and enterprise. The States lately in rebellion will again be gathered back into the fold, and the citizens of our common country again meet together as friends and wonder that anything could have so long and widely estranged them. The entire North is in a state of joyful intoxication. Copperheads and rebel sympathizers are as scarce as last year's roses. And now let us all do our utmost, in whatever way represents it, to hasten and consolidate our glorious re-union. Let us bear no grudges and indulge in no sneers or revengeful feelings. Let us welcome back our erring brethren and show them that we don't hate them for all the misery and suffering they have inflicted upon us.[33]

When this war shall cease what will be the story? It must be the grossest and unwarrantable barbarity of one side and the retaliation and humanity of the other.[34]

Richmond fell last Monday. The first troops to enter the fallen city were the colored troops of the 25th Corps. The soldiers in this hospital have not marched and suffered and bled in vain. And how the heart of our honest, excellent president swell with delight as he now sees his strait forward unswerving policy justified and rewarded. God bless him and be more resolved that the stars and stripes shall always wave over a free united and prosperous people.[35]

Lincoln

God Bless our noble President portrayed the instrument that ended the Rebellion. In death, Father Abraham was crowned for the ages, a towering figure honored, loved and even worshipped. He unselfishly became part of our lives, assuming the burden of his people. *The Last Chief* died to save the world, "his blood is freedom's Eucharist." His death was not in vain as the crime of slavery was ended and "God's holy work is done."

Story telling mixed facts with fiction and folklore with Aesop. Lincoln was a raconteur of jokes and stories drawn from Euclid, Shakespeare, the Bible and wood-stove banter. The political consequence of one battle was plainly explained in *A True Lincoln Story*.

He was asked how General Thomas victory before Nashville went. Hoods army was compared to Bill Sykes dog Yaller who was forever getting into the neighbor's house and chicken coops. They tried to kill it a hundred times. Got a bladder of a coon and filled it with powder and put it in a hot buttered biscuit. The dog swallowed it and exploded. The head of the dog lit on the porch, the forelegs on the fence, the hind legs in a ditch and the rest lay around loose. A neighbor proclaimed, "Bill I guess there aint much of that dog of yours left. "Well no," said Bill, "I see plenty of pieces but I guess that dog as a dog aint of much account now." Just so, the fragments of Hood's army aint of much account anymore.[36]

With malice towards none and mercy for all, he was magnanimous in forgiveness, offering pardons for deserters and hopeless enlisted men who were dying fast enough without him adding to the total. His penchant towards pardons was illustrated in *Reminiscences of Mr. Lincoln.*

> A distinguished citizen of Ohio had appointment with the President at 6 p.m. He entered the White House and saw a poorly clad young woman violently sobbing. She had been ordered away after waiting many hours to see the President about her only brother who deserted and was condemned to death. Both were foreigners and orphans. Lincoln's friend takes her to see the President. Lincoln exclaimed, "You have come here with no governor, Senator or Congressman to plead your cause. You seem honest and truthful and don't wear hoops-and I will be whipped but I will pardon your brother."

The pain of assassination was tempered by tales of Lincoln's nobility, kindness and fatherly love. *The Widow's Testimonial* and the Albany newsletter were such items.

> At the funeral of the President, a beautiful wreath of white roses graced the coffin sent from Boston by the sister of a young soldier who had been pardoned by the President when sentenced to be shot for desertion.[37]

> From a window in New York hangs a crutch shrouded with crape, and inscribed with the words "Our loss." Thereby hangs a tale. A woman sits at the window who has given her all to the country. No panoply catafalque covers the remains of her husband, yet she grieves with the emblem most expressive of her loss. She gave him up for her country's sake, and he lies on Gettysburg's bloody field. With a leg gone, he was slowly moving about, when he was struck again. Our late President visiting the hospitals, saw his death struggle and heard his last words, "Good-bye Carrie—meet me in heaven." The President's heart was opened. He stopped a moment, and wrote a letter of consolation to "the widow of John Dinsmore," to be sent with his crutch, and fifty dollars from his own purse. The widow has a sacred right to mourn such a loss.[38]

In Albany, when President Lincoln's remains passed through, it was said: "Four years ago, O' Illinois we took from thee and from among thy people an untried man; we return him to thee a mighty conqueror! Not thine any more, but the nation's—Not ours but the world's. Give him resting place, oh ye prairies! Make room for the ashes of the noblest man of all time." Father Abraham belonged to the ages, incomparable to mere mortals, bigger than life in death, etched forever in the heart, soul, and memory of the Grand Union he had preserved for generations to come.

The tone of reconciliation and hope for the future lasted one week. Lincoln's assassination changed the mood, intent, and direction of the country and would remain so for over a century. With one bullet, a very different world emerged: embittered, enraged with pain and seeking justice and revenge. The reconstruction of the union would be long, painful, and incomplete. Some wounds festered and did not heal.

> The hand of charity and friendship for the poor and afflicted was ready to pardon guilty rebels but now the whole loyal nation mourns a great and good man.... As their motto was in Latin "Sic Temper Tyrannies," ours is plain English. "War for revenge, death and annihilation to traitors and assassins." Because of this accursed rebellion, people cry out for vengeance. The calls for justice come from maimed and crippled soldiers now swarming the country. They demand it. Let every traitor beware the vengeance of an outraged people. Let every sympathizer with this accursed rebellion be marked and no mercy shown him. Let the traitors be exiled."[39]

In the hospital ward, a large portrait of Lincoln was draped in black crepe, reflecting feelings of the soldiers. How could this happen? Was it from the wickedness of evil, a natural result of the crime of rebellion, a dying gasp, a pitiless, venomous fling?

Per order of Grant—at 10 a.m., all troops parade. All labor of day cease. Flag is to be at half-staff. At dawn there will be a thirteen gun salute and afterwards every thirty minutes till sunset. At the close of day there will be a thirty-six gun salute. Army officers will wear badge of mourning on left arm and on swords for six months. Hospital officers will also wear badge of mourning.[40]

Attorney General Speed decisions: 1. Rebel officers who surrendered have no homes in loyal states and have no right of return. 2. Those rebels in civil service have no right to return to Washington. 3. Rebel officers have no right to wear their uniforms in any of the loyal states.[41]

Numerous references were made of the assassin Booth, whose name was soon immortalized in infamy.

The most venomous outlaw hunted and hated was trapped in a foul barn. Deserving the severest torture and intense agony, he remains beyond reach of human eyes. His dust is consigned to the unknown and his immortal soul to hell as all wicked men in proportion to wickedness. Authorities disposed of the body in secret so no martyrdom would follow. Where Booth lies: a small row boat received the carcass of the murdered body carried into darkness laden with shot and drowning manacles.[42]

Temperance

The notion "help yourself and God will help you," represented the bootstrap approach of overcoming alcoholism. Support services for the mind and soul of patients played an important role and comprised some of the material found in this newspaper. *Come from your roving* warned of sin, sorrow, loneliness and poverty sure to follow intemperance. Sainthood was not required to enter heaven, and sinners could be forgiven. Prayer and love could overcome temptation. *Mother to her son* warned that failure to shun the tempting goblet would produce the horror of madness, murder and everlasting woe. Fore sake the siren drink or perdition waits! Many of the Puritan persuasion avoided the drink but recognized the perfect rights of others to indulge. Others were absolute and would not support a political candidate unless he supported total prohibition.

Another vice thought remedial to discipline was profanity, a customary form of communication in all armies. Smoking and chewing tobacco was next on the hit list.

Profane swearing never did any man any good. No man is the richer or happier or wiser for it. It commends no one to any society. It is disgusting to the refined; abominable to the good; insulting to those with whom we associate; degrading to the mind; unforgiveable, needless and injurious to society.

Sermons

For many soldiers, prayer meetings and Sunday services were important parts of their life. Sermons were published for those unable to attend services. A New Hampshire soldier whose pen name was F. J. E. W. scribed *Brevities* covering Pride, Wealth, Love and Music as it affected the faithful.

The heart of man is like a sensitive plant expanding under God's smile but with the first rude touch bunches closed. God teaches the wandering bird to fly to warmer climate when the cold blasts of winter approach so he has taught the Christian to search the scriptures for comfort as adverse storms and bitter trials assail him.... Pride causes more misery and mishaps than any other fault but can lead to lofty and beautiful deeds.... It is worth and not wealth that ennobles.[43]

"Be not afraid for I am with you" derived strength from faith. Another shield against death and evil was the sanctuary and comfort of Mother and home. With great certainty, the heavenly shield was extended to the loyal defenders of the Constitution and Union while the rest were suffering damnation. A soldier wrote to his wife in *The Night before the Battle* that "the cannon's rage will stun the ear and fill the soul with fear. Blood may flow and I give myself to God's sweet care!" This sentiment was confirmed in another poem, "trust in God, land free from sorrow and pain and believe in heaven from this world to another." *The Lost Parent* imagined their son guided through the gates of heaven to a world everlasting and joyful.

Prisoners of War

Southern militias committing atrocities were widely reported. Captured union or rebel soldiers might be found hanged or with their throats slit. Reaction in kind or "shot in retaliation" was a virtual guarantee. The murder of a Union Major and his men in Little Rock, Arkansas, led to the shooting of a number of rebel soldiers in retaliation. "A rebel Major will be shot for Major Wilson as soon as one reaches here from among the prisoners recently captured."

A *New York Tribune* correspondent traveling with Sherman described a "horrible butchery." Thirteen Union foragers were found murdered, seven by the side of the road, all shot in the chest with a large placard pinned to each, "this is the way we treat Kilpatrick's thieves." Three were found in a house, shot down after they surrendered.

Three more were along the roadside with throats cut from ear to ear. One had a placard announcing "South Carolina's greeting to Yankee vandals." The next morning five more were found who had been murdered after surrendering and given up their arms. A rebel correspondent, after detailing the manner in which the dead Union soldiers were robbed and stripped, noted that "as a matter of course our boys cannot be condemned for robbing dead Yanks for they need all they can get."[44]

The foragers or "bummers" were assigned to find provisions for the army with little restriction. Confederates approached supply needs with similar desperation.

On December 1, 1862, we left for Fredericksburg with shelter tents found near a lunatic asylum and three days ration to last five. Miraculously poultry and cattle arrived as we visited a stately mansion boasting many acres. Enlisted men pretended to be officers and got fed in the mansion as foraging was not successful. Entering a farm-house with no living creature visible, a soldier commandeered a scared Negro.
"Where's your chickens?"
"All stole."
"Where's your master?"
"Locked up in de house."
"Bring him out."
"Him got de key.
"Then down goes the door!"
Three raps brought the secessionist master out, ordered to provide something to eat. The only livestock found was a calf butchered on the spot. As the calf gave an expiring bleat its owner protested: "The d—d Yankees have got another calf." The result was 300 chickens found in the garret were indiscriminately slaughtered by the advancing column before we left the premises. No rations were issued for days so men were obliged to live on the country and the above is about what living on the country means. It doubtless appears rough to persons unacquainted with the necessities of war, but the men were hungry and the people disloyal or if loyal only by necessity.

Treatment of prisoners described returning prisoners of war, emaciated with open wounds, the result of malnutrition and exposure. There were other stories illustrating moral outrage and anger over rebel barbarity overcome by heroic women and good Samaritans.

Rebel barbarity—A wife and her crippled husband were both arrested for feeding a deserter unknown to them until his death. Their three small children were now forced to be alone. She was compelled to join the prisoners lying on bare floor with no change of clothing afforded.

A contrast—Our citizens are contributing liberally to the fund for the relief of starving citizens of Savannah. The rebel authorities are starving our soldiers who are prisoners of war and endeavoring with demoniac malice to render them unfit for future service. The contrast is very great and it marks the moral difference between the people of the North and those of the South.

A heroic woman. The wife of seriously wounded Captain Ricketts went across enemy lines agreeing to become prisoner to take care of his badly shattered leg finding him in desperate condition. Her tender and continuous nursing skill over months avoided amputation and saw him completely healed. She nursed many other wounded officers and men and received no favor from the rebel authorities while sharing the same fate of the other prisoners. Ricketts was exchanged, joined another command and again was badly wounded at Cedar Creek with his right arm being paralyzed in part. He is now a Major General and a division commander.

A census of the dead at Andersonville prison was smuggled out by an unnamed Hartford soldier of the 16th Connecticut Volunteers. He was a prisoner for 17 months while detailed as a nurse, having lived in several prisons, escaped once and was recaptured. According to the *Record*, he attributed bad treatment to fiends and traitors "who ought to be made to serve out the rest of their days in the darkest dungeons." The total dead from March 1864 through January 1865 numbered 12,639. Most died in the stifling summer months in the absence of clean water and other necessities of life. [Private Durance Atwater of Terryville was paroled in March 1865, having smuggled the list in the lining of his coat which he later unsuccessfully tried to sell.]

"Richmond is starving; desertions from the rebel army are numerous." A chorus of a rebel song warned: "hard times coming, starvation now at hand; the officers eat the flour bread, and soldiers eat the bran." This was good news for the North except that some Union soldiers were facing similar prospects. The *Record* reported on December 21, 1864: "A soldier of the 16th Connecticut, formerly worked at Colt's armory, left home at two hundred pounds has recently arrived home in Hartford, from Andersonville. He weighs now but fifty-six pounds, looks ten years older, and is so emaciated that friends don't know him." The topic of mistreated Union prisoners had emotional and political legs, bringing demands for retaliation. A line item in *Record* declared, "The whole number of Union prisoners confined in Libby Prison during the war is estimated at 125,000." Another added, "A rebel correspondent at Florence, South Carolina states there are over 10,000 prisoners and 1,000 dead from scurvy."

Prison horrors decried 10,000 brave brothers dying under the traitors' law. "Beneath the scorched Georgian sun the dead line is watched under warden's guns. No food or water, no shelter, no humanity for the rag clothed volunteer with wasted limbs, surrounded by filth and channel ooze. This slow torment is evil in hell ruled by a craven hand." The same sentiment was reflected in *Oh ye who yet can save us, will you leave us here to die?* Men with shattered arms and missing legs, tattered, pale and gaunt, languished in dreary circumstances. In an ode on Jeff Davis, it was suggested that his proper fate be a cage "to repent for all the prisoners he sent to Andersonville in mud, to be unsheltered there to starve and die."

More Rebel Barbarity looked at the bleak and unforgiving conditions facing Union prisoners where "man's inhumanity to man" festered and continuation of war prevented wounds from healing.

> Many thousand prisoners were exchanged and those going south reached their destinations rugged and healthy and have told a story that should have shamed their government. From Libby, Andersonville and every other of their damnable prison-holes have returned to us thousands of emaciated beings, ready to die as they reach their native soil, while from thousands of our homes curses go forth upon the brutality which has laid low in filthy rebel dungeons so many of our sons.

The consequences of war were woven into the fabric of this newspaper. *The Anthem of Peace and War* foresaw an end to famine, red-eyed murder and hollow-eyed women weeping. Walls blackened and roofless could shelter no one. Severe desolation was *The Orderly's Lament*, where the noble steed's gay and prancing days were clearly over. There was no life, nor light or hope; only the crow who sang "caw, caw, and caw."

Northerners viewed the South as the poor man fighting a rich man's war. A clear-eyed Georgian depot master diagnosed the situation with clarity.

> They say they are retreating but it is the strangest sort of retreat I ever saw. They allers are whipping the Federal armies, and they allers fall back after the battle is over. I allers told 'em it was a dam humbug and now I know it. Right here on John Wells' place, hogs, potatoes, corn and fences all gone. As for the nonsense of splitting the Union, why dam it the state of Georgia is being split right through and through from end to end! It is these rich fellows who are making this war and keeping their precious bodies out of harm's way. There's many in the army running away, I could play dominoes on their coattails. There's my poor brother sick with small pox at Macon working for eleven dollars a month and has not got a cent of the dam stuff for a year. 'Leven dollars a month and 'leven thousand bullets a minute. I don't believe in it, sir."[45]

The Volunteer

Enlisted men were subject to the orders, whims, and moods of officers and NCOs alike, and appreciated jokes at their superiors' expense. Regionalism, army protocol, rank and privilege were fair game to inform, amuse and even the playing field.

> *A green private.* A soldier guarded a fort entrance while leaning against the wall with gun by his side. He failed to salute the lead General of the 5th Corps.
> "Who do you belong to? How long have you been in the service?"
> "The 101st New York sir; I came day before yesterday," answered the poor private.
> "Do you know what these are and what they show?" asked the general pointing to his shoulder straps.
> "No sir."
> "Well two stars stand for major general and is always entitled to a salute."
> A colonel emphasized the point, pointing to the eagle on his shoulder, and asked, "Do you know what these are?"
> "Yes sir; it's a pigeon, but I'll be darned if I know what it means."
> In addressing a jury on one occasion, the celebrated Mr. Jeffrey found it necessary to make free with the character of a military officer who was present during the whole harangue. Upon hearing himself several times spoken of as "the soldier," the son of Mars, boiling with indignation, interrupted the pleader: "Don't call me a *soldier*, sir; I'm an *officer*." Mr. Jeffrey immediately went on; "Well, gentlemen, this officer, *who is no soldier*, was the sole cause of the mischief that has occurred."
> A company of one of the Pennsylvania regiments was stationed on the banks of the Potomac as pickets. During the night an officer, in making the rounds, happened to come upon one of the posts,

when a picket suddenly brought his musket to "charge," and commanded the officer to "halt." He halted and they stood in silence when the officer tired of being pinned there, asked:
"Well, what's next?"
"Say Brandywine, d—n you or you can't pass!" was the answer.
The officer shouted "Brandywine!" and was allowed to pass.

A jester puts his belt on backwards with U.S. upside down.
"The Captain said I would have to stand on my head in order to right it."
As it happened he could stand on his head almost as well as on his feet and immediately took that position while holding his musket at parade rest, the muzzle resting between his feet. The Captain and all the enlisted men were convulsed with laughter but not the Colonel. "Sir, what do you mean by such conduct? Are you not aware that you are liable to punishment?"
"I don't know about that sir, I got a breastplate with the U.S. printed bottom upwards and the Captain told me I'd have to stand on my head and now if you can't read it I don't know what in thunder to do." The parade was dismissed.

Last winter, a Yankee soldier, out walking at Wheeling, while to himself a talking, experienced a feeling, strange painful and alarming from his cap up to his knees as he suddenly discovered, he was covered with bees! They rested on his eyelids and perched upon his nose; they colonized his peaked face, and swarmed upon his clothes. They explored his swelling nostrils and into his ears; they crawled up his trousers and filled his eyes with tears. Did he yell like a hyena? Did he holler like a loon? Was he scar't and did he cut and run? Or did the critter swoon? Ne'er a one. He wasn't scar't a mite; he never swoons—or hollers, but *he hived 'em in a nail keg, and sold 'em for two dollars!*

A soldier who went through Savannah with Sherman tells of the trip. The boys learned how to rob bee-hives without the penalty of stinging. The plan was to rapidly approach a hive, take it up suddenly, and hoisting it upon the shoulder, with the open end behind, run like thunder. The bees hustle out and fly back to the place where the hive stood. The honey belongs to the boys who win it!

The Volunteer is versatile, enduring and saint-like in suffering and deprivation. Winter quarters are made comfortable by his ingenuity and hard work.

Logs were split, notched and fitted taking sixteen to twenty-four slabs, four on each side with pin poles used for rafters and shelter tents placed over them, each squad working on their own house and streets made out. Tents or a cracker box taken apart made the door. A fireplace was made by digging a few inches making a chimney of sticks, barrels or cans piled eight feet high and plastering the outside with mud. Bunks were pine logs split four feet wide and accommodated two each. The slats were small pine trees five and half feet long lay close together and covered with pine boughs and blankets. With a bright fire and shelter, he was ready for winter.[46]

European officers saw remarkable qualities in the American soldier. One distinguished observer commented, "I had but a poor opinion of your troops when I first saw them in camp. They acted so little like the soldiers of the continent. And when I saw them on the march, I was doubly surprised and shocked at the loose manner in which they proceed on the route. But when the battle commenced, and the legions came up and began to form, then I saw the Army of the Potomac. Your soldiers drill on the battlefield."

In an editorial in *The Soldier*, the inevitability of sacrifice was detailed. "Who shall repay the brave soldier due him for the dangers and hardships he has to pass through in fighting." He battled for right and justice and to preserve the glorious union. Only soldiers knew the peril, hardships and dangers. "They sleep on damp ground, sustain long tiring marches in hot sun, and yet remain patient and endure. How many sacrifice their lives on the altar of their country, that you and your children may enjoy the blessings of Freedom."[47]

Another editorial, *How Soldiers Feel in Battle*, deflated the balloon of being "eager for the fray, burning to lead the fight against the foe, or longing for a short sleep and shortened limb under the surgeon's hands." Would he stand shoulder to shoulder with his peers, or fold? "The first battle does not distinguish the brave form the cowardly. It is the second one with recollections of the carnage and narrow escapes of the first that tries a soldier and tests his metal."[48]

A most important feature was the will to fight and persevere in an unflinching manner. For the *Record*, "the brave man is not he who fears not, for that is stupid and irrational; but he whose noble soul subdues its fear, and bravely dares the danger that ordinary nature would shrink from."

The bravery, endurance and willingness to sacrifice were noted by a *London Star* editorial in April 1865, celebrating the American experiment.

> The reckless bravery of those patriot soldiers fighting in the cause of freedom, the prodigality with which they shed their blood, the contempt which they manifest for toil, danger, death and the wonderful skill and fortitude of their leader, were made the objects of the most unceasing slander. The noble youth of New England resolved to grapple with the monster of slavery until it should perish or they fail in the attempt.... The spectacle is thus presented to the world of what an army of freemen can accomplish and the force with which a nation governed by free institutions can exert in its own defense.

Leaving home was no small sacrifice. In *The Soldier's Parting*, he bade farewell to his precious wife and little ones. His country called and he responded with a fervent wish that God protect them. In *Just before the Battle*, a family man asked, "I will not forget you, will you forget me?" In *Night before the Battle*, picket duty meant reclining on the chilled, dew-soaked ground, bedded with his grounded horse, struggling to be warm. Man and horse awaited the battle to come as darkness replaced light.

Each soldier's day started at dawn with *The Song of the Bugle*. Rousted from damp floor and blanket, the war horses were alerted and the soldiers readied their sabers. The gallant trooper believed heavenly trumpets would signal the end of war and hate, leaving peace for eternity.

Disabled

How would society respond to the wishes and needs of the returning volunteers? Who would hire them or take them into their loving homes?

> War has left ravages upon the country and upon the people. Generations will honor and revere the veterans of the war of emancipation. Thousands upon thousands of poor cripples must pass into eternity. These cripples are now in the country, in hospitals, and demand every attention that can be paid them. To be sure, glory is in every scar, and homage is theirs from all for their deeds of valor and their sacrifices. Let them be helped on and cheered through life and then their sacrifice is not worse perhaps than death to them.[49]

The End discussed the bitterness, isolation and finality many would experience. Some could no longer march, nor carry the flag or answer the bugle's call. Their "brothers" were gone or crippled, forlorn and useless, nursing shattered limbs, absent young ambition or dreams for the future. Some tried to forget but never would.

Society could not forget the maimed, whose missing limbs and crutches became ubiquitous to every town and village. *The Invalid Corps* praised the unretiring brave serving with limp and deformity, still contributing though not on the battlefield. They knew not of cowardice but of courage, honor and pride.

What became of the crippled and forlorn? Some brood, separated from society, never to sit a horse or march again. Peer encouragement gave the recovering patient an insider's view on performing activities of daily living without arm or leg. Many could still serve their country while maintaining a sense of self-worth despite physical disability.

Returning Veterans

The end was bitter for some and bittersweet for others. The bronzed heroes began returning with tattered flags and worn blue coats, in thinned-out regiments. As the boats landed, men and women, citizens of all ages and colors cheered. Bands played for each parade; speechifying was endless, and bouquets and wreaths were strewn before the feet of the victorious soldiers. As the *Record* stated, "we owe it to ourselves and to the country and memory of those who have fallen and to the widows and orphans left behind. A bountiful collation should be provided for every regiment on their arrival home and they should be received with the honors due them. It must be shown that we appreciate the services of our nation's heroes."[50]

The jumble of emotions and the social reality of war's end were prime topics of thought. *Our Boys Are Coming Home* offered welcome on behalf of mothers, sisters and star-gazed maidens. Only some vacant hearths would at last be filled.

Of great importance was obtaining a proper pension. Entitled for a lifetime annuity were the following: invalids disabled since March 1861 in the line of duty, widows of soldiers who died of wounds in service, children under 16 if no widow or if remarried, mothers dependent on the son for support, and sisters under 16 dependent in whole or part. Rates of pensions for enlisted men were $9 per month, Captain $20, Lieutenant Colonel and higher $30. The cost of supporting Civil War veterans was four times the cost of fighting the war, and by the turn the century was the leading expense for the U.S. government.

Warnings were posted in newspapers about "Exorbitant fees charged for collecting bounties and pensions due soldier's widows." The charges for such service ranged from $10 to $300. Arrests of recruiting officers, mustering officers, substitute brokers, internal revenue assessors and others connected with the enlisting business helped protect the volunteer from being swindled. Aid agencies moved in to provide services gratis. Paymasters were instructed to make payments directly to soldiers and not to agents, a notary or a lawyer.

One million men returned "from the public udder to obtain sustenance elsewhere. It is an immense accession of dependents and labor seekers to a country, and will be seriously felt in all departments of trade and business." Economics and morality demanded work places earned with the blood, sweat and tears of returning veterans. Volunteers needed assurance that they would not have to beg and would replace those who had stayed home. The stark reality of returning volunteers was summed up by an editorial certain to strike a welcome chord of resonance.

> Surely there is but one national debt we cannot pay and that is to the brave men whose chests have stood a wall of resistless fire to stop the rolling waves of treason. Let not the people's gratitude find its only expression in words. These men need employment. Their life in the field has greatly interrupted their opportunities and facilities for falling into remunerative occupation. Let every good citizen do

what he can to ensure these bronzed veterans permanent and profitable employment. Far better this than noisy reception or festival recognition, all well and proper in their way.[51]

Will You Remember Me?

Poems invoked battlefield grounds soaked in blood as grieving families sobbed, surrounded by the peal of church bells and a soulful choir. Some soldiers dreamed of death amidst the cacophony of battle or from the insidious cough of consumption. A calm and peaceful aura enveloped the stricken soldier, who was joined by other veterans, all very still with cold, marble faces and sunken, unblinking eyes. Courage in battle was defined as a duel with death. "Upon the first fire I immediately look upon myself as a dead man. I then fight the remainder of the day, regardless of danger, as a dead man should. All my limbs which I carried to the field I regard as so much gained, or so much saved out of the fire."

Death was the commonest theme for poems. The titles referred to chaotic darkness and the hereafter: "death, dying, fatal, missing, returning, un-returning, fallen, unknown, grave site, going to grave, after battle and coming home." The depth of sadness and drought of joy could not be flushed with ordinary tears.

What of the unidentified, unmarked, nameless soldier? Who should visit them? Some were hastily buried "to shield from sight of foe and careless tread" and were memorialized in *The Unknown Dead*. Headstones marked each martyr as the "Unknown Union Soldier, unknown on earth but not in heaven." The notion of mortality was distant and nebulous for those under 26 years, the average soldier's age. Those without blemish or bodily ache, a full head of hair, unlimited stamina, and bottomless urges did not give it much thought except when it occurred to others.

In the forests of Virginia was a grave for the unknown, with a wooden marker at its base inscribed: *A Union Soldier-Mustered Out*. It inspired a poem describing a symphonic din of battle wreathed in smoke and flame from the fiery rain of musket and cannon. When the shooting stopped, the only sounds were the moans of the dying, those who survived long marches and short rations for the final mustering out.

A soldier was mortally wounded at Gettysburg in *Kiss me, Mother, once Again*. The field of bloody carnage was blanketed with those once young and daring, now ghostly in appearance. The thin smile on an angelic face seemed sad and lonely amidst so many others in peaceful slumber, freed from earthly pain. He was not afraid to die and only asked for his mother's kiss, just once more.

The Fallen Soldier was to be married in a week and was found with a bloodied likeness of his accomplished fiancée in his vest. Love of country did not protect against the indifferent dagger of death. This youthful hero with fixed smile and stiff and clotted garments would never consummate a pledge of life-long companionship and happiness. He felt blessed and thankful to have her likeness and spirit with him at the end.

The sights, sounds and smells of war triggered images that could recur for life as dream-like remembrances of things past.

> In a hospital in Philadelphia, lay a soldier with dark eyelashes, and cheeks with hectic flush due to the insidious disease consumption. A painful cough is wearing away his life. He hears a soft sweet strain of music from an earthly choir. He recalls marching in blood stained southern soil and hears the sobs and tears of agonized parents and awakens to a calm and sweet peace near fellow sufferers. He is now

in a grave in Pennsylvania surrounded by black robed forms whose happiness fled along with his dying breath.[52]

As the sun set, the battlefield was a stew of a lifeless boy soldiers, fathers, husbands, sons and neighbors. Assurance was needed to answer the plea *will you visit me in my grave?* Will you mourn or even remember me? "Tell mother and sister not to weep, but remember me, if you will." He welcomed visitors any day or night, fearing being alone and forgotten.

A mother replied to an anxious son in *Answer to Just before the Battle Mother*. "No, I'll not forget you, darling," how strange he should even ask. He was defending what was right in a raging conflict and might not come home. But being brave and true, God would protect and not forget him and all welcomed him home."

The Unreturning Braves questioned if society would remember the fallen, the maimed, the prisoners, the widows and orphans. What of the betrothed and lovers whose fleeting memories were replaced with emptiness and heartache, a future blackened in ruins like many cities and towns.

> Now that all New England is being made happy with her returning soldiers, does she remember the "unreturning braves?" Does she think of the bleaching bones, the shallow graves—the hollow skulls protruding from their last resting places-the eyeless sockets glaring up at the scorching sun—the awful spectacle of unburied men, lying in their steps as they staggered and fell to raise no more? Does she think of the desolate homesteads—the mourning friends, the tearful wife and her babes striving in vain to find "papa" among returning brave? Does she mind how pale and silent are her maidens as they stand in the crowd who welcome with joyous faces and cheery voices the dear ones, the long tried and battle scarred brothers, fathers, husbands and lovers.[53]

Till we meet was published as the war ended. What once meant nostalgic joy and sweetness had become eyes dimmed with tears of sadness and pain, sobbing over the cold stillness of lips and eyes and hands folded on the chest. *Our boys are coming home* gave thanks to God for answering prayers for the dawn of peace and freedom amidst the ring of church bells and song in the warmth of golden jubilee bonfires.

After three long years, the tanned and battered soldier wondered if wife and children would remember them in *The Return*. A bronzed warrior with long and shaggy hair, a limp and absent arm or leg, might frighten the little boy never yet seen. An old robin with halting wing twittered a greeting for the returning pilgrim relieved of weary burden, summer's heat and winters snow.

Joyful hearts were beating under a bright, shining sun, the sweet air invigorating for the living. War and deadly strife had ended as cannon and rifle were silent, in *Willie's coming home*. With moon and stars as guide, his roaming days, pain, and sorrow were over. The cold ground was his blanket but his comrades need not mourn as the angels had taken him home.

In the summer of 1864, a published order declared, "every Man to the Front to strengthen our victorious armies. The ranks must be filled to finish off the reeling enemy." At war's end, the opposite was mandated. To save money, no goods were to be purchased and the hospitals would be emptied of patients no longer requiring treatment.

On June 3, 1865, the 14th Connecticut Volunteers of Norwich, the Governor's home town, arrived in New Haven. Some had been interred in Andersonville and would remain there.

> They arrived Saturday morning on a steamer Granite State from New York, the first of the returning regiments. It was organized under the President's call of May 1862 and left in August with 1,040 men.

Antietam, Gettysburg, Fredericksburg, Chancellorsville, Wilderness, Cold Harbor, Spotsylvania, and at Fredericksburg lost 100 men in ten minutes. At Gettysburg they captured five battle flags. The boat arrived at 10 a.m., Wharf and State Street was crowded with friends cheering lustily. Tattered battle flags were riddled with bullet holes and grimed with battle smoke. An escort was provided by City Guards and Governors Guard to the State House where arms were stacked. They marched to the U.S. Hotel for a fine breakfast and were escorted to camp grounds where new tents were ready. These honorable veterans embraced loved ones, many an eye dimmed because of those who never returned. Men cheered, windows crowded with fair ladies threw bouquets and wreaths to the bronzed soldiers whose path was strewn with flowers.

Celebrations and parades followed in many cities and towns, preparing for a grand celebration on the 4th of July. Troops returning through New York City were feted with cheering crowds for half a mile. Soldiers honorably discharged could retain their knapsacks, haversacks and canteens at no charge as well as weapons at the following rates: muskets with accouterments $6, carbines with accouterments $10, revolvers $8, sabers and swords $3.

For the last week in June, there were 104 sick patients and 48 wounded men admitted, leaving 547 patients still in the hospital. Some had unhealed wounds and other conditions for which there was no cure and only palliative treatment was available.

Several Connecticut regiments returned that summer, marching up New Haven's main avenue towards the town's green. The vast throngs cheered and shook the soldiers' hands while shedding tears of joy for the heroes come home. A little, golden-haired girl stood on tiptoes in the rear to see amongst these war-worn veterans the color sergeant, her father coming home. Earlier in the day, her mother received a letter saying he would not be coming home, that they had left him in the field. Such was the introduction of *the Fatal Letter*, published July 12, 1865. Who would mourn them? The maiden, wife and mother were destined to wait forever, offering loving caress in memory only.

With the war over and to keep busy, wards were cleaned and whitewashed. The examining board met daily with numerous clerks to prepare discharge papers, five per man. The hospital closed on January 1, 1866, and was then sold for building material.

The *Valedictory* thanked those responsible for the great victory over slavery and the maintenance of the Union: brave soldiers who maintained the brunt of battle and the doctors and their assistants who gave their all.

> We have endeavored to lay before its readers the most interesting and pleasing material ... and has always stood for the maintenance of the Union but now its mission fulfilled it sleeps. Its purpose was to relieve the monotony of Hospital life. The brave heroes who have fought so nobly can always say, "I fought for and helped to save the nation which traitors sought to destroy.[54]

The last issue reported on unchanging human nature in New Haven, Connecticut, no different from elsewhere. "The quartermaster building at this Hospital was broken into and a large amount of clothing removed. A large number of pants, coats, blouses, shirts, and other articles are gone. The culprits were not apprehended."

On the last page of the last issue was an ad from the U.S. Sanitary Commission, whose office was next to the army hospital, offering services of the Bureau of Employment for Disabled and Discharged Soldiers and Sailors, at no charge.

NINE

Voice of the Soldier

Sloan U.S. Army General Hospital in Montpelier, Vermont, was the largest of three state hospitals with a total capacity of 1,850 beds. [See Appendix V] It was a mile from town on an elevation 150 feet above the adjacent Onion River. The original octagonal plan with 12 wards and standard buildings begun in 1865 was not completed before the war ended. Eight plastered and clap-boarded wards were 108 feet long and 26 feet wide, holding 40 beds each. Standard windows and ridge ventilation were installed. Water was brought through wooden pipes from a spring in the hills to a receiving tank of 40,000 gallons. Separate, small privies attached a drainage system with 12 square inches of spruce plank surrounding the buildings and passed under them for reception of sewage. It discharged into a brook and was flushed from the tank periodically. This failed, as "foul odors penetrated the wards and caused its disuse."[1]

Volunteers published and edited the *Voice of the Soldier* as a triweekly for three months ending in June 1865. Its price was competitive at $1 a year or five cents per issue. Its crisp logo spoke of its contents. On each side was the flag, in the center a podium upon which sat a large bible with the words "Loyalty" and "No compromise with traitors." The *Hospital Register* in Philadelphia gave endorsement. "It contains a partial list of the patients in that hospital along with other interesting news, and like all other hospital papers is loyal to the core. We wish it success, and gladly give it a place on our exchange list." Only one issue survives.

Advertisements

Hospital admissions were listed by name and company along with returned to duty, transferred, admitted from furloughs and discharged. A hospital directory included the surgeon in chief, executive officer, acting assistant surgeons (two), medical cadet (one), quartermaster, commissary chief, hospital stewards (two) and the ward master. A City of Montpelier Directory offered a comprehensive description of goods and services available for the volunteer: attorneys at law (six), hotels (four), druggists and apothecaries (three), photographers (three), clothing (three), physicians (one), dry goods, grocery, restaurants, boot and shoe makers, hardware, dentists, harness makers, hardware, booksellers and stationers, meat markets, furniture and carpets, leather dealers, livery stables, baker, jewelry, book binding and frames.

Ads were typical for a hospital newspaper. A full column for a photographic studio with "elegance and beauty by artists" was most prominent. S. P. Redfield was a dealer in

VERMONT HISTORICAL SOCIETY.

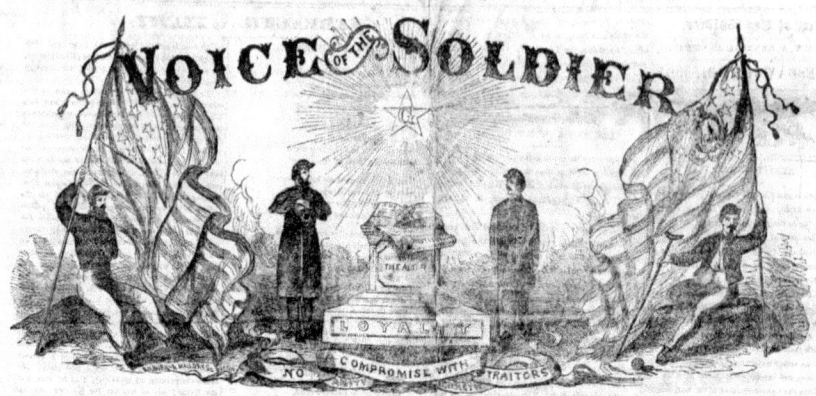

Voice of the Soldier

LOYALTY — NO COMPROMISE WITH TRAITORS

VOLUME 1.   SLOAN U. S. A. GENERAL HOSPITAL, JUNE 21, 1865.   NUMBER 14.

THE VOICE OF THE SOLDIER

Is published and edited by the Soldiers of Sloan U. S. A. Gen. Hospital, Montpelier, Vt.
Published bi-monthly.
Terms, one year, $1.00
Single copies, .05

ADVERTISING:
One column, one year, $50.00
One square, 5.00
(An average letter should be addressed to
Sergt. W. E. BLISS,
1st Bat. V. R. C.
Sloan U. S. Gen. Hospital, Montpelier, Vt.

Poetry.

Original.
ONE HUNDRED YEARS FROM NOW.

A PARODY BY THE PRINTERS.

Montpelier will be just as fair,
And girls as sweet I trow,
And soldiers just as jolly
One hundred years from now.
They'll sound along the Styx as then,
With all their winning ways,
And scan the right lip with smiles
As those of other days.

The Old Brick Church will still lift up
Its height to heaven view,
While Hopkins' trail descendants
Will venerate the clergy,
With well blocked shoes and white kid gloves
The "Vets" will bather roam,
And holy "beans" eat on the bridge,
By page of Mercantic's Rose.

Our Court House still will be o'ercrowded,
If verdant youths allow
The embroid'-tongued roomer to pasture them,
One hundred years from now.
The Lawyers then will lie and cheat,
And laugh and eat plea
Twas' it here, as one for all your woes,
An eye upon the fee.

2.40 nags and fast young men,
Will through our villages ride;
With flighty teams and right away pairs,
They'll manage 'tet' her side.
Green Country-lads and ''slouched up'' fops,
To black-eyed belles will bow;
But fairer forms won't flirt with us,
One hundred years from now.

We trust, our Tabor will still be heard,
The Soldier's right in view,
May patrons pat the printer well,
The Lord get his dues;
And when old Time his form shall lock,
Death knock him into pi;
To us may he bid a welcome home,
In realms beyond the sky.   S. F. K.

§ loan Hospital, Montpelier, Vt.

THE VOICE OF PEACE.

Lift up thy voice, America!
Thy enemies shall see
What glory, might, and Liberty,
There still remains in thee.
Upon thy brow, so beautiful,
I've set my holy seal,
And every foe that trod thee low
Shall for thy mercy kneel.

From God's pure presence I have come,
With power in my hand;
And I will wave my bow aloft
Till I have earned the land.
I bring thee rest—sweet, blissful rest—
And hope to cheer the sad;
And health, and wealth, and happiness,
With love to crown the whole.

"Fearless and independent" still,
America, arise!
Thy noble feet, blood-colored and torn,
Shall e'er to brighter skies,
Back to thy home, forgiving heart,
Thy wandering sons may come,
And in the land that gave them birth,
Shall find a new home.

ON AN UNEQUAL MATCH.

There is between Jane and Jim,
But one thing in common. I aver,
She is a fool to marry him,
And he's a fool to marry her.

Original Miscellany.

Written for the Voice of the Soldier.
THE GALLERY OF ART.

BY OUR ART-CRITIC.

No 1, hanging on the wall at the right of the Arch, is a very well made picture by Thos. Ham. It represents Dorset Life in St. Lawrence Co. N. Y. The principal figure is a square built, dark complexioned black whiskered man with a large whip in one hand, a plug of tobacco in the other, just before him several very fine looking oxen, cows, sheep, swine and calves. Just behind him is a long legged farmer driving some goats, look sickly looking cows which he wishes to sell. The driver is represented as looking rather contemptuously at those while at the same time a curious smile is seen creeping over his chin while he repeats the following stanza from Byron:—

"Keep your d—d old mahogany frames,
Until some Hospital Conqueror comes along."

The artist has exhibited a profound knowledge of "Drover habits" and a thorough acquaintance with profane history.

No. 2, on the left hand side of the Arch, by Brad Lee represents "Scene in the French revolution." The artist has thrown a great deal of life and animation into this picture. The scene is laid near a large fiery river which stands the Radius of Venice. The principle figure sits a Freedmen with a huge round axe, cutting his way through a pile of rubbish that lays between him and a gold mine worth $25,000 per year. Over the mine stands a Lutherian Cries which, if is necessary to remove, before he can handle the gold. The artist has here portrayed in vivid lines the doubts and fears of the man with the axe, or he for a moment hesitates with axe raised on high over the sacred Cross. At this moment a Page from the King cries out: "The Cross is to be taken down to-morrow." while a small man in V. R. C. uniform chews his whiskers and says "So that thing is settled." There is little else to be said in regard to this picture, save that the landscape looks rather dreary.

No. 3 on State Corridor by Mr. Frank represents Copperheads.

The scene is laid in a Field red with gore, while the earth seems alive with snakes. The men who are digging there bare copper caps on their heads. Wooden shoes on their feet, from their pockets protrude photographs of Davis, Lee, Beauregard, Toombs, Wigfall, Dr. Blackhearse, together with copies of the Argus. In the distance is represented a gloomy prison with thousands of starving prisoners holding out their emaciated hands for aid. The only attention these copper workers bestow upon them is to say: "Served you right, what did you go down there fighting for?" The sky, however, is very prophetic. It represents a gallows on which Davis hangs, while the skeleton fingers of the martyred dead point at the Red Field as though saying "Thou also."

No. 4, by Mathew Maties, is a very lively piece of great merit. It is called "Justice on Duty." The picture is emblematic in its nature. Thus Justice is represented as an old man with a long nose, grey hair and eyes, with a slightly stooping form standing in the middle of the street with a "Cad" behind him, and a miniature Bill in front, supposed to be symbolical of the Dignity of Office, and to imply that every "Cad," which deserves an experienced hand is sure to end still. In the right hand of Justice may be seen the scales of truth balanced with a piece of Deacon Starr's cheese and them newly laid eggs on the other, while the left hand holds a scroll on which you can read "Justicia ad tyrant arrivo."

No. 5, is a landscape by a Prussian officer. It is taken at sunset. A broad river flowing through a beautiful vale, lofty trees on each side, a few boys, and a merchant sized men are hunting for pearl nude in crystal waters. The Heavy greens and lighting loads salt harmony to the scene while the soft sunlight falls in a halo of glory around a beautiful Camp in the distance, and a flock of doves on the Wing flying from one police the monotony of the sky. There is a fine green Wood on side, and near by a bright little cluster is included, On the banks of the river entirely wrapped up in a Hyde sits a Fisher with well baited hook and silken line.

The piece is well conceived. Plans radically is perfect. To make it however such a picture as every mother would wish to place in her parlor it needs some covering to cast some beautiful Cross to show that the Lord is recognized as the one who joins all these stray atoms together in one harmonious globe.

FREE LOVERS.

"Hearken at Berlin Mines among the Free Lovers. I arrive here last Tuesday 6 bitterley. dog I case the Say Lover set fast to his rotched plans. I know tell of these Free lovers for some time & I thank likewise and see what kind of kritters they was. I lighted my tent in a field near the Lar Kens as they call it and unfolded my banner to the breeze. Shortly the people commenced to congregate into my show & I began to kongraterlate myself on doin a stavin bizness. But they wur a ornery looking set, gussal say. The name faces was all kivered with hair and they looked fust starved to deth. The w'imain was wus nor the men. They wore tresst'd, short gire odis an straw hats, with bodied green ribbons onto them, & they all havid blue cotton umbrells in their hands. Howbev a pefectly orful looking froude presented herself in the doar. Her grip wuz skank knotty short & her shears was dissfull to behold. Sez she, Arksrt line? yes its true. O its true. Sez I, 13 cents, marm. Sez she, I sn't ye found ye at heart—as heart. O at hart. Sez I, O's yere fnotr'l on at kins & ye would ker found to fnd if ye had sam course. See also air yer a man? Sez I, think I am, but if you doan't yer may address Mrs. A. Ward Belliteville, Injunny, postage paid, and she will dewliver give the required infurmashun. Sez she, then you air what the w'im'l calls marrid? I sed, yes marm, I be. The ch'ovr'r 'd could then grabbed me by the arm and set sh'. In a wild voice, you air mine, O ya air mine. Sikerely, sed I, as I releseed my self frum her graep—Sh'er agone elarizzed on by the arm & sod, yu ar my affinity. Sez I what ai aireh is doar? Doa's'hat thou n'd know as she. No marm, sez I, I doant. See the'r'r'steen, man & he tell ye. Fur years yre yernol for thore. I knowed thoo wair in the world somewheres altho I kuowd not thy name or plase of residunce. My hart sed homesald anne out I knew thy heriage. He has come. O ain't ye bene—yu air husband, air my affinity. O cum you tetch—two match, and she bust out cryin. Yes sor I think it is a durnat sita too much. Hast thou not yearned for met the yelled, ringing her hands like a fremle play actor. Sez I, not a yunce. It ain't bine a grate speead of fny boved hol hollerl'd around us, & they aul reioiced fer fur heller shame, brut, Scott, storebry, etutery. I was jest as snad as a Mareh hair. Sez I, ye jerk of ornery critters go dum hum. I bair hein retehd vemain along with yu. My nain is Artimas Ward and yur is the door buses. I nov if I took like me if I sex arove, man & thy chidren ill look like me if I sex aloveoman: I done gn in her swim the laws ofmy cowntry as defance. I aint in favor of pirutesmfig of cuition jere illegel. I think yure affsuity bizais is carpet-bonnase, besides being outrageous wicked. I poored my indignashun in thar way and I jirt ive my of brith when I stop: I took down my tent & shall tev town this eveun." —A. WARD.

Boast beef, serenity of mind, and a pretty wife will make ever an man healthy, wealthy and wise.

The two shortest words to pronounce, yes and no, are those which demand the most thorough examination.

There the rock upon which we split, as the man said to his wife when she asked him to rock the cradle.

Scandal will rub out like dirt when it is dry.

EDITOR DREAMING ON WEDDING CAKE.

A batchelor editor out West, who had received from the hand of a bride a piece of elegant wedding cake to dream on, thus gives the result of his experience:

"We put it under the head of our pillow, shut our eyes sweetly as an infant blessed with an easy conscience, and soon snored prodigiously. The God of dreams gently touched us and presently in fancy we were married. Never was an editor happier. It was 'my love,' 'dearest,' 'sweetest,' 'angel,' 'honor' every moment. Oh, that the dream had broken off here! But no, some evil genius put it into the head of our ducksey to have pudding for dinner, just to please her lord.

In a hungry dream we sat down to dinner. The pudding moment arrived, and a huge slice steamed from right the plate before us.

'My dear, did you make this yourself?' said we fondly.

'Yes, love; ain't it nice?'

'Glorious—the best bread pudding I ever tasted in my life.'

'Plum pudding, ducky,' suggested my wife.

'Ah, no, dearest, bread pudding. I was always fond of them.'

'Call that bread pudding?' said my wife, while her lips slightly curled with contempt.

'Certainly, my dear—reckon I know. I have had enough at the Sherwood House to know bread pudding, by any, by all means.'

'Husband! this is really too bad—plum pudding is twice as hard to makes as bread pudding, and is more expensive and a great deal better. I say this is plum pudding sir,' and my wife's now flashed with excitement.

'My love, my sweet, my dear love,' exclaimed we soothingly, 'do not get angry, I am sure it's very good. It is bread pudding.'

'You mean, low wretch, you know it is plum pudding,' said my wife, in a higher tone, 'you knew it's plum pudding.'

'Then, mi'am, it is meanly put together, and badly burned, but the devil himself would not know it. I tell you, madam, most distinctly and emphatically, and I will not be contradicted, that it is bread pudding—and the very meanest kind, at that.'

'It is plum pudding,' shrieked my wife, as she hurled a glass of claret in my face; the glass itself tapping the claret from my nose.

'Bread pudding,' gasped we pluckly to the last, and at the same time grasping a roasted turkey by the left leg.

'Plum pudding,' rose above the din, as I had a distinct recollection of two plates smashing across my head.

'Bread pudding,' we groaned in a rage as the chicken left our hand, and flying with swift wings across the table, landed in madam's bosom.

'Plum pudding,' resounded the war cry from the enemy, as the gravy dish took its whizz we had been depositing the first part of our dinner, and a plate of beets landed upon our white vest.

'Bread pudding forever,' shouted we in defiance, dodging the soup tureen, and falling beneath its contents.

'Plum pudding,' yelled the amiable spouse, nothing daunted misfortune, she determined to keep us down by pitying up our head the dishes with no gentleness. Then, in rapid succession, followed the tureen, 'Plum pudding,' the shricked with every dish.

'Bread pudding,' in smothered tones came up from the pile. Then it was 'plum pudding' in rapid succession, the last cries growing feebler and feebler—till just as we ran remember, it had grown to a whisper. Plum pudding resounded like thunder followed by a tremendous crash as my wife leaped upon the pile with her delicate feet and commenced jumping up and down—when, thank heaven we awoke—and thus saved our life. We shall never dream upon wedding cake again."

drugs and medicine, dye stuffs, perfumery, paints, and oils. There was the standard tailor of fashionable garments and military uniforms, pension agents and other apothecaries. To appeal to soldiers eager for non-hospital cuisine, there were offerings of country produce, fruits, oysters and "food for the hungry." Also available were cigars, tobacco, hats and caps, books, periodicals and stationary, doors sashes and blinds, paper hangers, curtains, beds, mattresses, feathers, and mirrors.

Hospital visitation was from 1 to 4 p.m. The Chapel held "Sabbath religious worships" at 2 p.m. and 7 30 p.m. Sermonizing and preaching was minimalized, noting that "Religion is the best armor in the world, but the worst cloak that can be worn."

Romance and Marriage

Humor was combined with wisdom to entertain and inform the convalescents understandably apprehensive of their future. A prospective groom realized what is important following a fierce argument with his fiancé over the momentous decision as to whether the wedding cake would be bread or plum pudding. The dispute was settled much to his relief as he awakened from a bad dream, or was it? Examples of the same genre follow.

> An exchange newspaper says the best cure for palpitations of the heart is to leave off hugging and kissing the girls. If this is the only remedy we say, "Let her palpitate."
>
> Roast beef, serenity of mind and a pretty wife will make most any man healthy, wealthy and wise.
>
> "Oh! She was a jewel of a wife," said Pat on the death of his wife. "She always struck me with the soft end of the mop."
>
> In the town of Hebron was a doctor enamored of a beautiful young lady, and were engaged to be married. He was a strong and decided Presbyterian and she a Baptist. They were discussing the upcoming nuptials.
> "I am thinking of two events which I shall number among the happiest of my life."
> "And pray what may that be?"
> "One is the hour when I shall call you my wife for the first time."
> "And the other?"
> "When I shall present our first born for baptism."
> "What, sprinkled?"
> "Yes, my dear sprinkled."
> "Never shall a child of mine be sprinkled."
> "Every child of mine shall."
> "They shall be, ha?"
> "Yes, my love."
> "Well sir, I can tell you then, that your babies won't be my babies, so good night sir!"
> The lady left the room and the doctor left the house. The doctor never married and the lady is an old maid.[2]

Politics

After four long years of conflict, a war-weary nation asked, "When will this war end? It will stop when all the dark clouds have passed. When will it stop raining? When the rebels have had enough they will quit."

Opposite: Voice of the Soldier. **Sloan U.S. Army General Hospital, Montpelier, Vermont (courtesy Vermont Historical Society).**

The Voice of Peace[3]
Lift up thy head,
Calm the land, bring thee rest
And health and wealth and happiness.
The noble flag, blood-stained and torn
Shall wave in brighter skies
Back to thy brave, forgiving heart,
Thy wondering sons may come,
And in the land that gave them birth
Shall find again a home.

Emptying the hospitals was a cost-saving priority but recent recruits and not veterans were the first to be mustered out and sent home. "Veterans in the service from the beginning are still armed and equipped and are made to wait," but while receiving full pay with little work and no fighting.

Disabled

Dealing with the issue of the disabled was a priority. A wounded survivor of Cold Harbor was pessimistic. "What happiness is there in this world for a man who has lost the use of his limbs? I have not sufficient education to employ my brains, or the power to use my hands to earn an honest livelihood. I am poor and will not beg. I would rather die here than be burden on my friends at home." This was painful truth, plainly stated. *The Voice* went on: "There are thousands with no visible means of support except a paltry pension. Justice and gratitude demand lucrative employment. Sound minds and shattered limbs should be the only recommendations required. Schools need be established. There must be no injustice for 'cripples' now being discharged."[4]

For the celebration of July 4, 1865, the *Voice* suggested squads of amputees marching in columns with appropriate signs and flags. "Let all the one-armed men get together and get up a banner with appropriate mottoes. Let all the one-legged men do the same. Let the remainder form in squads: all who were wounded in the same battle get together with the ancient and honorable old guard of revolutionary war days. Do a grand thing, one worthy of our genius as Yankees."[5] [A more sensible approach was to have veterans march together by regiment rather than by battle, disease or injury. A grand achievement would be providing them all with a future, regardless of deformity.]

Conclusions

The hospital was one episode in a soldier's life, sometimes painful and forbidding but always worthy of chronicle be it in their last hours of life, a return to field duty or a discharge home. Thousands of volunteers and draftees made a pilgrimage through the health care system, often challenging every fiber of their being. Unlike today, the average hospital stay was weeks and months, not hours or days. Keeping mind and body occupied was a therapeutic goal, and reading was an accessible form of entertainment, replacing outdoor activities for young men who were bedridden or ambulatory only with assistance. For those of a religious bent, physical life became a contemplative one of faith, prayer, and introspection with sermons remindful of Sunday services back home.

Hospital life was often dull and devoid of excitement. After exhausting reading material, answering letters, discussing every topic, yarn and joke, reviewing their wounds and how they occurred, they were still not home. Lying immobile in bed for months with open fractures, slow-healing wounds and stubborn fevers in summer heat amidst stifling odors and soulful moans required the inertia, fortitude and discipline of marble statues. The suffering and bravery of hospital patients was often a greater test of strength and determination than required on the battlefield. Healing some ailments required not only pills, potions and surgery, but also injections of encouragement and hope for the future and a transition to civilian life were essential.

Nineteen self-published military hospital newspapers were produced, nine of which still exist. They give a unique perspective in digital and hard-copy formats. Holding in hand the large edition paper offers a sensibility not discernable from the glowing screen of a laptop. The contents were composed and edited by soldiers reflecting their experiences, aspirations and beliefs. They were printed on-site, issued weekly and cost one to five cents. The authors were convalescents, surgeons, medical students, chaplains, and women volunteers. Those who experienced history wrote it.

Funding came from advertisements, newspaper sales and an occasional subsidy. *The Soldiers' Journal* was a voice for the U.S. Sanitary Commission and the Christian Commission, providing printing press and seed money along with paid, multi-page ads each week. Changes in publishers or editors sometimes altered the quality and content from tedious literary and morality discussions to current events and burning concerns of the soldier. Just as there were differences and similarities for each hospital, so there were for each newspaper, providing unique material for each chapter.

The stated purpose varied. They would support an elaborate library and reading room and solicit reports of the war and experiences of soldiers tested by the fire of battle. Partisan or political material was encouraged by some and excluded by others. Any article or item of news from soldiers in camp or hospital, or from family, surgeons, medical students, ladies societies and chaplains was welcome.

For the *Hammond Gazette* it was to "benefit the sick and wounded and entertain and relieve their suffering."[1] For *The Cripple* it was "to relieve the monotony of sick and wounded in hospitals and not to hurt anyone's feelings while providing a new source of energy pulling the hospital forward, fight error, throttle prejudice, and inspire confidence."[2] For *The Soldiers' Journal* the primary object was to "promote interests of the soldiers in the ranks and to keep good order in their accounts with the government." They would learn practical matters such as procuring pay and clothing, obtain furlough and proper settlements on discharge without the expense or bother of claim agents, and finance a fund for orphans of soldiers who had fallen in the defense of the Union. By adapting itself to the *needs* of the soldier, the paper would be an "indispensable companion, counselor, and friend."[3]

The Crutch defined itself as not just a record of weekly news but a literary paper open to "patriot and poet," entirely devoted to the interest of the soldiers in the hospital.[4] It was not just a hospital registry with the "sufferance of military authority." It would "cheer, comfort and support new ideas and dispatch false ones," and relieve the tedium of hospital life with good reading, getting new ideas in and false ones out while encouraging perseverance and hope.

The goal for the *Hospital Register* was support of an elaborate library and reading room to "distract from boredom and inactivity, from disease or injury."[5] Reports of the war and experiences of soldiers were solicited from those with experience as only they can know the real horrors of war. There was a gap between those who wrote about war but did not experience its danger or suffer its consequences and those destined to limp with deformity and pain.

The goals for *The Cartridge Box* were to "cheer them during their sufferings ... and afford a sounding board on subjects agitating the country, educate minds and souls ... and allow them to express their thoughts and opinions. Give them books to read, sermons to heed, and not be cheerleader for the administration; then hunt down those venomous snakes."[6]

For the *Armory Gazette* in Washington politics was inescapably linked to its overriding purpose: support the government and oppose copperheads and traitors with "hard blows." They encouraged the exchange of political ideas while rigidly maintaining their unassailable support of the Republican administration, the downfall of the rebellion and "the holiness of our mission in establishing universal freedom in America."[7] The paper was strictly for the "benefit of the soldiers and not private interest." Surplus funds were for the benefit of those maimed by bullets or diseased from exposure and fatigue.

Knight Hospital Record had as its goal "to place before the readers news gathered from any source, such as incidents of battles, marches and bivouac from eye witness, hospital events and news items including its patients that was of interest to their friends, family and the public at large."[8] The platform was "one glorious union" made of all 34 states. Their audience was the bedsides of sick and wounded, in homesteads, camp and fortress.

Arresting editors and reporters, closing newspaper offices and even destroying presses without formal charges was a feature of this era. At Hammond Hospital there was an *Outrage upon the press* when vandals (Union soldiers) smashed presses and windows and destroyed office material over non-complimentary accounts on the handling of blacks and "disloyal" volunteers. The response, to make Peter Zenger proud, was "as the only loyal paper in this county, we shall fearlessly continue to do our duty as impartial journalists!"[9]

Printers experienced from civilian life and disabled from field service did the type and press-work. Two sized papers were produced; large format tablecloth (11 by 16 inches) and the standard small (8 by 10), mostly four pages in length. Proposed submissions were sometimes critiqued in print. Cautions and recommendations for prose and poetry were commandments, not suggestions. Rules on writing and physical visits to the press room were rigidly regulated and discouraged. The missile of print was meant for the ages, a force for truth and advancement of the human race.

Admissions, Discharges

Absent modern privacy laws, each paper listed the names of patients admitted, including rank, company and often diagnosis: those returned to duty, furloughed, deserted, transferred to other hospitals, discharged or died. A national directory was established on the whereabouts of those who filled the never-ending trains of ambulances whose journey was a way station to recovery or burial. The listing would be of great interest to each state's regiments as to the status of friends and neighbors. Many hospitals were filled with hometown patients, encouraging family visits while demonstrating that state-of-the-art health care was being provided.

Health Care Delivery

Series of articles detailed how the medical system worked from wounding to convalescing back home, from day of injury to awakening like Rip Van Winkle in a hospital ward back home. Hospital construction and its water supply and septic systems varied in quality but not importance. Initial bandaging and splinting by a regimental surgeon was followed by transfer for more definitive treatment to divisional hospitals, where a team of surgeons determined the need and timing of surgery. Painful rides over rough, corduroyed roads in ambulances absent shock absorbers delivered patients to trains for the less severe and ship transport for the more desperate.

The ubiquitous amputations and their complications were graphically described by surgeon, student and patient alike. Fatal secondary hemorrhage, hopeless infections, tetanus and the frustration of nineteenth century medical science weighed heavily on the medical staff. Loud or muffled cries of "Doctor!" or "Help!" or "God!" punctuated the chorus of groans that announced the suffering. This was an era absent intravenous fluids, transfusions, antibiotics, antisepsis, asepsis and modern surgical techniques. Once infection set in, further surgery was futile or hastened death. Despite overwhelming odds, try you must in the face of 75 percent mortality of open fractures of the femur in the best of hands.

To encourage enlistments, newspapers told of an amputee waving a newly created stump like a flag-pole, pledging allegiance in a patriotic, fond farewell to his absent part. Volunteers did not regret the loss as long as the glorious goals of the Lincoln administration were accomplished, or so it was said. For the most part the "saw-bones," nurses and cadets were welcome visitors, sometimes receiving gifts from their patients and seeing their names in the rafters during holiday celebrations. Newspapers listed them by ward and announced their achievements.

Treatment failure and other issues might call for the services of an embalmer, whose story was detailed with informative articles and advertisement, incidentally giving birth to a national funeral industry.

Irish, Blacks and Humor

One-line jokes and stories often centered along ethnic lines, for the times both politically and socially correct. The most recent émigrés were the Irish, serving in the lowest paying jobs and portrayed as jovial, second class citizens, fond of drink and a bit slow-witted. Blacks were believed lazy and inferior physically, morally and intellectually. Kernels of truth and wisdom passed their lips to surprised audiences. It was harder to argue against former slaves who defended the homes of white men.

Humorists Josh Billings, Petroleum V. Nasby, and Artemus Ward had a wide following in national and local publications, offering political and social satire on the high and mighty, the pompous and the hypocrites. Those who made no sacrifice were skewered for the amusement of those who did.

Mail

A three-cent stamp facilitated communication with loved ones and was the treatment of choice for *nostalgia* or the blues and the social media of its day. Envelopes embossed with the hospital name or "soldier's letter" were available for recipients to pay postage. Armed guards sometimes accompanied the mailmen as it became known that packages and letters carried cash. The average letter covered the same topics: food, health, money, write me and going home. Forty-year-old Alvin Ozro Brigham was older than most, happily married and eager to return to Fitchburg, Massachusetts. He was wounded in an assault at Petersburg June 17, 1864, just five months after mustering in and was recuperating from his wounds in a Washington, D.C., hospital.[10]

> I was glad that you are well. They have taken our names for transfer to New York where I think I can get a furlough and go home. We got ready to go yesterday and a lot went but they took only those that were the worst off to go by water and those that could go without crutches and can help themselves, they sent by railroad. We don't know what will happen and may be disappointed. We don't know who to trust on earth but there is one that we can trust—our Father in Heaven. If it pleases Him to so arrange things so I go home, He will do it and if not, we must submit to His will. My health is good and my wounds are getting along as well as could be expected. I have been paid for the last two months $26. If I stop long at the sutlers I fear he will get it all. You know I think a great deal about something good to eat. I hope I shall be in your arms before I write again.

He was killed in March 1865, on Lee's breakout attempt at Petersburg, survived by a daughter and a wife who remarried five years later and died in 1901.

Library

A library and reading room provided food for thought and "medicine for the mind," supported by religious organizations, the lay public and newspaper sales. Modern fiction, poetry, history, travel, and especially religious tracts and texts made up collections varying from 800 volumes in New Haven to 2,500 in Alexandria and 4,500 in West Philadelphia. Hospitals exchanging self-published newspapers allowed cross-pollination of ideas. Each covered similar topics, offering complimentary and divergent views on current problems and solutions. National, foreign and out of state periodicals, along with games, and piano or organ music, changed hours of idleness into productive reading and communicating. Four hundred-seat reading rooms allowed organized sermons, lectures and vocational endeavors. The morbid tendency of boredom, inactivity, weakness and depression of disease or injury were symptoms readily relieved by a treatment at low cost and without toxic side effects.

Hospital literature included literary efforts of "interesting original material both lively and honest." Great literary content would "relieve tedium of hospital life with good reading."[11] There was limited excitement generated by nuances of modern art and obscure figures from the ancient past. For literary and debating societies, the burning issues included the "artificialness of modern art," "what has caused the most misery, intemperance or the war," the soldier's future, and the morality of war.[12]

Advertisements

The location of the hospital determined the number and type of ads that appeared on the back page. Those near a large city had numerous local businesses vying for the soldier's paycheck with "cheap" prices. The Sanitary Commission and all its departments were frequent flyers, offering free advice and assistance on receiving bonus, pension or other benefits for the soldier and his family. They offered gratis room and board and made transportation funds available. Attorneys and solicitors for claims against the government, including absence of back pay, bonus, pensions and death benefits, were common but for a fee often exceeding a year's salary. The U.S. Sanitary Commission and other aid societies furnished information on the whereabouts and status of soldiers and sailors. Also listed were a directory of the Sons of Temperance, merchant tailors, booksellers, hardware, military goods, drugs and medicines, military boots and shoes, watches, jewelry, hats and caps, restaurants, fashionable clothiers and gold fillings to save teeth! Photographic portraits, especially carte de visits, were popular, reasonably priced and could be obtained in the hospital.

Disabled

Intramural baseball games between hospitals were common. Imagine the cheers of "Let's Go Cripples," or "Go Crutches!" In their salutatory addresses, the appropriateness of those names was opened for debate. Institutions designed for sick and wounded soldiers held many disabled, deficient or otherwise flawed. In Annapolis, it was reasoned, *The Crutch* provided useful support for the lame and hence its use to cheer, comfort and support. "You are beautiful. If you are a crutch I honor thee and thy scars, thy beautiful maiming, and glorious infirmities! Never give up! It is wiser and better to hope than despair."[13]

A parallel was drawn between scarred, deformed veterans and beauty to be honored and revered. Miss Amy E. Dickenson described a wounded soldier *"made beautiful by a scar."*[14] The maimed heroes earned an exalted and glorified status. Beauty is in the eye of the beholder and the virtue of deformity played better in prose and poem than in reality. After the cheering and music stopped, returning veterans, especially those with disabilities, faced the obstacle of fitting back into society where skills of sword and musket had no value. The tide of patriotism receded along with flag-waving and enthusiastic welcome homes. Veterans with an empty sleeve or pants leg were an everyday occurrence no longer inspiring the appreciation or cheer prevalent during the early war years. Some saw a bright future, having survived the blast iron furnace of war. These soldiers asked, "for what am I making the sacrifices and enduring these privations and trials?"[15] Though maimed in body, "great character was precipitated from the reagents of war," the likes of which was the envy of the world. "The sacrifices and trials of war have been and still are a *blessing* and not a *curse.*"[16]

Others saw things quite differently. "What happiness is there in this world for a man who has lost the use of his limbs? I have not sufficient education to employ my brains, or the power to use my hands in earning an honest lively hood. I am poor and will not beg. I would rather die here than be burden on my friends at home."[17]

For those chronically ill or otherwise disabled, a critical question was how society would respond to their needs and wishes. Who would hire them? Who would marry them? Who would provide for health care or instill confidence and hope for a decent future? Hospitals sprang up specializing in problems of the amputee and offering peer group support. The helping hand extended to the subjugated race and defeated Confederates should be even more so for those who died in battle, their widows and orphans. For the veteran, sound mind and shattered limb should be the only recommendation required for positions in post-war society. "It should be the present and future policy of the government to employ its disabled veterans in or out of service to the exclusion of those who sacrificed nothing."[18]

Some hospitals installed night school, using reading rooms as lecture halls for benefit of patients wanting to improve or establish employable skills. Some states organized employment agencies designed to bring businessmen in contact with potential candidates. Public attention was focused on enabling the maimed with financial aid, books, and training. "Those who stayed home should be replaced by soldiers." A national debt was owed the brave who had fought. "These men need employment. Their life in the field has greatly interrupted their opportunities and facilities for falling into remunerative occupation."[19]

Thousands of cripples fell and passed into eternity. "Glory, valor and sacrifice is in every scar. Let them be helped on and cheered through life and then their sacrifice is not worse perhaps than death to them."[20] *The End* discussed the bitterness, isolation and finality many would experience. They could no longer march, carry the flag or answer the bugle's call. Their "brothers" were gone or crippled, forlorn and without hope, nursing shattered limbs, absent ambition and dreams for the future.[21]

Society could not forget the maimed whose missing limbs and crutches became ubiquitous to every town and village. The Invalid Corps was praised as the unretiring brave served with limp and deformity. Their battlefield days may have been over but not service to their country.

Lincoln's second inaugural address promised "to bind up the nation's wounds; to care for him who shall have borne the battle, and for his widow, and his orphan." And so the Veterans Administration was born. Consideration was given to confiscating Confederate property or providing millions of acres of public lands in the far west.

Politics

Newspapers were published on federal grounds, under federal regulations and hence with oversight by military authorities who supported the Lincoln administration. Despite assurances to avoid political discussions and partisanship, the soldiers' favorite military and civilian leaders always shined brightly. "We cannot make it a channel for discussion of questions relating to the government or candidates for presidency."[22] Like many campaign promises, remaining neutral and avoiding partisan politics was ignored or forgotten.

"Southerners are guilty of the highest crime that can be committed against any nation."[23] No compromise and unconditional submission were the only justice. In the deep-seated Puritan ethos, the rebellion was a crime described in biblical terms. The criminals needed to be apprehended and punished or the righteous would go unfulfilled. For some this was a holy war to be conducted to its end no matter how bloody or costly in life, limb, or coin. There were but two kinds of citizens, patriots and traitors.

The poisonous "copperheads" were to be loathed and exterminated for the vermin they were. This description applied not to the Confederates or even their local militia but to members of the Democratic Party in the North whose platform promised to end the war by leaving the states divided and slavery intact. Letters to the editor indicating a soldier could be loyal to the Union and belong to the Democratic Party were published but confined to the traitor column, proposing prison, extradition or the hangman's gallows.

The *Armory Gazette* noted that "Universal distrust is the rule in Washington. If there is a man here, who believes that his next door neighbor is an honest man, we wish he would step forward for inspection!"[24] As for Congress, cacophony and conflict reigned. "All is apparent confusion and excitement in a perfect Babel."[25]

The Soldiers' Journal was in close proximity to Washington, allowing observation of characteristics remaining unchanged 150 years later. Events that intensify partisan differences and poison political waters in the genetically contentious capital of Washington did not start or end with the Civil War. "There is a class of politicians in this country whose highest ambition is the defeat of any measure, however commendable, proposed by their opponents. They are willing to incur any risk in order that their end may be accomplished."[26] Party success trumped good of country. "Unpatriotic attempts to embarrass the government has forsaken every principle of political virtue and become the supple tools of their parent serpents; the devil and secession."[27] What was the solution to this dilemma? "By all means draft Congressmen. They might do a little good in the Army as they are of no possible good where they are now."[28]

No society was more polarized than that of the mid-nineteenth century. Divided they stood, passions easily aroused, taking sides rather than applying reason: appeal to the worst angels. States were grey or blue and were often exploited by politicians and other leaders to divide rather than unite, no less than today. Marching orders were given by the one percent who owned most of the slaves and property.

Patriotic fervor and love of country warmed the blood and strengthened convictions.

To think otherwise was selfish and short-sighted. Others saw patriotism as the last refuge for scoundrels: "a fungus of civilization," "a cowardly narrow minded feeling as popular as whiskey," "empty declamations and hypocritical protestations now respectable."[29] For some this system of self-government was a train wreck no matter who the engineers.

For the Europeans, the forbearance and generosity afforded the Confederates at war's end was astounding. Their insurrectionists were hanged or beheaded and the leaders incarcerated. The Union magnanimously offered pardons to those who returned to the fold. A government surrounded in its capital by partisans hanged no one (except post-assassination), allowed public meetings, speeches in the press and ballots for the enemy. Such leniency had no parallel in history.

Battle

Who better to discuss the maelstrom of battle than those who experienced it? "The list of casualties of battle is but one page of many in the history of war's desolation where lands are laid waste, homes destroyed and deaths met without glory."[30]

Poems reverberated with drums beating and bayonets gleaming amidst deafening roar and rattle. Who would survive the charge with a lion's courage and slaughter rife? Who would be torn and mangled? The battlefield for both defeated and victorious was a "wail of orphanage and widowhood, a chill of woe and death broadcast across the land. See the charred earth, pools of clotted blood, and festering heaps of slain. Nature has never made such horrors!"[31]

A most important feature was the will to fight and persevere in unflinching manner, which for success required the support of public sentiment. Some prospered financially while others suffered and sacrificed, much to the surprise of European observers. The patriot soldiers showed "reckless bravery," prodigality in shedding their blood, and contempt for toil, danger and death under the remarkable skill and fortitude of their leaders.

Mortality

Death was a common theme for poems and short stories. The titles were about chaotic darkness, timelessness, and the hereafter. The depth of sadness and drought of joy brought despair in the face of dogged determination.

As the sun set, the battlefield was a stew of lifeless figures. The field of bloody carnage was blanketed with once young and daring warriors.. The thin smile on an angelic face seems sad and lonely amidst many others in peaceful slumber, freed from earthly pain. Only the living could answer the plea, *Will you visit me in my grave?*[32] Would they be mourned and remembered? A mother reassured an anxious son, "No, I'll not forget you, darling, how strange he should even ask." He was defending what was right and God's will be done. Be brave and true, we would not forget and all would welcome him home bounded by eternal heartache.[33] And finally "*They are coming,*" the soldiers were coming home but not her Dad; not today or tomorrow or in this life.[34]

Women's Rights and Contributions

At the Sanitarian Fair in Washington, President Lincoln spoke of the role of women. "Nothing great or glorious was ever achieved in which women did not act, advice or consent to."[35] Nothing was more painful and despairing than becoming a widow or childless.

Romance and marriage were of keen interest for those languishing in hospital wards with most of their lives still ahead. How does one romance and capture the right mate and what traits should she have? Should he seek the large orbs of Dorchester, a radiant beauty, or the shy and self-effacing lass? Was it better that she have winning grace and pleasing face than be fat or stately and not rude or too bashful?

A recurrent theme was the notion that love conquers all and the faithful wife could heal that which the doctor could not. A white-hot romance and the love of a woman could breathe life into the driest of bones without need of a biblical prophet. The young ladies preferred not the rich man's son with soft hands and draft exemption but the rough-hewn, hard-working volunteer who risked all for God and country. On his death bed, with febrile brow he was grateful to give his arm or leg for the Union cause. He had suffered calamitous wounds and was written off as hopeless by surgeon and nurse, only to be rescued by an angel in the form of invincible love: the fiancé, newly married bride or mother, arriving just in time. She cheerfully proclaimed, "I will be your right arm."[36]

A private with a broken body vied for the heart of a hometown maiden, in competition with a wealthy officer. "I am a common private, now crippled for life. They should have let me die that dismal night in the hospital when the ligature slipped off and the red life stream drained me and fever throbbed in all my veins." She arrived providentially, declaring, "If you will only let me be your little wife, I will nurse and care for you. Don't send me away or I shall die."[37]

The need for volunteers never ended. Hospital newspapers ran stories urging young men to join, emphasizing romance if not patriotism as a reason for enlisting. The "sweet, pretty, enthusiastic girl" was a matrimonial prize devoutly to be wished but not likely to be won by the shirker who stayed safely home. Volunteers got the gal, so join the army, lads!

The heartbroken mother or widow touched with bitter grief remained a willing donor to the Union cause. Costly sacrifices were made by unheralded women who received no medals or cheers from the crowds. Death sometimes intervened, creating an *"every-day heroine!"*[38] A pale-faced young widow, on daily hospital rounds amongst the wounded, provided inspirational words and deeds in memory of her dead husband. Another heroine brought her invalid son home as patriot, martyr, and hero. She offered for sacrifice her husband and sons, being left with only memories, shirts stiffened and scabbards stained with blood. She was grateful to have a surviving child, embracing his scars and crutches. "Mother, you would rather have me as I am, then not to have me at all?" He returned home to cheering town folk and a new, happy and rewarding life, or so the story went.[39]

A young man sought his mother's approval to join the army. She replied, "Do your duty. I give him to his country and pray that God will make him equal to his duty. To lose him would be fearful but to find him a weak coward in the day of battle would be more fearful still."[40]

Who shall sacrifice? Some stories revolved around the search for food, often involving chickens. "If you take my livestock, I can't eat. Now I aint got nothing but this one chickin."[41] The volunteer was a burnt offering on the altar of sacrifice. For his loved ones, the price for victory was awful and steep.

Sermon

The chaplain was a government employee who served multiple masters: the government, the soldier, and the bible. "All you have suffered incident to the state of war, pray God to pardon and heal you and when recovered go back to the field and renew your compliments to the enemies of our blessed country!"[42] Just as it was the surgeon's job to keep soldiers in the field fighting, so it was for the officer with collar.

Army chaplains and visiting ministers offered inspirational sermons on life and religion. They cautioned against drink, tobacco and profanity. Sacrifice, hard work, and a holy patriotic struggle against the evil of slavery were the road to salvation. Keeping busy was the Lord's work, idleness the work of the devil leading to drinking and gambling. "Read, discuss, learn, make things and do not be listless and inactive that will be a curse to yourself and to everybody else because Uncle Sam foots the bill and furnishes rations."[43]

A common reference was the plight of the Israelites and flight from slavery. Moses called for a draft with no exemptions. None were too bald, edentulous or stiff jointed. It was clear whose side God was on. The rebels were doomed to Perdition. The calamity of war must at least in part be punishment for personal transgressions and failure to follow the gospel. In his second inaugural address, Lincoln attributed the war as God's punishment for the evil and sin of slavery.

There were always the "incessant grumblers" who seemed to resist change or notions of self-sacrifice. Anti-war sentiment was based on biblical notions of peace and good will towards men, opposed to hate and destruction and concluding that "all wars are wrong" and not all were heroes. Some had "cannon fever," an illness caused by the sight and sound of gunfire, cured by flight in the opposite direction.[44] Staying in the rear to avoid active duty was a full-time job. Some always seemed "too sic to go bak to the war," while suffering from "the excruciating torture of chronic rheumatism, malignant type."[45]

Accepted reasons for draft exemption were memorialized in satirical pieces. A "union man" claimed an interest to serve but alas was the sole support of an aunt requiring his full, devoted attention. Also he snored and marched backwards. Some needed to stay home, entertain the ladies, draw up battle plans to gain glory and win victories. Another was disappointed at being neither halt, lame, blind or without teeth. He was not a Quaker, clergy, coward, copperhead or drunkard but held a serious objection to being shot and becoming an "unwilling justifiable homicide."[46]

Optimists with opposing views urged faith, hope and continued sacrifice on behalf of the government as the best option for victory. "Never give up! It is wiser and better to hope than despair."[47] One correspondent took issue with the chaplain's views on how to be a Christian and do right. "How can a Christian engage in war and kill when the Bible says it is wrong to kill? *Why men do war* in the face of the Christian doctrines: peace on earth; thou shalt not kill, and love one another. Spending time and resources on fixing the social condition of man instead of physical destruction was more righteous, sensible and profitable."[48]

None knew more about the unfair and cruel realities of war than the volunteer who witnessed the carnage. For some, war meant valor, magnanimity, heroism, and a test of manhood.

Delusions of soldiering included glory, gallantry, fearless charges and carelessness of life.

> Do not ask returning soldiers about the propriety of war because they lie and do not ask mothers for their views as if it was their fault. The truth will not be found in speeches, posters, bounties or advertisements, which is sentimental, vain and unsubstantial. There was no special eagerness for the fray, inclination toward bullets, longing for short sleep and shortened limb or haste to enter the Promised Land.[49]

The volunteer left a happy fireside, threw aside his wealth, loaded himself with backpack, toiled daily on dreary marches, and slept under the stars, eating ill-cooked food to gain an opportunity to kill one another. Evil died hard, requiring hope, faith, courage and manly fidelity. "It is easy to glorify the national flag and the soldier's skill, devotion and valor, brave men living and dead with stout hearts and heroic deeds."[50]

Hope for the nightmare's end was the keynote of many sermons. "Four years after Lincoln's first election, thousands are now resting below the sod. Thousands are crippled crutching their way through life and widowed thousands bedew their cheeks with tears, while orphaned thousands bewail those who return not. Oh God how long!"[51]

Temperance

Consumption of alcohol is part of the American character, both praised and demonized in biblical passages. By the mid-nineteenth century, hundreds of temperance societies preached total abstinence or strict moderation, adding tobacco and profanity to the unwanted list. Financial and social ruin and damnation were the destiny of those falling prey to the grape! Delirium tremens was the work of the Devil, setting a final course for ultimate destruction. For some it was fate, bad luck, a crabby wife or business reverses that drove them to drink. "I couldn't help it. I am a wretched man! I am a victim and martyr."[52]

Lincoln

Society needs heroes. The exploits and victories of Sheridan, Sherman, and especially Grant commanded public interest. They represented the common man, plainly clad and spoken, courageous and decisive minus the affectations, fuss and feathers of high society and the antebellum South. And they brought victory.

The linchpin was Lincoln, a towering figure physically and metaphorically. His origin was frontier poverty, self-taught and plain spoken with the poetic prose of an American Shakespeare. His words were biblical, incisive with granite-like logic. Harriet Beecher Stowe described an honest, fatherly, patriotic man who upon leaving Springfield for Washington asked his townspeople "to pray for me." Lincoln was strong, tenacious and firmly grounded, "the most abused man of our nation."[53]

By May 1864, it was clear to some newspapers that Providence had provided a "man of steel" as pilot for the ship of state. There followed a painfully prophetic request; "May he live to see the end of his great work and receive the heartfelt thanks of a grateful and Christian people."[54]

During election season, a proud and patriotic stance was attributed to the volunteer. "They voted nobly. Those who lived in rain filled rifle pits and trenches were unable to sit during meals. Their face, hands, feet and musket was covered with mud. They sleep in mud, eat in mud, watch in mud, fight in mud and shiver in the autumnal wind."[55]

Democrats were determined to make Lincoln a one-term president and thwart him at every turn. They tried to defeat or delay his domestic and war agenda. Hospital convalescents were loyal and unconditionally idolized the Commander in Chief, with overwhelming support at the ballot box despite a grueling, endless war. Fear of defeat on Election Day 1864 was real though greatly diminished by Sherman's victory in Atlanta. Still, the iconic Lincoln was defeated in New Haven County, Connecticut, York County, Pennsylvania, and New York City by sizable margins thanks to the immigrant vote.

The event that seared the soul and heart of the nation was the assassination of America's Moses, who would not cross the Jordan into the Promised Land. Black crepe borders framed an outpouring of grief with intensity still aglow today. The prayers he had asked were returned by millions grateful for his wisdom, skill and great sacrifice. The mood of reconciliation, compromise and love for neighbor changed to revenge, hate and division.

Prisoners of War

There were several reports of "man's inhumanity to man," "rebel barbarity," and "horrible butchery" committed by Southern militias and army units whose intention was to inspire terror.[56] Sherman's foragers were sometimes captured and executed by rope, bullet or sword. Some militias left calling cards such as "this is the way South Carolina greet Yankee vandals."[57] Dead Union soldiers were stripped and robbed, guaranteeing retaliation. Confederates collected "Lincoln ears" which were harvested from black Union soldiers.

The ill treatment of prisoners of war produced a blistering anger. Returning cadaveric volunteers were the victims of extreme crowding, absent health care, exposure to the elements, contaminated water supply, and starvation. Those willing to allow the departure of the South could no longer offer a peace branch to barbarians whose inhumane behavior, deliberate or not, shocked a nation.

The grim tale unfolded in *Prison Horrors*. "Leagued in hate with hell, lies chained lions on southern sand, dying of slow torment in a Christian land. Their only food was rotten dole. No water! No breath!"[58]

Will you leave us here to die was a desperate plea not to forget those languishing in prison. "Meager, tattered, pale and gaunt," growing weaker daily from "cold and want," hopeless captives whose families wonder if both love and faith were dead at home. They lived in mud and iron cage "unsheltered there to starve and die."[59]

Sacrifice

The editorial boards expressed no doubts about the soldier's proper role. "Each and all should strive to bring this accursed rebellion to a speedy termination; the cause is noble, and just. The man who loves not his country is worthless and unchristian. An able man who will not fight and defend it is a coward."[60] Soldiers left home, surrounded by loved ones, hearts aching, children clinging, and received a parent's blessing and prayer, and a "God bless" from his partner in life. He endured privations, hardships and dangers, was self-reliant and disciplined, knowing what to do and then doing it.[61]

His key attributes were *true courage, willing obedience* and *patient endurance.* He received and inflicted wounds without rest and marched long distances under a heavy pack. He knew not why they were there, what they had done, where he was going, the distance to be traveled, or what he was going to do.

They wore leaky boots in cold, wet grounds, washed in a cold stream and had breakfast of bitter coffee, hard tack and cold pork. Guns were slung across shoulders, knapsacks over the back, to march through mud, frost and snow, erect bridges, and charge deadly rifle pits. "Our veterans should know they are appreciated but can't fail to note despairingly the contradiction of the silent and barren reception they now receive with that which they were formerly honored. Let us cheer the soldiers."[62]

The names and dates of wars change, but the needs of its workers stay the same. How did they maintain a stable and positive frame of mind while lying exposed and vulnerable on a ward of fevered brows and desperate wounds? Newspapers were the repository of period history, merging philosophy, religion, economics, science, politics, and humor. It was an instruction manual on the life of a soldier trapped in a fratricidal civil war.

The ability and will of society to absorb returning veterans has always been a vexing problem. The war experience made men "ennobled, more worthy, and put a little manhood into them." It developed what was there: humanity, generosity and courage.[63]

Hospital literature allowed the invalid to march again, to revel in heart-warming and soul-wrenching stories. It was a "medicine for the mind." The pen became mightier than the sword for the soldier who could no longer bear arms.

What is past is prologue. All these issues remain.

Appendices

I. Union General Hospitals, December 1864[1]

Department	Number of Hospitals	Total Beds	Occupied
Washington	25	21,426	13,865
Pennsylvania	18	18,709	13,412
East (N.Y., New England)	25	14,829	9,302
Northern (Ohio, Ind., Ill.)	23	11,421	10,735
Cumberland (Tenn.)	21	10,751	7,939
Ohio	17	8,535	6,970
Middle (Maryland, De.)	11	6,189	4,993
Gulf (La.)	8	5,808	1,991
Virginia and North Carolina	5	5,344	4,283
Missouri	8	3,462	2,638
Tennessee	10	3,055	1,263
West Virginia	5	3,038	1,978
Northwest (Wis., Iowa)	4	2,532	2,034
Arkansas	6	1,517	1,101
South (S.C., Fla.)	4	941	605
Kansas	2	500	300
Total:	192	118,057	83,409

II. Department of Washington, December 1864[2]

Hospital Name	Locality	Medical Officer in Charge	Beds	Occupied
1. **Armory Square**	**Washington**	**Surgeon D.W. Bliss**	**1,000**	**690**
2. Carver	Washington	Surgeon G. A. Judson	1,300	722
3. Campbell	Washington	Surgeon A. F. Sheldon	900	633
4. Columbian	Washington	Surgeon T. R. Crosby	844	538
5. Douglas	Washington	Assist. Surg. W. F. Norris	400	203
6. Emory	Washington	Surgeon N. R. Mosely	900	645
7. Finley	Washington	Surgeon G. L. Pancoast	1,061	755
8. Freedman	Washington	Act. Ass. Surg. A. R. Abbott	72	72
9. Harewood	Washington	Surgeon R. B. Bontecou	2,000	1,207
10. Judiciary Square	Washington	Assist. Surg. E. E. Griswold	510	311
11. Kalorama	Washington	Act. Assist. Surg. R. Thomas	434	54
12. Lincoln	Washington	Assist. Surg. J. C. McKee	2,575	2,012
13. Mount Pleasant	Washington	Assist. Surg. A. Allen	1,618	898
14. Ricord	Washington	Surgeon C. W. Hornor	120	107
15. Stanton	Washington	Surgeon B. B. Wilson	420	266
16. Stone	Washington	Assist. Surg. P. Glennan	170	139
17. Seminary	Georgetown	Surgeon H. W. Ducachet	121	13
18. Augur	**Near Alex.**	**Surgeon G. L. Sutton**	**668**	**443**

Hospital Name	Locality	Medical Officer in Charge	Beds	Occupied
19. Claremont	Alexandria	Surgeon E. Bentley	164	34
20. L'Ouverture	Alexandria	Surgeon E. Bentley	717	617
21. 1st Division	Alexandria	Surgeon E. Bentley	753	669
22. 2d Division	Alexandria	Surgeon E. Bentley	993	856
23. **3d Division**	**Alexandria**	**Surgeon E. Bentley**	**1,350**	**1,198**
24. Fairfax Seminary	Virginia	Surgeon D. P. Smith	936	373
25. Hammond	Point Lookout Maryland	Surgeon A. Heger	1,400	450
Total:			21,426	13,865

III. Department of Pennsylvania[3]

Hospital	Locality	Medical Officer in Charge	Beds	Occupied
1. Broad Street	Philadelphia	Assist. Surgeon T. C. Brainerd	525	411
2. Citizen's Volunteers	Philadelphia	Surgeon R. S. Kenerdine	236	48
3. Convalescent	Philadelphia	Surgeon T. B. Reed	766	590
4. Haddington	Philadelphia	Surgeon S. W. Gross	1,320	970
5. Islington	Philadelphia	Act. Assist. Surg. J. Patterson	60	15
6. McClellan	Philadelphia	Surgeon L. Taylor	1,089	1,089
7. Mower	Philadelphia	Surgeon J. Hopkinson	3,100	2,311
8. **Satterlee**	**Philadelphia**	**Surgeon I. I. Hayes**	**3,519**	**2,464**
9. South Street	Philadelphia	Act. Assist. Surg. R. J. Levis	288	288
10. Summit House	Philadelphia	Surgeon J. H. Taylor	1,204	845
11. Turner's Lane	Philadelphia	Surgeon R. A. Christian	285	211
12. Officers'	Cammack W.	Assist. Surg. A. A. Storrow	92	20
13. Chester	Chester	Surgeon T. H. Bache	878	536
14. Cuyler	Germantown	Assist. Surg. H. S. Schell	646	380
15. U.S. General	Pittsburgh	Surgeon Jas. Bryan	723	584
16. White Hall	White Hall	Assist. Surg. W. H. Forwood	1,369	776
17. **York**	**York**	**Surgeon John W. Mintzer**	**1,600**	**1,003**
18. Beverly	Beverly, N.J.	Assist. Surg. C. Wagner	1,000	841
Totals:			18,709	13,412

IV. Middle Department Hospitals[4]

Name	Location	Medical Officer	Beds	Occupied	Vacant
1. Convalescent	Baltimore	Surgeon T. Sims.	380	302	78
2. Jarvis	Baltimore	Assist. Surg. D. Peters	1,213	959	254
3. National Hotel	Baltimore	Surgeon Z. Bliss	400	303	97
4. Newton University	Baltimore	Surgeon R. Pease	260	248	12
5. McKim's	Baltimore	Surgeon L. Read	300	213	87
6. West's Buildings	Baltimore	Surgeon A. Chapel	425	305	120
7. **Division No. 1**	**Annapolis**	**Surgeon B. Vanderkieft**	**1,562**	**1,545**	**17**
8. Division No. 2	Annapolis	Surgeon G. Palmer	600	482	118
9. Officers' Hosp.	Annapolis	Surgeon B. Vanderkieft	409	169	240
10. USA Gen. Hosp	Annapolis Jct.	Assist. Surg. C. Bacon	290	273	17
11. Tilton	Wilmington	Surgeon E. Baily	350	194	156
Total:			6,189	4,993	1,196

V. Department of the East[5]

Name	Location	Medical Officer in Charge	Beds	Occupied
1. Ladies Home	New York City	Surgeon A. B. Mott	402	345
2. St. Joseph	New York City	Surgeon B. A. Clements	325	220
3. Transit	New York City	Surgeon A. H. Hoff	62	0
4. David's Island	New York City	Assist. Surg. W. Webster	1,700	870

Name	Location	Medical Officer in Charge	Beds	Occupied
5. Ft. Columbus	New York City	Assist. Surg. P. S. Connor	100	19
6. Grant	Willet's Point	Surgeon A. H. Thurston	1,203	393
7. McDougall	Ft. Schuyler	Assist. Surg. S. H. Orton	1,184	506
8. Officers'	Bedloe's Island	Surgeon J. Simons	103	20
9. Albany	Albany	Assist. Surg. J. F. Cogswell	482	428
10. Buffalo	Buffalo	Dr. J. M. Brown	150	91
11. Sisters of C.	Buffalo	Surgeon A. Crispell	200	69
12. Elmira	Elmira	Act. Assist. Surg. J. Stanchfield	325	231
13. St. Mary's	Rochester	Act. Assist. Surg. A. Backus	680	536
14. Troy	Troy	Surg. G. H. Hubbard	300	219
15. Ward	Newark, N.J.	Assist. Surg. J. T. Calhoun	927	723
16. **Knight**	**New Haven, Ct.**	**Surgeon P. A. Jewett**	**607**	**510**
17. Webster	Manchester, N.H.	Surgeon A. T. Watson	475	258
18. Brattleboro	Brattleboro, Vt.	Surgeon E. E. Phelps	725	415
19. Baxter	Burlington, Vt. Act.	Assist. Surg. S. W. Thayer	500	336
20. **Sloan**	**Montpelier, Vt.**	**Surgeon H. Janes**	**469**	**421**
21. Mason	Boston, Mass.	Act. Assist. Surg. W. E. Townsend	60	59
22. Readville	Boston, Mass.	Surgeon F. H. Gross	1,000	765
23. Dale	Worcester, Mass.	Surgeon C. N. Chamberlain	480	370
24. Lovell	Portsmouth G. R.I.	Surgeon L. A. Edwards	1,464	713
25. Cony	Augusta, Me.	Act. Assist. Surg. G. E. Brickett	816	816
Totals:			14,829	9,302

VI. Hospital Newspapers

Newspaper	Hospital	Location	Beds	Publication Dates	Cost/Year
Hospital Register	Satterlee	Philadelphia	3,519	Feb. 14, 1863– June 24, 1865	$1.00
Armory Square Hospital Gazette	Armory Square	Washington	1,000	Jan. 6, 1864– Aug. 21, 1865	$1.00
The Soldiers' Journal	Augur	@ Alexandria	668	Feb. 17, 1864– June 21, 1865	$2.00
The Cripple	Division No. III	Alexandria Virginia	1,350	Oct. 8, 1864– April 29, 1864	$1.00
The Crutch	Division No. I	Annapolis Maryland	1,562	Jan. 9, 1864– May 13, 1865	$2.00
Hammond Gazette	Hammond	Point Lookout Maryland	1,400	Nov. 1863–1865	$2.00
The Cartridge Box	York	York Pennsylvania	1,600	March 5, 1864– April 22, 1865	$2.50
Knight Hospital Record	Knight	New Haven	607	Oct. 5, 1864– July 12, 1865	$1.50
Voice of the Soldier	Sloan	Montpelier Vermont		April 1865- June 21, 1865	$1.00

Chapter Notes

Introduction

1. MSHWR. Vol. 1, Part 3, p. 964.
2. Ibid. p. 896.
3. Ibid. p. 897.
4. Ibid. p. 908.
5. Ibid. p. 908.
6. Ibid. p. 943.
7. I. Spar. *New Haven's Civil War Hospital.* Jefferson, North Carolina. 2014.
8. MSHWR. p. 957.
9. Ibid. p. 960.
10. Ibid.
11. Ibid. p. 962.
12. Ibid. p. 961.
13. D. Reynolds. *Lincoln's Selected Writings. On Discoveries and Inventions.* W.W. Norton, 2015. pp. 184–187.
14. G. Prescott. *History, Theory, and Practice of the Electric Telegraph.* Boston: Ticknor and Fields. 1866.
15. I. Spar.
16. H. Holzer. *Lincoln and the Power of the Press.* Simon and Schuster. 2014.

Chapter One

1. MSHWR. Part III, Volume I. p. 926.
2. Ibid. p. 928.
3. *Hospital Register.* August 29, 1863.
4. *Army Medical Bulletin*, Number 47, 1939. pp. 1–3.
5. Nathaniel West. *History of Satterlee U.S. Army General Hospital.* p. 27.
6. *Satterlee U.S. Army General Hospital General Order Books 1862-4.*
7. Ibid.
8. Ibid.
9. Ibid.
10. Ibid.
11. N. West. *History of Satterlee Hospital.* p. 9.
12. MSHWR. Vol. 3. Part III. pp. 926–930.
13. *Armory Square Hospital Gazette.* August 21, 1865. No. 75.
14. Satterlee Order Books.
15. Ibid.
16. Ibid.
17. Ibid.
18. Ibid.
19. Ibid.
20. *Hospital Register.* Aug. 29, 1863.
21. Ibid. February 14, 1863. Vol. 1 No. 1.
22. *Hospital Register.* May 30, 1863.
23. Ibid. November 14, 1863.
24. Ibid. March 7, 1863.
25. Ibid. June 4, 1864.
26. Ibid. Sept. 14, 1864.
27. Ibid. May 6, 1865.
28. N. West. *History of the Satterlee Hospital.*
29. N. West. *Catalogue of Library, Satterlee Hospital.* 1863.
30. *Satterlee General Hospital Order Books 1862-4.*
31. N. West. *History of the Satterlee Hospital.* p. 36.
32. *Hospital Register.* June 6, 1863.
33. Ibid.
34. Ibid. March 18, 1865.
35. Ibid. August 1, 1863.
36. Ibid. September 3, 1864.
37. Ibid. June 25, 1864.
38. Ibid. July 25, 1863.
39. Ibid. February 14, 1863. Vol. 1, No. 1.
40. Ibid. March 14, 1863.
41. Ibid June 6, 1863.
42. Ibid. July 4, 1863.
43. Ibid. May 2, 1863.
44. Ibid. August 1, 1863.
45. Ibid. March 18, 1865.
46. Ibid. March 4, 1865.
47. Ibid. May 2, 1863.
48. Ibid. March 19, 1864.
49. Ibid July 24, 1864.
50. Personal collection.
51. Personal collection.
52. N. West. *History of the Satterlee Hospital.* pp. 10–13.
53. Ibid.
54. *Hospital Register.* August 1, 1863.
55. Ibid. August 29, 1863.
56. Ibid. February 4, 1865.
57. Ibid. June 7, 1863.
58. Ibid. March 14, 1863.
59. Ibid. February 14, 1863.
60. Ibid. March 14, 1863.
61. Ibid. March 4, 1865.
62. Ibid. January 23, 1864.
63. Ibid. July 9, 1864.
64. Ibid. November 12, 1864.
65. Ibid. March 26, 1864.
66. Ibid. June 17, 1865.
67. Ibid. April 18, 1863.
68. Ibid. June 20, 1863.
69. Ibid. June 27, 1863.
70. Ibid. July 12, 1863.
71. Ibid. April 11, 1863.
72. Ibid. February 28, 1863.
73. N. West. *History of the Satterlee Hospital.* p. 35.
74. *Hospital Register.* April 11, 1863.
75. Ibid. February 21, 1863.
76. *Satterlee General Hospital Order Books 1862-4.* Circular 3, Sept. 1862.
77. *Hospital Register.* June 13, 1863.
78. Ibid.

Chapter Notes

79. Ibid. August 29, 1763.
80. Ibid. November 14, 1863.
81. Ibid. January 9, 1864.
82. Ibid. July 30, 1864.
83. Ibid. May 7, 1864.
84. Ibid. November 12, 1864.
85. Ibid. June 25, 1864.
86. Ibid. April 18, 1863.
87. Ibid. March 21, 1863.
88. Ibid. February 21, 1863.
89. Ibid. April 25, 1863.
90. Ibid. June 27, 1863.
91. Ibid. February 20, 1864.
92. Ibid. August 1, 1863.
93. Ibid. June 27, 1863.
94. Ibid. July 12, 1963.
95. Ibid. March 7, 1863.
96. Ibid. June 25, 1864.
97. Ibid. March 18, 1865.
98. Ibid. March 18, 1865.
99. Ibid.
100. Ibid. May 6, 1865.

Chapter Two

1. MSHWR. pp. 936–7.
2. *Armory Gazette.* July 2, 1864.
3. Ibid.
4. Hospital letter. Personal collection.
5. *Armory Gazette.* January 14, 1865.
6. MSHWR. pp. 936–7.
7. *Armory Gazette.* October 22, 1864.
8. Ibid. October 29, 1864.
9. Ibid. September 24, 1864.
10. Hospital letter. Personal collection.
11. Ibid.
12. *Armory Gazette.* January 20, 1864.
13. Ibid. June 18, 1864.
14. Ibid. June 4, 1864.
15. Ibid. January 7, 1865.
16. Ibid. January 6, 1864. Vol. 1, No. 1.
17. Ibid. October 22, 1864.
18. Ibid. January 7, 1865.
19. Ibid. January 14, 1865.
20. Ibid.
21. Ibid. January 7, 1865.
22. Ibid. January 7, 1865.
23. Ibid. January 28, 1865.
24. Ibid. January 21, 1865.
25. Ibid. May 28, 1864.
26. Ibid. August 20, 1864.
27. Ibid. June 4, 1864.
28. Ibid. April 9, 1864.
29. Ibid. January 21, 1865.
30. Ibid. May 14, 1864.
31. Ibid. August 13, 1864
32. Ibid. April 30, 1864.
33. Ibid. July 2, 1864.
34. Ibid. August 13, 1864.
35. Ibid. January 27, 1864.
36. Ibid. December 10, 1864.
37. Ibid. July 2, 1864.
38. Ibid. January 7, 1865.
39. Ibid.
40. Ibid. May 28, 1864.
41. Ibid. February 3, 1864.
42. Ibid. January 20, 1864.
43. Ibid. February 3, 1864.
44. Ibid. October 29, 1864.
45. Ibid. April 2, 1864.
46. Ibid.
47. Ibid. September 10, 1864.
48. Ibid. September 3, 1864.
49. Ibid. October 15, 1864.
50. Ibid. January 14, 1865.
51. Ibid.
52. Ibid. October 22, 1864.
53. Ibid. July 23, 1864.
54. Ibid. April 29, 1865.
55. Ibid. April 30, 1864.
56. Ibid.
57. Ibid. June 4, 1864.
58. Ibid. April 23, 1864.
59. Ibid. July 30, 1864.
60. Ibid. August 13, 1864.
61. Ibid. June 25, 1864.
62. Ibid. Hospital letter. Personal collection.
63. Ibid. September 10, 1864.
64. Ibid. January 6, 1864.
65. Ibid. February 10, 1864.
66. Ibid. July 9, 1864.
67. Ibid. February 10, 1864.
68. Ibid. February 10, 1864.
69. Ibid. April 30, 1864.
70. Ibid. June 25, 1864.
71. Ibid. July 23, 1864.
72. Ibid. June 25, 1864.
73. Personal collection.
74. Ibid. October 15, 1864.
75. Ibid.
76. Ibid. December 31, 1864.
77. Ibid. January 6, 1864.
78. Ibid. January 27, 1864.
79. Ibid.
80. Ibid. April 9, 1864.
81. Ibid. September 17, 1864.
82. Ibid. January 14, 1865.
83. Ibid. July 9, 1864.
84. Ibid. April 16, 1864.
85. Ibid. January 7, 1865.
86. Ibid. August 21, 1865.
87. Hospital letter. Personal collection.

Chapter Three

1. *The Soldiers' Journal.* April 6, 1864.
2. Ibid. February 24, 1864.
3. Ibid. September 14, 1864.
4. Ibid. May 25, 1864.
5. Ibid. December 7, 1864.
6. Ibid. February 24, 1864.
7. Ibid. March 2, 1864.
8. Ibid. August 25, 1864.
9. Ibid. March 2, 1864.
10. Ibid. August 10, 1864.
11. Ibid. June 21, 1865.
12. Ibid. April 20, 1864.
13. Ibid. July 6, 1864.
14. Ibid. March 23, 1864.
15. Ibid. April 20, 1864.
16. Ibid. October 5, 1864.
17. Ibid. August 10, 1864.
18. Ibid. July 6, 1864.
19. Ibid. March 30, 1864.
20. Ibid. March 23, 1864.
21. *The Soldiers' Journal.* August 17, 1864.
22. Ibid. April 27, 1864.
23. Ibid. August 17, 1864.
24. Ibid. December 21, 1864.
25. Ibid. August 3, 1864.
26. Ibid. November 16, 1864.
27. Ibid. March 9, 1864.
28. Ibid. May 4, 1864.
29. Ibid. March 9, 1864.
30. Ibid.
31. Ibid. December 21, 1864.
32. Ibid. January 4, 1865.
33. Ibid. December 21, 1864.
34. Ibid. January 18, 1865.
35. Ibid. April 30, 1864.
36. Ibid. July 20, 1864.
37. Ibid. September 28, 1864.
38. Ibid. February 1, 1865.
39. Ibid. August 17, 1864.
40. Ibid. March 16, 1864.
41. Ibid. November 16, 1864.
42. Ibid.
43. Ibid.
44. Ibid.
45. Ibid. March 16, 1864.
46. Ibid. June 29, 1864.
47. Ibid. February 17, 1864.
48. Ibid. April 6, 1864.
49. Ibid. May 11, 1864.
50. Ibid. February 23, 1864.
51. Ibid. June 29, 1864.
52. Ibid. March 9, 1864.
53. Ibid. July 6, 1864.
54. Ibid. November 16, 1864.
55. Ibid. August 10, 1864.
56. Ibid. October 26, 1864.

57. Ibid. May 25, 1864.
58. Ibid. May 4, 1864.
59. Ibid. March 30, 1864.
60. Ibid. October 5, 1864.
61. Ibid. July 20, 1864.
62. Ibid. July 6, 1864.
63. Ibid. May 18, 1864.
64. Ibid.
65. Ibid.
66. Ibid. March 16, 1864.
67. Ibid. December 14, 1864.
68. Ibid. March 16, 1864.
69. Ibid. June 22, 1864.
70. Ibid. March 23, 1864.
71. Ibid. August 3, 1864.
72. Ibid.
73. Ibid. June 22, 1864.
74. Ibid. December 14, 1864.
75. Ibid. July 13, 1864.
76. Ibid. October 26, 1864.
77. Ibid. October 26, 1864.
78. Ibid. October 26, 1864.
79. Ibid. March 16, 1864.
80. Ibid. June 29, 1864.
81. Ibid. August 3, 1864.
82. Ibid. October 19, 1864.
83. Ibid. March 16, 1864.
84. Ibid. November 2, 1864.
85. Ibid. August 3, 1864.
86. Ibid. November 16, 1864.
87. Ibid. June 7, 1865.
88. Ibid. June 21, 1865.
89. Ibid. August 3, 1864.
90. Ibid. December 21, 1864.
91. Ibid. February 24, 1864.
92. Ibid. March 2, 1864.
93. Ibid. September 28, 1864.
94. Ibid. March 2, 1864.
95. Ibid. March 16, 1864.
96. Ibid. July 13, 1864.
97. Ibid. August 3, 1864.
98. Ibid. July 6, 1864.
99. Ibid. June 15, 1864.
100. Ibid. May 11, 1864.
101. Ibid. October 26, 1864.
102. Ibid. May 25, 1864.
103. Ibid. September 21, 1864.
104. Ibid. May 25, 1864.
105. Ibid. June 21, 1865.
106. Ibid. January 11, 1865.
107. Ibid. January 4, 1865.
108. Ibid. December 21, 1864.
109. Ibid. June 7, 1865.

Chapter Four

1. MSHWR. Part III. Vol I. p. 960.
2. *The Cripple*. October 22, 1864.
3. Hospital letter. Personal collection.
4. Ibid. October 8, 1864. Vol. 1. No. 1.
5. Ibid. January 14, 1865.
6. Ibid.
7. Ibid. December 31, 1864.
8. Ibid.
9. Ibid. April 22, 1865.
10. Ibid. December 10, 1864.
11. Ibid.
12. Ibid. October 29, 1864.
13. Ibid. January 7, 1865.
14. Ibid. February 4, 1865.
15. Ibid. January 7, 1865.
16. Ibid. November 26, 1864.
17. Ibid. April 29, 1865.
18. Ibid. November 5, 1864.
19. Ibid. November 19, 1864.
20. Ibid. November 26, 1864.
21. Ibid. January 28, 1865.
22. Ibid. February 25, 1865.
23. Ibid. February 18, 1865.
24. Ibid. October 29, 1864.
25. Ibid. March 4, 1865.
26. Ibid. October 22, 1864.
27. Ibid. April 1, 1865.
28. Ibid. November 26, 1864.
29. Ibid. November 19, 1864.
30. Ibid.
31. Ibid. February 18, 1865.
32. Ibid. March 11, 1865.
33. Ibid. December 31, 1864.
34. Ibid. March 4, 1865.
35. Ibid. January 21, 1865.
36. Ibid. January 28, 1865.
37. Ibid. February 4, 1865.
38. Ibid. October 22, 1864.
39. Ibid. March 25, 1865.
40. Ibid. December 3, 1864.
41. Ibid. January 28, 1865.
42. Ibid. April 8, 1865.
43. Ibid. April 1, 1865.
44. Ibid. October 15, 1864.
45. Ibid. April 22, 1865.
46. Ibid.
47. Ibid. February 4, 1865.
48. Ibid January 14, 1865.
49. Ibid.
50. Ibid. December 24, 1864.
51. Ibid. March 4, 1865.
52. Ibid. April 29, 1865.
53. Ibid. March 11, 1865.
54. Ibid. January 28, 1865.
55. Ibid. March 4, 1865.
56. Ibid.
57. Ibid. January 21, 1865.
58. Ibid. November 19, 1864.
59. Ibid. April 8, 1865.
60. Ibid. December 3, 1864.
61. Ibid. April 29, 1865.
62. Ibid. October 8, 1864.
63. Ibid. April 8, 1865.
64. Ibid. November 19, 1864.
65. Ibid. March 18, 1865.
66. Ibid. April 15, 1865.
67. Ibid. April 22, 1865.
68. Ibid. February 11, 1865.

Chapter Five

1. *The Crutch*. July 9, 1864.
2. Ibid. January 9, 1864.
3. Ibid.
4. Ibid. March 25, 1865.
5. Ibid. March 19, 1864.
6. Ibid. February 6, 1864.
7. Ibid. October 22, 1864.
8. Ibid. February 20, 1864.
9. Ibid. January 21, 1865.
10. Ibid. February 6, 1864.
11. Ibid. April 30, 1864.
12. Ibid. May 7, 1864.
13. Ibid. April 1, 1865.
14. Ibid. May 7, 1864.
15. Ibid. July 16, 1864.
16. Ibid.
17. Ibid. September 17, 1864.
18. Ibid. April 8, 1865.
19. Ibid. January 16, 1864.
20. Ibid. October 15, 1864.
21. Ibid. May 7, 1864.
22. Ibid. June 11, 1864.
23. Ibid. October 1, 1864.
24. Ibid. April 9, 1864.
25. Ibid. March 26, 1864.
26. Ibid. April 8, 1865.
27. Ibid. September 10, 1864.
28. Ibid. October 1, 1864.
29. Ibid. October 29, 1864.
30. Ibid. April 22, 1865.
31. Ibid. April 23, 1864.
32. Ibid. October 1, 1864.
33. Ibid. December 31, 1864.
34. Ibid. July 30, 1864.
35. Ibid. February 6, 1864.
36. Ibid. October 1, 1864.
37. Ibid. February 6, 1864.
38. Ibid. June 11, 1864.
39. Ibid. March 25, 1865.
40. Ibid. April 22, 1865.
41. Ibid. May 21, 1864.
42. Ibid. Feb. 13, 1864.
43. Ibid. September 3, 1864.
44. Ibid. June 11, 1864.
45. Ibid. July 30, 1864.
46. Ibid. March 19, 1864.
47. Ibid. May 12, 1863.
48. Ibid. May 14, 1864.
49. Ibid. May 7, 1864.

50. Ibid. August 27, 1864.
51. Ibid. February 4, 1865.
52. Ibid. April 15, 1865.
53. Ibid. February 6, 1864.
54. Ibid. May 14, 1864.
55. Ibid. April 16, 1864.
56. Ibid. August 13, 1864.
57. Ibid.
58. Ibid. October 22, 1864.
59. Ibid. September 10, 1864.
60. Ibid. November 5, 1864.
61. Ibid. February 11, 1865.
62. Ibid. October 1, 1864.
63. Ibid. November 19, 1864.
64. Ibid.
65. Ibid. November 26, 1864.
66. Ibid. December 31, 1864.
67. Ibid. April 8, 1865.
68. Ibid.
69. Ibid. December 31, 1864.
70. Ibid. May 14, 1864.
71. Ibid. February 6, 1864.
72. Ibid. June 11, 1864.
73. Ibid. May 14, 1864.
74. *Harper's Weekly.* June 18, 1864.
75. Ibid.
76. *The Crutch.* July 30, 1864.
77. Ibid. December 10, 1864.
78. Ibid. December 3, 1864.
79. Ibid. March 25, 1865.
80. Ibid.
81. Ibid. May 6, 1865.
82. Ibid. April 8, 1865.
83. Ibid.
84. Ibid. May 28, 1864.
85. Ibid. July 23, 1864.
86. Ibid. May 13, 1865.

Chapter Six

1. MSHWR. Part III. Vol. I. p. 942.
2. Ibid. p. 943.
3. Ibid.
4. *Hammond Gazette.* April 13, 1864.
5. Ibid. March 3, 1863.
6. Ibid. March 16, 1864.
7. Ibid.
8. Ibid. September 8, 1863.
9. Ibid. March 16, 1864.
10. Ibid. April 6, 1864.
11. Ibid. July 7, 1863.
12. Ibid.
13. *Armory Gazette.* Aug. 20, 1864.
14. Ibid.
15. *Hammond Gazette.* March 3, 1863.

16. Ibid. Aug. 24, 1864.
17. Ibid. March 3, 1863.
18. Ibid. February 10, 1863.
19. Ibid. May 4, 1864.
20. Ibid. July 7, 1863.
21. Ibid.
22. Ibid. July 7, 1863.
23. Ibid. June 9, 1863.
24. Ibid. July 7, 1863.
25. Ibid.
26. Ibid.
27. Ibid.
28. Ibid. September 8, 1863.
29. Ibid. September 7, 1864.
30. Ibid. May 4, 1864.
31. Ibid. April 6, 1864.
32. Ibid. May 18, 1864.
33. Ibid. February 10, 1863.
34. Ibid.
35. Ibid. March 3, 1863.
36. Ibid. August 24, 1864.
37. Ibid. June 9, 1863.
38. Ibid. May 4, 1864.
39. Ibid. March 16, 1864.
40. Ibid. June 9, 1863.
41. Ibid. March 16, 1864.
42. F. Esmarch. *Verbandplatz und Feldlazareth.* p. 122. Appendix II.

Chapter Seven

1. Letter Dr. A. J. Blair, March 1865. Personal Collection.
2. J. McClure. *East of Gettysburg.* p. 136.
3. Ibid. June 18, 1864.
4. *The Cartridge Box.* December 17, 1864.
5. Ibid. March 5, 1864.
6. Ibid.
7. Ibid. April 16, 1864.
8. Ibid. April 30, 1864.
9. Ibid. April 8, 1865.
10. Ibid. December 3, 1864.
11. Ibid. March 4, 1865.
12. Ibid. September 10, 1864.
13. Ibid. April 30, 1864.
14. Ibid. December 17, 1864.
15. Ibid. April 8, 1865.
16. Ibid. February 25, 1865.
17. Ibid. November 26, 1864.
18. Ibid.
19. Ibid. April 8, 1865.
20. Ibid. December 10, 1864.
21. Ibid. April 9, 1864.
22. Ibid. January 21, 1865.
23. Ibid. November 26, 1864.
24. Ibid. March 12, 1864.
25. Ibid.

26. Ibid. April 22, 1865.
27. Ibid. December 24, 1864.
28. Ibid. February 4, 1865.
29. Ibid. August 20, 1864.
30. Ibid. April 15, 1865.
31. Ibid. December 10, 1864.
32. Ibid. March 11, 1865.
33. Ibid. December 3, 1864.
34. Ibid. July 23, 1864.
35. Ibid. December 17, 1864.
36. Ibid. April 16, 1864.
37. Ibid. May 14, 1864.
38. Ibid. May 26, 1864.
39. Ibid. June 4, 1864.
40. Ibid. June 11, 1864.
41. Ibid. August 6, 1864.
42. Ibid. November 19, 1864.
43. Ibid. December 10, 1864.
44. Ibid. October 1, 1864.
45. Ibid. May 13, 1865.
46. Ibid. December 24, 1864.
47. Ibid. January 21, 1865.
48. Ibid. April 9, 1864.
49. Ibid. August 13, 1864.
50. Ibid. July 30, 1864.
51. Ibid. January 21, 1865
52. Ibid. August 27, 1864.
53. Ibid. March 11, 1865.
54. Ibid. June 18, 1864.
55. Ibid. December 24, 1864.
56. Ibid. April 9, 1864.
57. Ibid.
58. Ibid. April 16, 1864.
59. Ibid. April 23, 1864.
60. Ibid. December 24, 1864.
61. Ibid. April 22, 1865.
62. J. McClure. *East of Gettysburg.* pp. 34–35.
63. Ibid. p. 112.
64. Ibid. p. 114.
65. *The Cartridge Box.* August 20, 1864.
66. Ibid. September 10, 1864.
67. Ibid. February 18, 1865.
68. Ibid. November 19, 1864.
69. Letter Dr. Blair. Personal collection.
70. *The Cartridge Box.* November 19, 1864.
71. Ibid. May 13, 1865.
72. Ibid. July 30, 1864.
73. Ibid. April 29, 1865.
74. Ibid. May 13, 1865.
75. Ibid. July 2, 1864.
76. Ibid. October 22, 1864.
77. Ibid. December 10, 1864.
78. Ibid. September 3, 1864.
79. Ibid. June 18, 1864.
80. Ibid. September 3, 1864.
81. Ibid. August 13, 1864.

82. Ibid. April 1, 1865.
83. Ibid. September 24, 1864.
84. Ibid. March 12, 1864.
85. Ibid. April 9, 1864.
86. Ibid. November 19, 1864.
87. Ibid. May 7, 1864.
88. Ibid. April 2, 1864.
89. Ibid. October 8, 1864.
90. Ibid.
91. Ibid. September 24, 1864.
92. Ibid. November 19, 1864.
93. Ibid. November 26, 1864.
94. Ibid. March 11, 1864.
95. Ibid. March 5, 1864.
96. Ibid. Sept. 10, 1864.
97. Ibid. Nov. 5, 1864.
98. Ibid. July 9, 1864.
99. Ibid. December 17, 1864.
100. Ibid. June 24, 1865.
101. Ibid. May 7, 1864.
102. Ibid. April 22, 1865.
103. Ibid.
104. Ibid. April 29, 1865.
105. Ibid.
106. Ibid. May 20, 1865.
107. Ibid. June 17, 1865.
108. Ibid. June 24, 1865.
109. Ibid. August 27, 1864.
110. Ibid. July 8, 1865.

Chapter Eight

1. I. Spar. *New Haven's Civil War Hospital*. p. 93.
2. Ibid. p. 105.
3. Ibid. p. 21.
4. *Knight Hospital Record*. October 5, 1864.
5. I. Spar. *New Haven's Civil War Hospital*. p. 62.
6. *Knight Hospital Record*. July 12, 1865.
7. Ibid. p. 113.
8. Ibid. October 12, 1864.
9. Ibid. December 31, 1864.
10. Ibid. November 2, 1864.
11. Ibid. November 23, 1864.
12. Ibid. January 18, 1865.
13. Ibid. June 14, 1865.
14. Ibid. May 3, 1865.
15. Ibid. June 14, 1865.
16. Ibid. May 10, 1865.
17. Ibid. May 17, 1865.
18. Ibid. June 14, 1865.
19. Ibid. December 7, 1864.
20. Ibid. January 18, 1865.
21. Ibid. May 3, 1865.
22. Ibid. January 18, 1865.
23. Ibid. January 16, 1864.
24. Ibid. November 9, 1864.
25. Ibid. November 2, 1864.
26. Ibid.
27. Ibid.
28. Ibid.
29. Ibid. October 26, 1864.
30. Ibid. June 28, 1865.
31. Ibid. June 21, 1865.
32. Ibid. December 21, 1864.
33. Ibid. April 12, 1865.
34. Ibid.
35. Ibid.
36. Ibid. February 8, 1865.
37. Ibid. May 24, 1865.
38. Ibid. May 31, 1865.
39. Ibid. April 19, 1865.
40. Ibid.
41. Ibid. April 26, 1865.
42. Ibid. May 3, 1865.
43. Ibid. March 15, 1865.
44. Ibid. April 5, 1865.
45. Ibid. January 25, 1865.
46. Ibid. January 4, 1865.
47. Ibid. January 11, 1865.
48. Ibid.
49. Ibid. February 1, 1865.
50. Ibid. June 21, 1865.
51. Ibid.
52. Ibid. June 14, 1865.
53. Ibid. July 12, 1865.
54. Ibid.

Chapter Nine

1. MSHWR. Part III. Vol. I. p. 950.
2. *Voice of the Soldier*. June 21, 1865.
3. Ibid.
4. Ibid.
5. Ibid.

Conclusion

1. *Hammond Gazette*. April 13, 1864.
2. *The Cripple*. December 24, 1864. No. 12.
3. *The Soldiers' Journal*. Feb. 17, 1864. Vol. 1. No. 1.
4. *The Crutch*. May 13, 1865.
5. *Hospital Register*. September 10, 1863.
6. *The Cartridge Box*. March 5, 1864.
7. *Armory Square Hospital Gazette*. February 3, 1864.
8. *Knight Hospital Record*. July 12, 1865.
9. *Hammond Gazette*. February 10, 1863.
10. Personal collection.
11. *Hospital Register*. September 3, 1864.
12. Ibid. February 20, 1864.
13. *The Crutch*. March 19, 1864.
14. *Armory Gazette*. September 10, 1864.
15. *The Crutch*. August 20, 1864.
16. Ibid. August 13, 1864.
17. *Voice of the Soldier*. June 21, 1865.
18. *The Soldiers' Journal*. January 11, 1865.
19. *Knight Hospital Record*. June 21, 1865.
20. *Armory Gazette*. Sept. 10, 1864.
21. Ibid. February 1, 1865.
22. *The Crutch*. February 20, 1864.
23. *The Soldiers' Journal*. March 2, 1864.
24. *Armory Gazette*. Jan. 27, 1864.
25. *The Soldiers' Journal*. October 26, 1864.
26. Ibid. June 29, 1864.
27. Ibid.
28. *Armory Gazette*. October 22, 1864.
29. *Hospital Register*. June 6, 1863.
30. Ibid. April 18, 1863.
31. *The Soldiers' Journal*. July 13, 1864.
32. *Knight Hospital Record*. April 5, 1865.
33. Ibid.
34. *Knight Hospital Record*. Website Hartford Medical Society Library.
35. *The Soldiers' Journal*. June 29, 1864.
36. *Hospital Register*. January 9, 1864.
37. *Armory Square Hospital Gazette*. June 25, 1864.
38. Ibid. July 2, 1864.
39. Ibid. December 31, 1864.
40. *The Soldiers' Journal*. June 15, 1864.
41. *Hospital Register*. July 12, 1863.
42. *Hospital Register*. July 25, 1863.
43. *The Soldiers' Journal*. March 23, 1864.
44. *Armory Gazette*. January 27, 1864.
45. Ibid. February 21, 1863.

46. Ibid. June 21, 1863.
47. *The Crutch.* February 6, 1864.
48. *The Cripple.* April 1, 1865.
49. *Hospital Register.* August 1, 1863.
50. *The Soldiers' Journal.* March 9, 1864.
51. *The Cripple.* March 4, 1865.
52. Ibid. November 19, 1864.
53. *The Soldiers' Journal.* Harriet Beecher Stowe. March 16, 1864.
54. *The Cartridge Box.* May 7, 1864.
55. *The Crutch.* November 5, 1864.
56. *Knight Hospital Record.* April 12, 1865.
57. Ibid. April 5, 1865.
58. Ibid. March 1, 1865.
59. *Knight Hospital Record.* December 31, 1864.
60. *The Cripple.* December 24, 1864.
61. *The Crutch.* April 16, 1864.
62. *The Soldiers' Journal.* August 3, 1864.
63. Ibid. February 24, 1864.

Appendices

1. *Medical and Surgical History of the War of the Rebellion.* Part III. Volume I. Medical History. p. 964.
2. Ibid. p. 960.
3. Ibid.
4. Ibid. p. 962.
5. Ibid. p. 961.

Bibliography

Armory Square Hospital Gazette. Armory Square U.S. Army General Hospital. Washington, D.C. January 6, 1864–August 21, 1865. Vol. 1. No. 1–75. Library of Congress. http://civilwardc.org/texts/newspapers.

The Cartridge Box. U.S. Army General Hospital. York Pennsylvania. March 5, 1864–April 22, 1865. York County Heritage Trust, York Pennsylvania.

The Cripple. U.S. Army General Hospital, Third Division. Alexandria Virginia. October 8, 1864–April 29, 1865. Volume 1, No. 1–30. Connecticut State Library. Hartford, Connecticut.

The *Crutch.* U.S. Army General Hospital, Division 1. Annapolis Maryland. January 9, 1864–May 13, 1865. Vols. 1–2, nos. 1–71. Maryland State Archives http://aomol.msa.maryland.gov/megafile/msa/speccol/sc2900/sc2908/crutch/html/index/html

Esmarch, F. *Verbandplatz und Feldlazareth: Vorlesungen für Angehende Militairarzte.* Berlin, 1868. Verlag Von August Hirschwald.

Hammond Gazette. Hammond U.S. Army General Hospital. Point Lookout, Maryland. Feb. 10, 1863–Aug. 29, 1863. Historical Society of Pennsylvania, and personal collection.

Hammond, William. *Treatise on Hygiene with Special Reference to Military Service.* Philadelphia. Lippincott. 1863. Pages 324–386.

Harper's Weekly. Vol. III, No. 390. June 18, 1864.

Holzer, Harold. *Lincoln and the Power of the Press.* Simon & Schuster, 2014.

Hospital Register. Satterlee U.S. Army General Hospital. Philadelphia, Pennsylvania. Feb. 14, 1863–June 24, 1865. Vol. No. 1–52. Vol. 2. No. 1–44. Historical Society of Pennsylvania and personal collection.

Knight Hospital Record. Knight U.S. Army General Hospital. New Haven, Connecticut. October 5, 1864–12 July 1865. Vol. 1. No. 1–40. Hartford Medical Society.

Lincoln's Selected Writings. Editor David S. Reynolds. W.W. Norton. 2015. Address to the Washington Temperance Society of Springfield, Illinois. February 22, 1842. Lecture on Discoveries and Inventions. Bloomington, Indiana, April 6, 1858. Lecture on Discoveries and Inventions, Jackson, Illinois. February 11, 1859.

McClure, James. *East of Gettysburg: A Gray Shadow Crosses York County, Pa.* York Country Heritage Trust. 2003.

The Medical and Surgical History of the War of the Rebellion (1861–65). Part III, Volume 1. Washington, D.C. Government Printing Office. 1888. Pgs. 896–966.

Phalen, James. "Richard Sherwood Satterlee, Brevet." *The Army Medical Bulletin,* Number 47. (January 1939). Pgs. 1–3.

Prescott, George. *History, Theory, and Practice of the Electric Telegraph.* Boston: Ticknor and Fields. 1866.

Satterlee General Hospital Order Books 1862–4. Archives and Special Collections. A.C. Long Health Sciences Library of Columbia University. N.Y., N.Y.

The Soldiers' Journal. Augur U.S. Army General Hospital. Near Alexandria Virginia. Feb. 17, 1864–June 21, 1865. Volume 1, No. 1–50. Volume 2, No. 1–18. Library of Congress. http://civilwardc.org/texts/newspapers.

Spar, Ira. MD. *New Haven's Civil War Hospital. A History of Knight U.S. General Hospital, 1862–1865.* McFarland, 2014.

Voice of the Soldier. Sloan U.S. Army General Hospital. Montpelier, Vermont. June 21, 1865. Vermont Historical Society.

West, Nathaniel. *Catalogue of Library, Satterlee Hospital Reading Room.* 1863. Philadelphia, King and Baird, printers on Sansom Street.

____. *History of the Satterlee U.S. Army General Hospital, at West Philadelphia, Penn.* October 8, 1862, to October 8, 1863. Printed by Hospital Press 1863.

Index

Numbers in ***bold italics*** indicate pages with photographs.

advertisements 21, 22, 60, 61, 81, 127, 138, 160, 161, 178, 179, 193, 217, 219, 225
Alexandria, Virginia 72, 78, 111, 114, 115, 132
amputation 3, 37–38, 40–41, 66, 68–69, 98, 126, 143–144, 194–195
apothecary 12, 41

baseball 46, 225
battlefield 35–36, 42–43, 107–109, 129–130, 164–165, 185–186, 194, 206, 212–215, 228
Beecher, Henry Ward 57, 84, 146
Billings, Josh 118–***119***, 123–124, 145–146, 169, 180, 196, 200
blacks 31–32, 64–65, 88–89, 115–116, 139–140, 161, 166–167, 181–182, 197–199
Brown, John 106, 122
Buckingham, William 3, 54, 74, 161
Butler, Benjamin 94, 160

chaplain 5, 12, 22–23, 25, 28, 30, 83, 230
Christmas 28, 36, 57–58, 75, 138, 150, 152
copperheads 44, 61–62, 104, 166, 182, 187–188, 201–203, 227
correspondents 17–***18,*** 19–20, 81, 112–113, 139, 174–175, 192–193

Davis, Jefferson 105–106, 201
delirium tremens 56, 63, 118, 231
desertion 95–97, 102, 203
Dickenson, Amy 59, 66, 226
disability 39–40, 66, 70–71, 109, 114, 127, 144–145, 181, 187, 212–213, 220, 225

draft 43, 63–64, 128, 164, 181, 200–201, 230

editor 20, 79, 138, 174–5
embalming 22, 59–60, 99, 115
Esmarch, Friedrich 170

fire hazards 13–14; *see also* general anesthesia

general anesthesia 37–38
Germans 14, 32–33, 117, 171
Grant, Ulysses S. 45, 94, 99–100, 155, 204–205

Hammond, William 4, 9, 11, 39, 162–163
Hayes, Isaac Israel ***10,*** 13–14, 24, 28, 39
hospital directory 12, 21, 53, 136
hospital guards 15–16
hospital pass 14–***15***
hospital pavilions 4, 5, 11–13, 157, 171, 217
hospital stewards 50, 124, 125
hospital wards 4–5, 11, 14–15, 47–***48***, 140–141, 168, 184, 221

Indians 87, 115–116
Irish 32, 37, 69, 87, 117, 140–141, 166–167, 181–182, 199

Jews 65, 87–88, 167
journalism 7–8, 17, 79, 168

library 12, 22–25, 59, 83, 173, 176, 193, 225
Lincoln, Abraham 6–7, 44–46, 51, 57, 64, 89, 100–***101***, 102–103, 132–133, 149–150, 165–166 189–190, 205–206, 231–232

mail 30–31, 51, 82, 173–***174***, 193, 224
malingerer 39, 72, 230
medical cadets (students) 6, 12
medical records 11, 111
mortality 47, 65, 98–99, 114, 130, 185, 191, 214–215, 228
mothers 38, 71, 93–94, 142–143, 185–186, 229

Nasby, Petroleum V. 116, ***121***–122, 181
nuns 10, 16, 136, 157
nurse 34, 50–51, 58, 97, 99, 136, 142, 146, 156

patent medications 41–42, 126–127, 194
patient letters 50, 70, 75–76, 112, 224
patriotism 19, 27–28, 44, 58, 108, 147, 200, 228
pensions 81–82, 91, 209, 138, 163, 179, 193, 201, 213
pets 35, 108, 131, 155–156, 180–181
phrenology 88
politics 20, 44–45, 61–63, 103–105, 121, 148–149, 164–165, 188, 219, 227
printers 16, 51, 53, 61, 112–113, 138–139, 175, 223
prisoner of war 74–75, 93–95, 131, 150, 152–***153***, 154–155, ***159***, 186, 208–209, 210, 232
profanity 85, 118, 147, 177, 197, 207
prosthetic limb 98, 126

quackery 50, 126–127

returning home 73–74, 100, 197, 213–216

245

Index

romance and marriage 33–35, 57–58, 89–*90*, 91–93, 123–124, 145, 169–170, 179–180, 195–197, 218, 229

sacrifice 58, 106, 109, 127, 208, 211–212, 230, 233
salutatory goals *17*, 51, 53, 79, 112, 133–4, 136–*137*, *172*–173, 221–222
sanitation 5, 9, *49*, 112, 157, 160, 185, 217
Satterlee, Richard 10, 29, 30
sermons 25–30, 56–57, 85–87, 118–120, 142, 146, 164, 176–178, 197–198, 230
Sherman, William T. 45, 120, 188
specialization 38
Stanton, Edward 159, 161
submission of writings 81, 112–*113*, 139, 174, 192–193
surgeons 5, 12, 36, 49, 66–67, 97–98, 125–126, 168, 184–185, 192
surgery 67–68

telegraph 7
temperance 24, 29–30, 53–56, 84, 117–118, 146–147, 177, 197, 207, 231
tetanus 40, 41
Thanksgiving 150, 172
tobacco 56, 84–85, 118, 177

U.S. Sanitary Commission *17*, 82, 85, 138, 177, 196, 216

Vallandigham, Clement 105, 186, 202
volunteers 73, 84–87, 106–107, 110, 121, 128–130, 131, 164, 185, 187, 195, 210,-211, 231, 233

Ward, Artemus 87, 91–*92*, 122, 132-2, 145–180
water supply 5, 9, 47
women's contributions 58–59, 91, 93, 172, 195, 229
Wood, Fernando 103–104, 165–166
wound complications 40, 69, 70, 98

www.ingramcontent.com/pod-product-compliance
Lightning Source LLC
Chambersburg PA
CBHW081550300426
44116CB00015B/2826